OP 87-81

PSYCOLOGY.

6.50

*Dynamic Psychiatry*

*Edited by* FRANZ ALEXANDER, M.D., *and* HELEN ROSS

# Dynamic Psychiatry

FRANZ ALEXANDER, M.D.

THERESE BENEDEK, M.D.

HENRY W. BROSIN, M.D.

THOMAS M. FRENCH, M.D.

MARGARET W. GERARD, M.D.

MAURICE LEVINE, M.D.

DAVID M. LEVY, M.D.

JOHN W. LYONS, M.D.

MARGARET MEAD

LEON J. SAUL, M.D.

DAVID SHAKOW

LOUIS B. SHAPIRO, M.D.

THOMAS S. SZASZ, M.D.

EDOARDO WEISS, M.D.

JOHN C. WHITEHORN, M.D.

THE UNIVERSITY OF CHICAGO PRESS

*Subscription Edition Distributed by*

J. B. LIPPINCOTT COMPANY

PHILADELPHIA · MONTREAL

THE UNIVERSITY OF CHICAGO PRESS, CHICAGO 37
Cambridge University Press, London, N.W. 1, England
W. J. Gage & Co., Limited, Toronto 2B, Canada

# PREFACE

THIS volume offers to students of psychiatry a comprehensive view of dynamic psychiatry. The dynamic trend in psychiatry is the result of the impact of psychoanalysis, its theory, its method of investigation, and its therapy, upon the whole of psychiatry. Essentially this trend can be defined as the advancement of the study of psychiatry from a descriptive into an explanatory phase.

Through the application of the principle of psychological motivation to seemingly irrational psychopathological phenomena, it became possible to understand the deterioration of behavior as seen in neuroses and psychoses. This understanding was blocked so long as only the nature of conscious mental processes was known, since psychopathological phenomena do not follow the rational principles of conscious thought-processes. Psychopathology is characterized by regression to the primitive forms of unconscious processes similar to those which appear in dreams. The similarity between schizophrenic thought-processes and dreams was first noticed by Bleuler; the universal significance of unconscious processes and their peculiarities was first recognized by Freud and his followers.

Before Freud made known his discoveries and theories, the most that psychiatrists could do was to give a valid and detailed description of the symptomatology of psychiatric conditions, just as Cuvier and Linné did in the fields of zoölogy and botany. It was only after the principle of evolution was discovered by Darwin that their descriptive systems could be replaced by a dynamic concept and the differences between species understood.

The influence of Freud upon psychiatry was similar. In Europe, this influence was at first retarded by the feud which grew up between Freud and academic psychiatry and later by the deterioration of scientific activities, which followed the world wars. In the United States the emotional conflict between psychoanalysis and academic psychiatry was more remote and did not interfere substantially with the penetration of psychoanalytic concepts into psychiatry.

This penetration began about thirty years ago. The pioneers of this scientific movement were William A. White, Smith Ely Jelliffe, and Adolf Meyer. During the last two decades the assimilation of psychoanalysis by American psychiatry has gained momentum, and in recent years there has been a trend toward academic incorporation.

The impact of psychoanalytic concepts upon scientific developments is to be observed on six frontiers. (1) In clinical psychiatry proper, there have developed a psychopathology, based on dynamic concepts, and a psychotherapy, based on etiology. (2) On the border line between psychiatry and anthropology the study of personality development in different cultures has broadened the concept of basic human nature. The influence of parental attitudes in various cultures upon the formation of personality has become a focus of interest for a number of anthropologists who operate primarily with psychoanalytic concepts. Their work offers an opportunity for the comparative appraisal of cultural factors in the life-story of the individual. This psychoanalytic trend in anthropology has led to a new orientation within psychiatry itself, often referred to as "social psychiatry," a discipline still in its infancy. (3) In experimental psychology another cross-fertilization has taken place, particularly in the field of clinical tests. The intimate relation between psychoanalysis and Rorschach's original work was the historical starting point of this mutual influence. There followed in this country the experimental work of Henry A. Murray, whose Thematic Apperception Test rests entirely on psychoanalytic concepts. (4) In animal psychology, particularly with the American disciples of Pavlov, another point of contact with psychoanalysis was made. While at the beginning the animal experimenters were on the receiving side, their experimental study of animals promises an increasingly profound influence for the understanding and formulation of basic laws of organismic behavior. (5) On medicine as a whole the influence of psychoanalytic concepts and methods is shown in a new orientation: the psychosomatic approach to physiology, general pathology, and therapy. Essentially, this is the systematic co-ordination of somatic and psychological points of view, of somatic and psychological techniques for the study and cure of diseases, whether or not they manifest themselves primarily in somatic or in psychological symptoms. Because of this synthetic tendency, psychiatry is rapidly losing its earlier extra-territorial status in medicine, which came about because of the fact that psychiatry, in the study of psychopathological phenomena, had to adopt methods different from the physico-chemical methods universally accepted in medicine. (6) In child psychiatry perhaps the greatest influence of psychoanalysis has taken place. The child-guidance movement under the pioneering influence of Herman Adler and William Healy had developed a liberal and experimental outlook and had paved the way for the assimilation of psychoanalytic concepts. In therapy with children, psychoanalytic techniques have great possibilities, and in this particular area psychiatry can exercise a preventive function, the cherished aim of all medical disciplines.

The outgrowth of this sixfold scientific cross-fertilization is what may be termed "dynamic psychiatry."

Because of the multidisciplinary nature of our subject, we decided to publish a multi-author book in which the mutual interactions of psychoanalysis with allied fields are discussed by experts in their respective disciplines.

We have divided the book into three parts. The first deals with the basic concepts which have influenced the growth of psychiatry proper and the border-line subjects; the second, with clinical application of these concepts; and the third, with the extended influence of psychoanalytic theory on the current development in allied fields. In the third part we have included medicine with the social sciences. The last chapter is a panoramic view of the influence of Freud on the subjects which pertain to man.

The advent of dynamic psychiatry is liquidating the isolated existence of psychoanalysis. As a therapy, psychoanalysis is being reunited with medicine, where it originated as a method of psychiatry. As a body of theory, it is becoming recognized as a basic science both in psychiatry and in the social sciences.

The making of a multiauthor book has its tribulations, in which the authors perforce share. We wish to thank our collaborators for their efforts in behalf of this volume and for their patience in awaiting its appearance. We acknowledge with gratitude the untiring and careful help of Roberta Collard in the preparation of the manuscript.

Franz Alexander, M.D.
Helen Ross

Chicago, Illinois

# CONTRIBUTORS

FRANZ ALEXANDER, M.D. Director, Institute for Psychoanalysis, Chicago, Illinois; Clinical Professor of Psychiatry, University of Illinois College of Medicine, Chicago, Illinois

THERESE BENEDEK, M.D. Staff Member, Institute for Psychoanalysis, Chicago, Illinois

HENRY W. BROSIN, M.D. Director, Western Psychiatric Institute and Clinics; Professor and Chairman, Department of Psychiatry, University of Pittsburgh School of Medicine, Pittsburgh, Pennsylvania

THOMAS M. FRENCH, M.D. Associate Director, Institute for Psychoanalysis, Chicago, Illinois

MARGARET W. GERARD, Ph.D., M.D. Staff Member, Institute for Psychoanalysis, Chicago, Illinois; Professorial Lecturer, Department of Psychiatry, University of Illinois College of Medicine, Chicago, Illinois

MAURICE LEVINE, M.D. Professor of Psychiatry and Director of the Department, University of Cincinnati College of Medicine, Cincinnati, Ohio

DAVID M. LEVY, M.D. Attending Psychiatrist, New York State Psychiatric Institute, New York, New York

JOHN W. LYONS, M.D. Associate in Psychiatry, University of Pennsylvania School of Medicine, Philadelphia, Pennsylvania.

MARGARET MEAD, Ph.D. Associate Curator of Ethnology, American Museum of Natural History, New York, New York

LEON J. SAUL, M.D. Professor of Clinical Psychiatry, Chief of Section of Preventive Psychiatry, University of Pennsylvania School of Medicine, Philadelphia, Pennsylvania

DAVID SHAKOW, Ph.D. Professor of Psychology, University of Illinois College of Medicine, Chicago, Illinois; Professor of Psychology, University of Chicago (Faculty Exchange), Chicago, Illinois

LOUIS B. SHAPIRO, M.D. Staff Member, Institute for Psychoanalysis, Chicago, Illinois

THOMAS S. SZASZ, M.D. Staff Member, Institute for Psychoanalysis, Chicago, Illinois

EDOARDO WEISS, M.D. Staff Member, Institute for Psychoanalysis, Chicago, Illinois

JOHN C. WHITEHORN, M.D. Henry Phipps Professor of Psychiatry, Johns Hopkins University School of Medicine; Psychiatrist-in-Chief, Johns Hopkins Hospital, Baltimore, Maryland.

# TABLE OF CONTENTS

## PART III. INFLUENCE OF PSYCHOANALYSIS ON ALLIED FIELDS

## INDEX

# PART I
# CONCEPTS OF DYNAMIC PSYCHIATRY

# I

# DEVELOPMENT OF THE FUNDAMENTAL CONCEPTS OF PSYCHOANALYSIS

Franz Alexander, M.D.

## Discovery of the Dynamic Unconscious

THAT the human personality embraces more than the traditional concept of the conscious mind is a fundamental discovery of Freud. Many of the psychological functions of everyday life, such as fantasy, dreaming, and parapraxias as well as neurotic and psychotic symptoms and impulsive behavior, cannot be understood in terms of conscious motivation. They become intelligible only when unconscious motivation is reconstructed or made conscious.

The discovery of unconscious motivation had a profound influence upon psychiatric thought. It terminated a strange double standard which characterized the scientific approach to human behavior before the discoveries of Freud. Rational behavior had always been explained through conscious motivation, which could be established by introspection or by verbal communication. The moves of a chess player, for example, were explained not on a chemical or electrophysiological basis but on logical reasoning. But when the medical man was confronted with neurotic symptoms and psychotic behavior which appeared irrational and unexplainable with common-sense psychology, then he abandoned psychological causality and postulated some unknown changes in brain physiology as ultimate causes. When an adult experienced fear in high places or when crossing the street or when he had the urge to count every object in a room, this was called "psychasthenia," and certain changes in brain physiology were assumed. When a person driven by hunger killed someone in order to take away his possessions, this was considered a legitimate problem of psychology. One had only to understand the murderer's motivation to explain his deed. But if a person driven by paranoid delusions committed murder, attempts at psycho-

3

logical explanation were abandoned, and unknown changes in brain structure or physiology were hypothesized. The answer of Freudian psychology to this dichotomy was that both normal and pathological mental processes have their physiological side and are still largely unknown functions of the brain. Both normal and pathological mental processes can be explained, however, from psychological motivations. There is no fundamental difference between psychology and psychopathology: both follow the same basic principles. The reason that psychopathological processes appear irrational, that is to say, do not make sense, lies in the fact that they are determined by *unconscious* processes, which are more primitive than the conscious processes.

The nature of unconscious processes is revealed in dreams, in children's play, in free-floating fantasy, and in neurotic and psychotic symptoms. Unconscious processes can be understood on the basis of psychological causality only when their primitive nature is recognized. This primitive psychology is preverbal. Psychological maturation consists, to a large degree, in learning how to substitute mental processes, adjusted to reality, for wishful and preverbal thinking. Freud maintained that these primitive thought-processes and emotional reactions do not dissolve completely at maturation or become entirely transformed in well-integrated rational processes, but remain latent in the unconscious. The conscious mind defends itself against this latent influence through the mechanism of repression. Repression is responsible for the fact that personality is not a homogeneous entity.

Mental functions can be divided into two groups: rational well-integrated functions adapted to reality, and unconscious processes which make themselves noticeable directly in dreams, pathological symptoms, and errors of everyday life and indirectly through their influence on all mental processes. Their influence upon overt behavior is not obvious; but overt behavior can never be explained from conscious motivation alone. By means of a process called "rationalization," everyone covers up his unconscious motives to some degree with conscious ones, which are often of little dynamic significance. Recognition of this self-deceiving trend in man had a revolutionary influence upon contemporary thought and has gradually transformed the whole outlook of our era, just as the theories of Copernicus and Darwin influenced thinking in the past.

In the first phase of his scientific career, Freud's main concern was to demonstrate the existence of the dynamic unconscious through a study of hypnotic phenomena, hysterical symptoms, dreams, and parapraxias of everyday life. Gradually he developed techniques by which these unconscious processes could be studied by the physician and eventually brought into the consciousness of the patient. This brings us to the second phase in the development of psychoanalysis.

### DEVELOPMENT OF METHODS FOR THE STUDY OF UNCONSCIOUS PROCESSES

After hypnosis was abandoned by Freud, his first significant methodological discovery was that the spontaneous, uncontrolled, so-called "free associations" offer an approach to the study of the unconscious. He considered the method of dream interpretation, which was based on free association, the most effective technique. According to Freud, the dream is the royal road to the unconscious mind. It represents the intrusion into the conscious mind of unconscious processes; it reflects in an almost pure fashion the psychology of unconscious processes and offers an unparalleled opportunity to study their peculiarities. Neurotic and psychotic symptoms are in their dynamics identical with dream processes and therefore offer a similarly suitable wedge through which the psychological laws of the unconscious mind can be explored.

The fruitfulness of the psychoanalytic technique is amply documented by the theoretical and therapeutic exploits of the first two decades of psychoanalytic history, during which Freud and his growing number of followers explored the characteristics of unconscious thought-processes. This amounted to learning a new language, the symbolic language of unconscious processes, which differs considerably from the words of conscious thinking. During these early years the fundamental dynamic processes were discovered—repression, overcompensation, substitution and displacement, projection, rationalization, sublimation, turning impulses against the self. Through the discovery of the modes of emotional expression and thought on the preverbal level, the sense of all psychopathological phenomena revealed itself. Psychological common sense was applied to psychopathology, a field where this had not been possible before. Common-sense psychology, however, had to undergo certain modifications in order to become useful in deciphering the meaning of unconscious processes. This is the essence of what is known as "psychoanalytic interpretation."

The methodological significance of the procedure of interpretation is so fundamental that we shall interpolate a brief discussion.[1]

## Psychoanalytic Method of Investigation

Every science is based on the systematic development and refinement of the methods of observation and reasoning used in everyday life. Psychoanalysis, unlike earlier psychological methods, has refined the methods of common sense used to understand another person's motivations and actions.

Common sense itself is a complex faculty. It is based primarily on the fact that the observer and the observed are similar to each other. Both are human personalities. Through speech, they can convey their motivations to each other. This similarity allows identification. Knowing one's own motivations, one can easily extrapolate them to another person. This similarity between observed and observer obtains in no other science; it is characteristic of psychology alone. All psychological methods which fail to recognize and exploit this unique advantage have only a limited value for the study of human personality. So long as psychologists tried to imitate the methods of the experimental sciences and neglected to use and develop the natural faculty for understanding the mental processes of another person, psychology as a science of human personality could not develop.

Understanding another individual's mental situation through common sense alone, however, is not a reliable method. It is not sufficiently precise for scientific inquiry because of several sources of error. One of the main contributions of Freud's psychoanalysis was to improve and enlarge common-sense understanding. Four sources of error are inherent in psychological common sense:

1. Under ordinary conditions a person has no special reason to disclose his real motivations to another by verbal communication.

2. It is impossible to give a full account of one's motivations because many of them the individual himself does not know.

3. The vast extent of individual differences makes identification difficult, sometimes impossible. This is best seen if one tries to understand the mental situation of another person whose language one does not understand. The greater the difference be-

1. This methodological contribution of Freud's psychology was discussed by the author in an address given before the Harvey Society in 1930.

tween two minds, the greater the difficulty of mutual understanding. Difficulties in understanding the behavior of young
children, savages, psychotics, and neurotics are due to just these
divergences in mentality.

4. Every observer has some blind spots due to his own repressions. Either he will overlook in the other person those motivations which he tries to exclude from his own consciousness, or he
will project them into the other person, discovering the mote
in his fellow-man's eye while not noting the beam in his own.
The obstacle which one's own repressions constitute against understanding others can be appreciated if one realizes that the uni-
formity and harmony of the conscious mind are guaranteed by
repressions. To become an adult, it is necessary to "forget" infantile ways of thinking. The latter is to a much higher degree subject to the pleasure principle than is adult mentality, which has to
adjust itself to reality. The difficulty in understanding children,
savages, neurotics, and psychotics is therefore due not only to the
difference between their mentality and ours but also to the repressing forces within ourselves. In order to become a rational
adult, the primitive functions of the mind must be transformed
into co-ordinated rational processes. The phenomenon of dreams
alone shows clearly, however, that the substitution of rational
functions for more primitive processes is not complete. The conscious mind has to defend itself against following the universal
trend to regress to primitive forms of thought. Every night such
a regression takes place during sleep. Under external stress as a
result of traumatic experiences, such a regression shows itself in
neurotic or psychotic symptoms or in unrestrained behavior.

By means of the psychoanalytic technique, these four sources
of error, if not eliminated, have been reduced to such a degree
that psychology has become a science of the personality. The dis-
inclination of a person to give a full account of his mental state
is reduced in psychoanalysis because of the therapeutic situation.
The sick person, in the hope of being cured by the help of the
physician, is more willing than the well person to put aside the
usual restraints against revealing his most intimate feelings, as is
required by the method of free association. In free association,
thoughts and ideas can emerge which are usually forced out of
the focus of attention. The patient's desire to be cured is an almost
indispensable factor in psychological investigation, for it alone
guarantees a willingness for unreserved self-revelation. As a pre-

requisite of the methodical study of another person's mind, this type of patient-physician relationship has not been replaced by any other human situation. It is matched only by religious confession in respect to its frankness and the desire to reveal one's self. Religious confession, however, does not utilize the confessional situation for scientific study but for giving relief to the distressed mind.

The second source of error—the inability to reveal one's self completely because of repressions—is met by the analytical technique in two ways. Through free association the conscious control of mental processes is eliminated, thus allowing a more spontaneous expression of ideas which otherwise would not appear in the stream of consciousness. Abandoning conscious control, however, does not mean that the patient is freed from his repressions. The effectiveness of the repression is diminished, since conscious control and repression work in the same direction—to keep repressed thoughts out of the conscious mind. With the elimination of the one factor, the equilibrium between the tendency of repressed mental content to appear in consciousness and the opposing force which excludes it from consciousness is changed in favor of the former. Another factor which favors the process of self-revelation lies in the emotional rapport between patient and therapist. As soon as the patient becomes convinced that he is not being judged by the therapist, that the latter wants only to understand him, frank communication becomes possible.

It is most difficult to eliminate the third source of error—the difference between observer and observed. Differences of language and culture as well as of sex and age can be bridged, however, by consistent and prolonged study in frequent and continued interviews over a long period of time. The fact that neurotic symptoms, like dreams, are manifestations of unconscious processes makes them difficult to understand by rational common sense. Painstaking study of these more primitive preverbal mental processes has resulted in a knowledge which allows their translation into verbal thought-processes used by common-sense psychology.

The last source of error—the observer's own repressions—is reduced by the training analysis which is required in every psychoanalyst's training. Through his own analysis, the physician clears up those "blind spots" which result from repression.

With these measures, psychoanalysis has developed a technique of investigation which is adapted to the special nature of psychological phenomena. By this method it has produced a theory of personality which made possible the treatment of mental disturbances on an etiological basis.

The dynamic principles established by the psychoanalytic method are valid in themselves and independent of the generalizations and speculations concerning the ultimate nature of psychological forces. The laws of optics are valid, although physicists still disagree concerning the ultimate nature of light. The dynamic principles of psychoanalysis are independent of theories concerning the ultimate nature of the instincts. Without a brief sketch of what is called the "theory of instinct," however, the history of psychoanalytic thought would not be complete. This will be presented later in the chapter.

## FUNCTIONS OF THE EGO

Before the publication of *The Ego and the Id* (1923), Freud and his followers focused their attention chiefly upon the interpretation of repressed psychological content. Through a relentless study of dreams and other psychological phenomena in which the nature of unconscious processes is revealed, they developed the art of interpretation to a fine and precise instrument. In *The Ego and the Id*, Freud made the first attempt to visualize the total structure and functioning of what he called the "mental apparatus." He distinguished three structurally different parts: the id, the ego, and the superego (chap. iv). The *id* is the original power-house of the mental apparatus; it contains the inherited instinctive forces which at birth are not yet organized into a co-ordinated system. The *ego* is conceived as a product of development which consists in the adaptation of the inherited instinctive drives to one another and to the environment. The *superego*, too, is the precipitate of adaptation; it represents the incorporation of parental attitudes which are determined by the existing cultural standards. After maturation the ego becomes the dynamic center of behavior. Most important in this theory was the conception that mental functions have relationship to the total organism. The ego's function, according to Freud, is to carry out what is ordinarily considered co-ordinated rational behavior and is aimed at maintaining a constant condition (level of excitation) within the organism (stability principle). It is a homeostatic function. The homeostatic equilibrium is constantly disturbed by the life-process itself, by biological needs which arise within the organism, and by external stimuli. In satisfying biological needs and in defending the organism against excessive external stimulation, the ego performs its homeostatic task with the help of four basic faculties: (1) internal perception of instinctive needs, (2) external perception of existing conditions upon which the gratification of subjective needs depends, (3) the integrative faculty by which the ego co-ordinates instinctive urges with one another and with the requirements of the superego and adapts them to the environmental conditions, and (4) the executive faculty by which it controls voluntary behavior. Through the latter, the ego can implement the results of its integrative function, which consists fundamentally in the rational cognitive faculty.

In performing this function (homeostasis), the ego has to struggle continually against the primitive dynamic trend existing within the organism, namely, the tendency of every psychological urge to seek immediate gratification. This tendency, characteristic of the infant, is what Freud called the "pleasure-pain principle." He assumed that the gratification of every subjective need is connected with pleasure; its frustration, with pain. To relieve immediately any painful tension and to obtain immediate pleasure is the fundamental primitive motivating force within the organism.

This pleasure-pain principle, however, eventually causes more pain for the organism than pleasure, since immediate gratification often has painful consequences and may endanger survival. Under the influence of adverse experiences, the ego gradually develops the capacity to co-ordinate psychological impulses with one another and to adapt them to external conditions in a way that assures the best possible outcome in a given situation. The ego learns to postpone certain desires when satisfaction might endanger more important urges. It learns to compromise, to modify the desires, to subordinate less important to more important needs. In other words, the ego learns what is considered rational behavior. Because rational behavior appears to most adults as something natural, requiring no further explanation, its study has been neglected for many years.[2]

2. Recently, Thomas French has focused his main interest on analyzing the principles of rational behavior and describing in more detail what Freud called the "reality principle" (see *The Integration of Behavior*, Vol. 1: *Basic Postulates* [Chicago: University of Chicago Press, 1952]).

Well co-ordinated rational behavior is acquired by an arduous process of learning. Through continual groping experimentation the ego finds adequate behavior patterns, and through repetition their performance becomes routinized, automatic, and hence less energy-consuming. This tendency to accomplish the homeostatic task with a minimum expenditure of energy through repetition is the *economy principle*. Because the organism constantly changes during the process of growth and because conditions in the environment also change, it is necessary for the ego constantly to modify adaptive behavior patterns acquired earlier in the individual's life. Each change requires renewed experimentation until new adaptations are learned. Because of the economy principle, however, there is a tendency to keep old behavior patterns and to resist learning new ones. This manifestation of the economy principle can be aptly termed the "inertia principle." The phenomena of fixation, regression, and repetition compulsion are all based on the inertia principle. "Fixation" designates the tendency to retain previously successful behavior patterns. "Regression" is the tendency to return to them whenever new adjustments are required which are beyond the ego's integrative capacity. Regression is most common under experiences so traumatic that there follows a disintegration of the arduously acquired adaptive pattern into its constituent parts. These "parts" are patterns acquired earlier and gradually woven into more complex integrated behavior. "Repetition compulsion" is the propensity to repeat previously acquired patterns in accordance with the general principle of economy (inertia) instead of undertaking the energy-consuming task of finding new ways of behavior through the integrative process.

The human being does not learn everything through trial and error. "Identification" is another method of learning, a process by which the growing child takes over behavior patterns and attitudes from adults.

For the understanding of psychopathology, it is important to note that co-ordinated rational behavior can be maintained only through a constant struggle on the part of the ego, because the instinctual tendencies retain their original inclination for immediate gratification. This is the original basis of Freud's structural concept of differentiation between ego and id. He assumed that a tendency toward nonco-ordinated, isolated gratification is always present and manifests itself in all those psychological phenomena which are not rational or co-ordinated, such as dreams, free fantasy, impulsive behavior, and all that is known as "psychopatho-logical." Whenever the ego is threatened by impulses which are not in harmony with its accepted standards or reality, a conflict and concomitant anxiety arise. To anxiety the ego reacts by defenses which are erected against these tendencies threatening from within. These defenses are partly bulwarks which favor repression, such as overcompensation or rationalization, and partly vents by which the repudiated tendencies can find an outlet, such as projection, substitution, displacement, or turning impulses directed against external objects against the self. Mental disease represents a failure of the ego to secure gratification for subjective needs in a harmonious and reality-adjusted manner and a breakdown of the defenses by which it tries to neutralize impulses that cannot be harmonized with internal standards and external reality.

### Defenses of the Ego

1. *Repression.*—Whenever the ego fails in its integrative task of co-ordinating impulses with one another and with the existing environmental conditions, it adopts one or more of the defensive mechanisms it learned in earlier years. The basic mechanism consists in excluding from the consciousness the psychological content which it is unable to include harmoniously in its scope. This is called "repression" and was considered by Freud as the principal defense of the infantile ego, which has not the capacity to withstand temptation, postpone, or modify by compromise the gratification of an impulse. Whatever impulse appears in consciousness has to be converted into action immediately. Repression remains, therefore, the only effective defense. Repressed impulses, however, do not cease to exist merely by exclusion from consciousness and thereby from motor expression. To deal with the tension of these pent-up impulses the ego has to resort to further defenses, which can be classified in two groups: (*a*) further reinforcements of repression or (*b*) substitute vents by which the original impulses can find at least a partial, modified ego syntonic release and by which their pressure is decreased.

2. *Overcompensation.*—The ego may make use of an acceptable attitude to help an ego-alien attitude stay repressed. Thus pity may cover up unconscious cruelty, shyness can serve as a defense against exhibitionism, temerity against timidity, and boastful conceit against a feeling of inferiority. The conscious attitude

in these instances is the polar opposite of the repressed ego-alien tendency.

One of the most important overcompensations is that of love by hate or hate by love. This is observed when either love, such as homosexual desire, or hate directed against a benefactor becomes unacceptable to the ego. This attitude is based on the clinically important phenomenon of ambivalence—love and hatred toward the same person. A certain amount of ambivalence is universal, because the narcissistic nucleus of the personality "hates" every loved object which depletes the ego's self-love. The utilization of one component of the ambivalent conflict in order to keep the other in repression is therefore a very common phenomenon.

3. *Rationalization.*—This is a common technique by which the ego keeps certain tendencies repressed. Rationalization means the selection from coexisting motivations of those most acceptable to the ego. Emphasis upon the acceptable motivation allows the ego to keep the unacceptable repressed, since the selected motives can sufficiently explain the act in question ("I attack him because he is wrong and not because I envy him").

4. *Identification.*—Under certain conditions the mechanism of identification which plays such an important role in the healthy growth of the ego may become a defensive measure. Most common is identification with an object (a person) lost in bereavement or by separation or rejection. The ego in a way re-establishes the lost one by identifying itself with that person. Identification with a powerful enemy is another use of identification as a defense. By assuming the qualities of the opponent, anxiety is mastered.

5. *Substitution and displacement.*—Another common defensive measure consists in displacing an emotional attitude from one object to another. In this way hatred can be diverted from the person, whom to hate would cause conflict, to someone else, who may be justifiably disliked. Sometimes not the person but the act which is objectionable is replaced by another less objectionable one. This defense is characterized as "substitution." A murderous impulse may be replaced by a minor aggression or released by some impersonal destructive act, such as wood-chopping or boxing at the punch ball.

6. *Sublimation.*—The defense most important to society consists in substituting for an unacceptable tendency another one

which is appropriate for relieving the original tendency and at the same time has a socially useful aspect. Common examples are the substitution of all forms of creativity for sexual impulses or certain activities by which inanimate nature can be mastered for hostile aggressive tendencies.

7. *Projection.*—When a repressed tendency can no longer be kept out of consciousness, a radical defense may become necessary. An example is attributing a repressed tendency to another person. The ego can neither accept the subjective tendency as its own nor repress it. The only solution is then to deny its belonging to the scope of one's own personality. Through projection the ego abandons, to some degree at least, its reality-testing function by misinterpreting reality and thus returns to a primitive stage of development when external reality and internal (psychological) reality were not yet differentiated.

8. *Provocative behavior.*—In provocative behavior a person may express his original hostility against another person by inducing the other person to attack first. One's own aggressive behavior then appears as self-defense; this allows one to express one's hostility without internal conflict and at the same time keep one's motivations repressed.

9. *Turning feelings toward one's self.*—Another defense against unacceptable tendencies which threaten to break through the barrier of repression is turning them against one's self. Instead of expressing hostility or hatred against another person, the hatred is turned against the own self in the form of self-criticism and self-accusation. By the same mechanism, the feeling of love can be withdrawn from another person and turned into self-love.

10. *Isolation.*—Isolation is a technique mainly restricted to compulsive neurosis. Ego-alien tendencies which appear in consciousness are separated from the rest of the mental content and thus made innocuous. The patient may master his neurotic anxiety by carefully separating acceptable psychological content from the objectionable. This is the basis of many compulsive rituals—touching, washing, and all kinds of avoidances of trivial activities.

11. *Regression.*—Already described is the universal trend toward regression. An ego-alien tendency—for example, a sexual urge toward a tabooed person—can be replaced regressively by some pregenital, less objectionable attitude toward the same per-

son. Sexual desire may then be evaded by means of a dependent attitude, which has no obvious sexual connotation.

Regression is a universal mechanism. It is accentuated in neurosis. In fact, every neurotic symptom has a regressive connotation, inasmuch as adequate co-ordinated behavior is replaced by activities in fantasy, the content of which always shows a return to previous modes of gratification.

12. *Defense against guilt feelings.*—Defense mechanisms by which guilt feelings are prevented from becoming conscious are the most complex of all. Most phenomena qualified by the expression "masochistic" belong to this type of defense. By inflicting punishment upon one's self or provoking suffering, guilt feelings can be reduced or eliminated without the person's becoming conscious of their nature.

Like regression, these masochistic defenses have an outstanding significance in psychopathology because they are ubiquitous in neurotic processes. Regression to earlier modes of gratification—pregenital and oedipal fixations—creates of necessity either guilt feelings or feelings of inferiority or both. Owing to the deep-rooted emotional syllogism that suffering atones for guilt, guilt feelings and anxiety can be temporarily removed from consciousness through atonement by means of suffering.

13. *Defenses against inferiority feelings.*—Regression to earlier dependent states creates inferiority feelings (shame) which many patients try to repress and keep repressed by overcompensatory bravado (counterphobic behavior). This is particularly noticeable in delinquent behavior. Many wanton violations of law are motivated by deeply repressed inferiority feelings, which the delinquent denies by flaunting his independence and courage in destructive and aggressive behavior (see above, Sec. 2, "Overcompensation").

14. *Conversion.*—Ego-alien tendencies may be thoroughly repressed and find no expression on the psychological level or in co-ordinated behavior. The pent-up tension may then be relieved by changes in the field of the skeletal and laryngeal muscles or in the sense organs. These changes (paralyses, muscular contractions, spasms, convulsions, different kinds of sensory symptoms, such as anaesthesia and paresthesia or blindness and deafness) have a symbolic meaning and serve both the expression and the negation of the repressed ego-alien tendencies.

In the foregoing pages we have discussed the dynamic processes underlying the functions of the ego and its ways and means of dealing with instinctual forces. As stated before, these dynamic formulations are independent of speculations concerning the ultimate nature of the instinctual forces. Now we shall attempt to outline briefly the development of psychoanalytic views about the nature of the instincts.

## THEORY OF INSTINCTS

Originally, Freud assumed the existence of two basic instincts, the instinct of self-preservation and the sex instinct. He referred to them as "ego instinct" (*Ich-triebe*) and "libido." All observed psychological forces motivating behavior were considered as derivatives of one of these basic instincts. An antagonism between the two categories was assumed because sexual strivings were those commonly found to be repressed. Neurotic symptoms could be explained as substitute expressions of repressed, and thus frustrated, sexual strivings. The ego instincts tend to preserve the integrity of the organism, which is often threatened by sexual strivings not in accord with existing social standards. Incestuous cravings of the child and hostile feelings directed against the parent of the other sex are commonly repressed tendencies.

The distinction between ego instincts and sexual libido soon led to theoretical difficulties. When the existence of infantile sexuality was recognized, the concept of libido had to be extended to include not only race preservation but also the infantile manifestations of sexuality which have nothing to do with propagation. The latter center around the vegetative functions, which are in the service of self-preservation—pleasure sensations during sucking, the excremental act, and the exercise of muscles. In fact, most biological functions are the source of pleasure sensations which resemble the later sexual gratifications. Oral, anal, urethral, and muscular eroticism are connected with nutrition, excretion, grasping, and locomotion, which ultimately become subservient to self-preservation. Moreover, the emotional content of infantile sexuality is completely self-centered. Since the main object of these erotic interests is the child's own person, Freud called this form of libido "narcissistic." As soon as it was recognized that the first object of love is the self, the distinction between self-preservation and sexuality became contradictory.

The distinction between narcissistic libido and object libido called attention to the fact that love may be directed toward the self or toward other objects. The self-centered libido, however, could no longer be distinguished from self-preservation. Essentially, all functions of self-preservation were included in libido except aggression, which was relegated to the category of ego instincts. In the form of sadism, however, the aggressive hostile impulse also assumes a libidinous connotation. This made obvious the inconsistency of the original distinction between self-preservative and sexual instincts. Hostility remained the only manifestation of the ego instinct, and even this could not be claimed as nonsexual, at least certainly not on a phenomenological basis. Jung proposed a solution to this by abandoning Freud's dualism and attributing everything to libido. The Jungian "libido" became similar to Bergson's "élan vital" or to the notions of the German vitalists.

Freud was fully aware of the theoretical difficulties of the original libido theory, but only in 1920 did he revise his theory. He then introduced a new dualistic concept of instincts: life and death. He assumed an erotic principle which is a binding force and corresponds basically to the anabolic phase of metabolism. The upbuilding tendency is a manifestation of the erotic life-instinct. This force is opposed by the death instinct, which is a disintegrating force and appears biologically in biochemical catabolism. The two tendencies, according to Freud, are always mixed in their actual psychological manifestations. The erotic instinct has a narcissistic phase when it is self-preservative. In mature organisms it attracts the sexes to each other, and it then becomes race-preservative.

It is obvious that the theory of life and death instincts was no longer an attempt to describe instinctual forces but rather a philosophical abstraction. It contained, however, a valuable nucleus in distinguishing two basic vectors in the life-process—one upbuilding (anabolic) and one disruptive (catabolic). This paved the way for the psychosomatic view of the instinctual life which developed with increasing knowledge of the integrative functions of the organism as a whole.

This psychosomatic theory of sexuality attempts to reconcile both the psychology and the physiology of all those widely diversified behavioral phenomena which have one feature in common—that they yield erotic gratification. This common feature was what induced Freud to consider physical pleasure sensations, such as thumbsucking or the excitation of the anal zone, as sexual in nature. The most convincing observation was that a child may induce an erection by thumbsucking. Further studies have shown that many other functions of the body can yield erotic pleasure, such as urination, locomotion, looking, etc. Equally significant is the fact that all intense emotions can become the psychological content of sexual excitation. The craving to be loved and to love others, which is accompanied by the desire for bodily contact, is by no means the only content of sexual desires. The sadistic impulse to hurt, the inclination to suffer pain and humiliation, curiosity about sexuality, vanity about one's own body, with the wish to expose it in order to become the center of attention—all these may be emotional sources of the sexual impulse but may be expressed also without physical sexual connotation. On the basis of such observation, Freud concluded originally that sexuality is not dependent on a special emotional quality but has a quantitative basis; it is a special form of emotional discharge. Later he abandoned this view and attributed to sexuality a specific quality.

The fact that the same emotional tension, such as love or hate, can be discharged both in a sexual and in a nonsexual manner strongly supports the view that sexuality should be considered a specific form of discharge for any psychological tension. The peculiar nature of the sexual discharge can be understood from the psychological characteristics of sexual phenomena and from their biological function. Hostile aggressive behavior against a person who threatens one's security differs in many respects from wanton cruelty carried out as a form of sexual gratification. The first type of aggressive behavior is subservient to the practical goal of defending one's own interest. In the second type inflicting pain is a goal in itself, not subordinated to the interest of the total organism.

The same difference obtains in all other forms of sexual discharge. In scoptophilia, which is an erotic phenomenon, watching, observing, and satisfying curiosity are aims in themselves and are not substitutes for another goal. Learning about something, the knowledge of which is essential for self-preservation, is the nonsexual counterpart of scoptophilia. In the latter form of curiosity, self-preservation is the main goal; watching and finding out something are subordinated to it.

The same obtains to masochism. Carrying a heavy knapsack is a form of suffering the tourist has to endure in order to be comfortable when he reaches the mountain peak. It is not a source of pleasure but a necessary evil. This is not masochism but rational well-adjusted behavior. As soon as suffering becomes an aim itself, however, it assumes the concentration of sexual gratification. This is called "masochism."

Likewise, the early erotic preoccupations of the infant, such as thumbsucking or retention of excrement, are independent of the vegetative functions to which they are related: eating and the excremental act. Thumbsucking is not subservient to the utilitarian function of eating. It is carried out entirely as a source of pleasure, without serving any physiological function in the interest of the whole organism. Psychoanalysis postulated that the exercise of voluntary muscles may yield erotic gratification which is called "muscle eroticism." In early infancy the unco-ordinated movements of the child are not yet subordinated to any utilitarian goal and probably have the sole function of erotic discharge.

The psychosomatic view of sexuality here proposed attempts to assemble all the above observations into a comprehensive picture. The outstanding feature characteristic of all those phenomena which have an erotic connotation is that they discharge an *excess of excitation*. The nature of the excitation may be love, hate, curiosity, suffering, vanity—in fact, it includes the whole gamut of human emotions. Sexuality discharges any excess excitation, regardless of its quality. The sexual discharge of impulses is not integrated with other functions in the service of self-preservation. The same impulses, if co-ordinated into utilitarian functions, lose their sexual connotation.

The biological function of mature sexuality is propagation. When the organism reaches the limit of its growth, it can no longer increase and must divide. Cell division—the prototype of propagation—can be considered as the continuation of the process of growth beyond the limits of the individual unit, the cell. Surplus organic matter which cannot be integrated in a single biological unit is expelled and becomes a new organism. In multicellular organisms the same basic process takes place in a more complex manner. Propagation, then, results from surplus generated by growth. The psychological counterpart of this process is mature love. After the maturing organism becomes saturated with narcissistic love, there is an overflow of emotion, and other persons become the objects of this love: narcissistic love gives way to object love.

The pregenital manifestations of sexuality can be understood as manifestations of excitation which is in excess of what is needed for self-preservative aims. An excess of the incorporative urge which is no longer serving the utilitarian aim of satisfying hunger appears in thumbsucking or some other oral play (oral eroticism). Likewise, the anal manifestations of sexuality are not subservient to the excremental functions but serve mainly to relieve an excess of excitation (anal eroticism).

Erotic phenomena have a playful quality—in fact, all play activities are erotic in nature. For this reason, Eros is personified as a child. Most of the infant's self-preservative needs are met by the help of adults; many of his body functions are exercised mainly for the discharge of surplus excitation and for no utilitarian goal. From birth on, only the basic vegetative functions serve the vital needs of the organism. The sense organs and the muscles are not yet co-ordinated to serve utilitarian needs. The unco-ordinated movements of the infant are not suited for grabbing or locomotion and are carried out only for pleasurable discharge of tensions, as in the form of muscle eroticism. The racing colt exuberantly uses his accumulated energies, serving no purpose. The sense organs also are used for the sake of pleasurable activity alone. The eyes see for the sake of scoptophilic pleasure, and the hands touch for the sake of experiencing pleasant tactile sensations. Gradually, with growth toward independence, the functions which originally were practiced in a playful fashion become integrated for the utilitarian goals of existence. Now the eyes are used to find the food, the extremities to approach and to grab it. Erotic play gives place gradually to self-preservative functions; yet surplus energy in excess of the needs of self-preservation may be discharged in an erotic manner also in adult life. Finally, after the organism has reached the limits of growth, surplus intake in excess over expenditure is discharged in the form of propagation or its sublimated equivalents: in productive and creative activities.

This surplus theory of sexuality receives its strongest support from physiology. In the mature organism sexual excitation is discharged primarily through the genitourinary system, the physiological function of which consists precisely in discharging body products and emotional tensions which are no longer useful for the self-preservation of the organism. Physically, it discharges either waste or germ cells, which are not integrated with the rest of the organism. Psychologically, the manifestations of sexuality consist in discharging tensions for their own sake, tensions which are not subordinated to the needs of the total organism. Sexuality, with its physiological and psychological manifestation, can be considered as a drainage system of all energies which are not needed for the preservation of individual life and are in excess of the needs of the organism. The specific organ of this kind of discharge is the genitourinary tract.

The significant role of sexuality in neurotic disturbances becomes evident in the light of this view. Whenever the ego cannot carry out its homeostatic function of finding adequate gratification for subjective needs in harmony with the total personality, tensions accumulate which are not integrated with the total needs of the organism. Such unintegrated tendencies seek expression through sexual channels. When mature expression of the genital level is inhibited, the pent-up tensions seek regressive sexual expressions, which are in conflict with the accepted ego standards. In perversion they find direct pregenital expression, whereas in neurosis the ego defends itself against these infantile sexual strivings. As a result, substitute expressions are created as vents, in the form of neurotic symptoms. The latter are expressions of regressive strivings and of the ego's defenses against these unacceptable tendencies. In this view, Freud's original formulation, that neurotic symptoms are the negatives of perversions, finds a new confirmation.

## DYNAMICS OF EGO DEVELOPMENT

Growth and maturation are fundamental attributes of all living organisms. Lifeless machines, no matter how ingenious in performance, become old and rusty with time. Before the human organism becomes old and rusty, it passes through a cycle that is basically the same in every living being: growth until maturation characterized by the faculty of propagation, then decline until death. In the human organism this cycle consists of prenatal growth until birth, then infancy, childhood, pubescence, maturity, senescence, and death.

One of the features of this cycle specific for man is the prolonged biological helplessness of the infant. For this, there is no parallel in the animal kingdom. This comparatively long duration of dependent infancy offers a clue to many riddles of human development. The human infant, unlike most animals at birth, is not fully equipped with inherited automatic behavior patterns needed for independent existence; consequently, he must learn these functions through trial and error. The biological symbiosis between infant and mother continues for a while after birth but gradually yields to independent existence. First in nutrition, later in locomotion, and still later in his orientation to the world, the child becomes more and more independent, an achievement attained through the process of learning. In this process his identification with adults is of the greatest importance. This comparatively prolonged period of dependence, during which the infant, under parental guidance, gradually learns the ways and means of independent existence, accounts for the great variety of personalities found in the human species. The infant represents an extremely pliable yet unfinished substratum, upon which environmental influences, primarily the personalities of the parents, exert their molding impression.

Scientific recognition of the formative influence of early family life is the contribution of Freud and his followers. As a result of their studies, it was concluded that not only heredity but also the conditions of infancy determine our destiny.

It is only recently that students of personality have become impressed by the fact that personality development does not stop at a certain age, that significant changes take place in all phases of the life-curve, and particularly that the formative experience of early years do not necessarily leave irreversible effects. Many of the adverse influences of early childhood can be corrected by later experiences in life. Indeed, psychoanalytic therapy is based on this view. We try by methodical treatment procedures to bring about changes in personality structure, by undoing those unfavorable patterns established in an earlier period. All psychoanalysts conform implicitly to this view, in that they practice a therapy by which they endeavor to bring changes into personality structure. Yet many psychoanalysts are strangely inconsistent, in that they underestimate the influence of later experiences in life, to which they ascribe only a precipitating significance. While this often may be the case, profound experiences in later life, such as migration from one culture to another, continued contact with certain persons, as well as many vicissitudes of life, may produce deep changes in personality. If this were not the case, psychoanalytic therapy of adults, in itself a form of later experience, could not alter a patient's personality.

Today most psychoanalysts have reached a more balanced view, which recognizes the significance of three categories of factors in respect to the personality of the individual: heredity, early experiences within the family, and events of later life.

### FACTORS INHERENT IN PERSONALITY DEVELOPMENT

Heredity supplies the ground pattern that determines not only certain basic qualities but the whole rhythm of the life-span. With certain variations, the main phases of growth are rather uniformly predetermined by hereditary factors. Dentition, myelinization of certain nerve tracts, learning to speak and walk, the maturation of the sex glands, and, finally, the degenerative changes of senescence, take place—with individual variations—at about the same age and in every individual in the same sequence. This fundamental pattern of the life-curve cannot be changed by later influences.

Each phase of biological growth is characterized by well-defined psychological attitudes. Except for oxygen supply, the newborn infant is completely dependent upon the mother biologically, and consequently seeks gratification for his needs from the mother. His security is based on being loved and cared for. Gradually the child learns to use his biological equipment independently. The eye learns to focus, the hands to grab, the legs to walk. Interest in the vegetative functions of the body and curiosity regarding its anatomy are further characteristics of the first six years. Later this curiosity is replaced by an investigative interest in the external environment. Now the phase of biological mastery of body functions is followed by a period in which the development of intellectual functions predominates, gradually allowing an independent orientation to the surrounding world (chap. iv).

The next important phase, the period of adolescence, is again determined by biological factors, the maturation of the sex glands. By now the growing organism has developed all its functions, to which finally the faculty of propagation is added. Although biologically the adolescent organism has reached the end of its growth, its psychological state can be sharply differentiated from maturity. In our culture biological growth is ahead of psychological maturation. This fact offers a clue to the understanding of most of the peculiarities of the adolescent. The salient feature of this period is the novelty of the new state of being grown-up, particularly in respect to the propagative faculties. In adolescence, the biological ability to procreate is as if foisted upon an emotionally unprepared and inexperienced organism. A full-grown body is intrusted to an inexperienced mind. The main characteristics of the adolescent—his proverbial awkwardness and insecurity—follow this discrepancy. The adolescent impresses us as not knowing what to do with himself in his newly attained state. Adolescent competitiveness can be traced back to the same basic circumstance. The adolescent feels as if he were constantly in a test situation; he must prove to himself and others that he is already a man. The only way to do this is to measure himself against others.

This competition demands a continuous practice of the adolescent's full-grown capacities. During the period of adolescence the young person gradually grows emotionally into the advanced mature status that he had reached biologically several years before. The self-confident attitude of the mature person is based on taking himself and his capacities for granted. This is in sharp contrast to the insecurity of the infant and the adolescent. As a consequence of this inner security, the mature adult's interest no longer centers around the self but can be turned outward toward the environment.

The psychological attributes of maturity, like those of other age periods, can best be understood from the biological conditions of maturity. As long as the organism grows, intake and retention of substance and energy outweigh their expenditure. Otherwise growth would not be possible. The psychological manifestation of this state of affairs is that in the immature organism the wish to receive outweighs the wish to give. When the organism reaches maturity, it can no longer add anything to its own size; growth has reached its natural limits. The body cannot organize more living matter within its own system. Therefore, individual growth stops, and propagation serves as a means of releasing surplus energy. Propagation in this light can be understood as development beyond the limits of individual growth.

As stated before, all energy that is not needed to maintain life can be considered surplus energy. This is the source of all sexual activity; it is also the source of all productive and creative work. This surplus energy shows itself in the mature person in generosity, the result of overflowing power which the individual can no longer use for further growth and which therefore can be spent in creative pursuits. The mature person is no longer primarily a receiver. He receives, but he also gives. His giving is not subordinated primarily to his expectation of return; it is giving for its own sake. Just as receiving love and help are the main sources of pleasure for the growing child, so for the mature person pleasure consists in spending energy productively for the sake of others and for purposes beyond himself. This generous, outwardly directed attitude is what in ethics is called "altruism." In the light of this view, altruism, the basis of Christian morality, has a biological foundation; it is a natural, healthy expression of the state of maturity.

It is important to emphasize that the platonic ideal of emotional maturity is never reached by most persons in its complete form; it is only approached. Individual differences are enormous and account for the existence of the leader and follower types, the latter the more numerous. Whenever life becomes difficult and presents situations beyond the individual's capacity to solve, there is a tendency to regress toward less mature attitudes, in which a person may still rely on the help of parents and teachers. In our hearts we all regret having been expelled from the Garden of Eden by eating from the tree of knowledge—a symbol of maturity. In critical life-situations, most persons become insecure and seek help even before they have exhausted all their own resources.

### RELATION BETWEEN PERSONALITY DEVELOPMENT AND SOCIAL STRUCTURE

Every form of social organization requires of its members the capacity to replace self-interest to some degree with an interest in others. This is the reason why no society could be run by children or adolescents. Different forms of social organization, however, require different degrees of maturity. In all authoritarian governments, the status of the majority of the people resembles that of children more than that of independent adults. Virtue consists in obeying the existing rules and in being subordinate to the rulers, whose obligation is to take care of their subjects. In such societies people express their mature state only by taking care of their progeny. All social manifestations of individual productivity are absent. With the exception of two short periods in history, humanity has always lived under some form of authoritarian system, be it feudalism, absolute monarchy, fascism, or communism. Free societies have existed for a short period in ancient Greece and during the last three hundred years in some parts of Western civilization. These two brief periods in the history of Western civilization were undoubtedly the richest in artistic, scientific, and literary productivity. There is danger that under the paralyzing threats of global wars our present experiment with freedom may be relegated to history and free societies may be engulfed by the rising tide of authoritarianism.

Social attitudes, however, are not good or bad in themselves; they are organic parts of each culture and can be evaluated only in the framework of different social organizations. Educational attitudes and methods of child rearing do not develop in a vacuum; they are determined by the total social structure. Recent anthropological studies have shown that national charcteristics are primarily due to certain uniform paternal influences, which are determined by the total social configuration.

For example, Japanese worship of authority was the precipitate of century-long feudalism. Not only was it the reflection of the feudal ideology in the mind of the individual, but it was also an indispensable guaranty for the survival of the feudal system. Similarly, the American emphasis on individual accomplishment and depreciation of authority worship are expressions of the American social structure and at the same time the guaranties of its survival. Such attitudes, transmitted to each child by family influences, have a social function. They are adaptations of the individual to the social structure in which he lives. It is clear, then, that no educational philosophy can be foisted upon a nation which does not spring organically from that nation's cultural soil. In this perspective, the naïveté of plans much discussed in postwar years to re-educate foreign nations according to our own ideals becomes transparent. The social attitudes of a nation can be changed only by changing its whole social structure.

A self-governing, free democracy requires greater independence of its citizens than does any other social system. The question is how such emotional independence can be achieved—independence that can withstand the regressive pressure of adversity.

It is obvious from what has been said that emotional independence is achieved gradually during the process of growth. The child will assume independence if he has opportunity in each phase of development for self-expression, by which he learns to make use of the faculties that correspond to his age. He will learn to assume responsibility for his own activities if his self-control is not based on fear of external authorities but is rooted in his own conscience. This conscience develops through positive identification with adults. If the socialization of the child is achieved primarily through fear of punishment, only a grudging type of conformity will develop. Rigorous discipline, enforced by corporal and other forms of punishment, is suited to bringing up a militant aggressive youth, as exemplified by ancient Sparta, Hitler's Germany, and Soviet Russia. All the hatred generated in the punitive atmosphere of the playroom, the school, and the military barracks is channelized toward foreign societies or minority groups. It is held from expression against the internal authorities of the state by terror. This form of society, therefore, must always be a police state. It goes with the complete deterioration of internal standards of self-responsibility and independence.

The process of social adjustment in free democracies must be based on favoring the development of standards that become integral parts of the personality. In the technical language of psychoanalysis, the boundary between ego and superego disappears in such a person. This type of personality structure will develop only if the process of social adjustment is based on positive identification—on love, trust, and admiration felt by the child for those who are intrusted with his upbringing. As Freud has recognized, love is a unifying force, hatred a dividing one. If social adjustment is based on hate and fear, the internal image of the external authorities—the conscience—will remain a foreign body within the personality. Only if the child loves those whose social attitudes he incorporates during his development, only if he has confidence in them, can the image of these persons become one with the rest of the personality.

In such education the emphasis is not merely on restraining the original impulses but in directing them into socially valuable creative expression. Full expression of individuality has been the chief source of every step in social progress. The major problem of our time is to produce socially minded, co-operative adults, without sacrificing individuality.

## PSYCHODYNAMIC PRINCIPLES OF THERAPY

In its main phases, psychoanalytic therapy has followed the development of theory. When the dynamic influence of unconscious tendencies was discovered, the therapy consisted in bringing repressed psychological content into consciousness. Cathartic hypnosis was such a procedure, a device by which the ego's rejection of repressed material was circumvented by the artificial hypnotic state. Freud soon realized that the mobilization of the repressed is not sufficient to cure neurotic symptoms but that the ego must undergo changes in order to become capable of integrating repressed material into its system. The therapeutic aim must therefore consist in achieving changes in the ego. With this new orientation, the center of interest shifted from the understanding of the unconscious, the knowledge of symbolism, the art of translating the archaic picture language of the unconscious into verbal thinking, to the study of the defenses of the ego. The crucial discovery concerning the ways and means by which the ego's defenses can be influenced was that of the transference phenomenon. Its therapeutic significance was only gradually recognized.

In cathartic hynosis the therapeutic factor consisted in an intensive emotional experience, in the dramatic reliving of repressed traumatic experiences of the past. Freud soon recognized that the traumatic experience in itself was not the most important pathogenic factor, but those preceding experiences which had made the patient vulnerable. What the patient felt as a trauma in itself was often a quite trivial occurrence. For example, Anna, Breuer's patient, developed her aversion to drinking water when she saw her English governess' little dog drink from a dish used by the family. When she recalled this episode in hypnotic trance, she burst out with violent hatred against the governess and abused her profanely. After this, her symptom—aversion to water—disappeared. Freud correctly concluded that this trivial event in itself could not account for the symptom. Anna must have been sensitized by previous experiences in order to react so violently. Today, with our knowledge of the typical tragedies of childhood, it is not difficult to conclude that the dog for Anna represented another child with whom she had had to share the governess' attention. Her hatred of the governess was due to her inability to share love, a quality which she must have acquired in her early development.

After Freud recognized the importance of the genetic exploration of the individual's early history for the understanding of the precipitating factors in neurosis, his therapeutic efforts became focused on the reconstruction of early emotional development. This required filling in gaps of memory caused by repressions. Free association in the emotionally permissive atmosphere of psychoanalytic interviews was an ideal device for the systematic study of the patient's past. A period followed in which the genetic re-construction of personality development became the aim of ther-apy. Gradually, however, the importance of the patient's emo-tional experiences in the transference relationship to the analyst became more and more appreciated. The most consistent evalua-tion of the therapeutic significance of the transference was con-tained in a pamphlet published by Ferenczi and Rank in 1926, in which they expounded the thesis that not remembering but re-living the traumatic experiences in the transference is the effective therapeutic factor. Memory gaps may never be filled; yet a patient may be cured if he learns a new solution for his past emotional conflicts when these reappear in his emotional involvement with the analyst. This significant publication was unfavorably received and remained buried for more than fifteen years, until in the Chi-cago Institute for Psychoanalysis a systematic re-evaluation of therapeutic factors was undertaken.[3] This project required ex-perimentation with the technique of treatment. The routine of daily interviews and the so-called "passive" attitude were aban-doned, and every detail of the treatment, the frequency of inter-views, interruptions, and as much as possible of the patient's life-situation were planned according to the nature of the therapeutic problem.

The significance of the therapist's attitude toward the patient has also been explored. The phenomenon of countertransference in recent years has received increasing recognition. Originally, Freud conceived the analyst's role as a neutral one. The therapist was supposed to serve merely as a screen upon which the patient projected the emotional reactions that originated in childhood in relation to his parents. In the light of precise scrutiny this postu-late turned out to be a theoretical construction. The analyst's per-sonality and his reactions, in spite of his efforts to remain imper-sonal, influence the course of the treatment. The patient senses these reactions, although he frequently misinterprets them ac-cording to his own emotional needs. The Chicago studies paid particular attention to the mutual emotional relationship between patient and physician; the concept of the patient's corrective emo-tional experience as the central factor in psychoanalytic treatment has evolved.

The essence of this theory can be summarized as follows: The

3. Franz Alexander, T. M. French, *et al.*, *Psychoanalytic Therapy* (New York: Ronald Press, 1946).

neurotic condition is the result of the ego's failure to accomplish its function, which consists in finding gratification for subjective needs in a way that maintains harmony between the various aspects of the personality and the environment. This function of mediation between conflicting or partially conflicting needs and desires and their adaptation to environmental conditions are essentially problems of integration. Every person has his own integrative capacity. French subjected the integrative function to a careful study, in which he tried to evaluate its quantitative variations. The integrative faculty varies from person to person, and in the same person it is influenced by different factors. Excessive intensity of an emotional need, for example, interferes with effective integration. Postponement of immediate gratification was recognized by Freud as one essential feature of reality-adapted behavior. Intense and urgent emotions tend to seek immediate gratification and thus interfere with effective integrative functioning. Low intensity of motivations may also decrease the integrative faculty. A person not keenly interested in what he has to accomplish will be less inclined to undertake the arduous task of appraising the whole problem and trying to solve it. Anxiety, too, depending on its intensity, may either favor or paralyze the integrative functions. Past successes and resulting hope increase integrative ability; consistent failure impairs it.

Another factor which interferes with adaptive behavior is related to the basic mechanism of repression. Repression is the characteristic defense measure of the weak ego of the child, who cannot control those desires which appear in his consciousness and which are in conflict with the requirements of the environment or with other subjective needs. He has only one way to save himself from the painful experiences he was subjected to in the past when he gave in to such impulses: he has to exclude them radically from his consciousness. This saves him from a conflict with reality and/ or internal conflict but, at the same time, creates a frustration. Eventually the repressed impulse will seek outlet in symptoms. Through repression the ego is deprived of dynamic force, which it could utilize if it were able to integrate the force within its system. The highest form of integrative function requires conscious deliberation. Everything excluded from consciousness is beyond the reach of the ego's integrative functions. Neurotic symptoms are like foreign bodies and represent isolated substitute gratifications which are the source of conflict and suffering.

Psychoanalytic therapy aims at the extension of the ego's scope by making repressed tendencies conscious. For this purpose it attempts to mobilize unconscious material. In order to overcome repressions by systematic psychological maneuvers, one must know the causes of repression. As shown above, the child represses those tendencies the expression of which caused him pain, such as physical suffering, punishment, withdrawal of parental love, and resulting insecurity. The emergence of such a tendency constitutes a danger to which the ego reacts with anxiety. According to Freud, anxiety is the signal for the ego to repress such dangerous impulses. Essentially, this process is similar to conditioning. The sequence of events has three links: (1) emergence of the impulse, (2) acting upon it, and (3) painful results. Originally the anxiety was aroused by the memory of a painful experience; it reappears whenever the impulse involved emerges. In order to avoid the associated anxiety, the impulse is repressed and excluded from motor expression.

Psychoanalytic therapy in this light reveals itself as a process of reconditioning. The ego is induced to face a repressed impulse by eliminating the anxiety which induced repression. This is achieved by reproducing the original situation but changing the conditions so that they lose their anxiety-producing effect. As soon as the patient senses that the analyst's response to expression of his impulses is different from that of the parents, the intimidating effect is removed. The aim of the therapy consists, first, in reviving the interpersonal situation which led to the original repressions and, second, in supplying a new kind of experience which is suitable for undoing the effects of the parental responses. Accordingly, the analyst's response to the patient's expression should be different from the parental ones: they should perhaps be the opposite of the parental reactions. This can be achieved only if the analyst is able to reconstruct the pathogenic parental influences and respond to the patient's emotional manifestations in a manner appropriate to the counteracting and neutralizing of the disturbing influence of the parents. Essentially this is nothing but emotional reconditioning.

The objective attitude of the therapist which Freud recommended is different from anything the patient has experienced before, because complete objectivity does not exist in ordinary human relationships. The corrective influence of this objective attitude can be further enhanced if the therapist's reactions are

specifically calculated to counteract the effect of parental reactions.

The practical conclusion from all this is that, in place of his
spontaneous countertransference reactions, the therapist must
assume an attiude toward the patient which in the light of the
patient's history appears appropriate to the undoing of the pathogenic influences of the parents. In this way the emotional experiences in the therapy will have a corrective influence, resulting in
the lifting of repressions. The patient will be able to face what he
formerly repressed because of parental censure.

It would be an oversimplification, however, to assume that repressions are always due to intimidating parental attitudes. Permissive parental behavior may create guilt and favor repression of
aggressive impulses. The therapist, therefore, cannot always assume a permissive attitude. Often a strong-hand atmosphere is
needed, as in cases where parental overindulgence has caused intensive guilt feelings which lead to the repression of the guilt-
provoking impulses.

The emphasis on the therapeutic importance of the emotional
experience during treatment is essentially a vindication of Ferenczi's postulate, that the patient's reliving of the original conflicts in
the transference situation is the primary tool of psychoanalytic
therapy.

All this does not disprove, however, the value of insight. By his
interpretive work, the analyst assists the patient's ego in integrating the new material liberated from repression. Making conscious
what was hitherto repressed requires the reduction of anxiety.
This is achieved by the corrective emotional experience and by
the insight which in itself has an anxiety-reducing effect. The
ego's function is mastery through insight. The integrative function is based on the appraisal of the total situation—both internal
and external. Hence interpretive work increases the ego's self-
confidence in dealing with newly uncovered material. Something
a person understands loses its threatening quality; understanding
means mastery. Properly devised attitudes and correct interpretive
work together constitute psychoanalytic therapy.

Recently special attention has been given to the dependent
cravings of the patient which tend to prolong the treatment. The
neurotically impaired ego, to some degree, relinquishes its basic
function of sustaining emotional equilibrium by its integrative
and executive functions. It eliminates by repression all those im-

pulses with which it cannot deal. Instead of using independent judgment, the ego is under the influence of incorporated parental images (superego reactions). Analytic therapy tries to substitute for this automatic regulation independent judgment appropriate to the mature state. It tries to replace parental precepts by conscious judgment which is flexibly adjusted to the ever changing situations. This is the essence of self-reliant rational behavior. In the transference situation the original parent-child relationship is re-established as the analyst replaces the incorporated image of the parents. The intra-psychic conflict between ego and superego is now converted into its original pattern through the relationship between patient and therapist. While the aim of the analytic therapy consists in replacing the automatic superego regulations with conscious control by the ego, the patient's tendency is to prolong the dependent relationship and rely on the analyst's aid instead of assuming responsibility for himself. This is essentially true for all neurotics and to a lesser extent for everyone. The trend toward dependence is deeply rooted in all human beings. It is only in degree that people differ from one another in this regard. The function of analytic therapy is to counteract this trend and induce the patient's ego to accept self-government. This entails persistent effort to counteract the dependent urge. Failure in self-government increases regression toward dependence; success encourages it. Every independent and successful accomplishment of an adaptive ego function means a step toward mental health. Yet the trend toward regression because of the inertia of the organism is ever present. It is one of the most difficult tasks of psychoanalytic therapy to dislodge the dependent relationship which gives the patient so much relief in his neurotic stress. By its very nature the analytic technique necessitates the establishment of a dependent relationship between patient and therapist, in order to allow the patient to relive and face again the old unresolved interpersonal relations with the parents. Inasmuch as it encourages dependence, the analytic technique which is devised to cure the neurosis carries in itself a factor which prolongs the neurotic condition. In order to resolve infantile reactions, one feature of which is always dependence, one must reproduce them in the transference; only then can one combat them. Much of the recent technical experimentation concerns this inherent difficulty in the analytical technique. Prolonged uninterrupted daily interviews in many cases favor the development of an intensive dependent relationship and consequently postpone recovery. To overcome this weak spot in the analytic technique is one of the crucial technical issues.

From the therapeutic studies of the Chicago Institute for Psychoanalysis, a series of technical recommendations resulted. The essence of them is that, from the beginning, the therapist must be aware of the danger inherent in the regressive tendencies of the patients. To counteract this danger, the analyst must consistently give the patient as much independence as possible. Interpretations alone cannot accomplish this. The dependent tendencies can often be counteracted by reducing the contact with the patient to that minimum which is necessary to preserve the continuity of the treatment. Properly timed reduction of the frequency of interviews, shorter and longer interruptions, are indispensable in every case. Encouraging the patient to new life-experiences outside the treatment suitable to increase self-confidence and encourage hope are also potent devices in weaning the patient from dependence on the therapist.

Our present technique of psychoanalytic treatment should by no means be considered as final and in need of no further improvements. In addition to numerous successfully treated cases, there are many failures and "interminable" analyses in which the treatment has become an emotional crutch which the patient can no longer dispense with. Not all these cases should be lightly dismissed as incurables. The long duration of many analyses should also serve as an incentive to explore further the possibilities for modifications by which the treatment procedure can be made more economical. Such advancement can come only from relentless experimentation, from the constant re-examination of the psychological processes during treatment and the re-evaluation of theoretical views, and particularly of those habits in treatment which stem neither from theory nor from controlled observations but which have been preserved merely through adherence to tradition.

# II

## DREAMS AND RATIONAL BEHAVIOR[1]

### Thomas M. French, M.D.

#### Freud's Analysis of the Significance of Dreams

NEARLY everything significant that we know about dreams today we owe to Freud's classical study, *The Interpretation of Dreams* (6). From Freud we learn that dreams protect sleep from disturbing wishes by creating the illusion that these wishes are fulfilled. Dreams are not the nonsense that they seem to be. They impress us as meaningless only because another part of the mental apparatus, which Freud calls the "dream censor," distorts and disguises the wish-fulfilling fantasies so as to make them unrecognizable. The wishes that threaten to interrupt sleep are usually unacceptable to the socially adjusted parts of the personality. Usually they are wishes that have been excluded from consciousness, "repressed" as Freud calls it, during waking life. The dream censor continues to struggle to keep them repressed while we are asleep. Only a few dreams, especially those of very young children, are undisguised wish-fulfilling fantasies. In contrast to the simple wish-fulfilment dreams of young children, the dream of an adult is usually a "disguised fulfilment of a repressed wish."

#### Freud's Analysis of the Dream Work

To get data for finding the hidden meaning of a dream, Freud utilized the method of free association. Starting, one by one, with each of the details of the dream text, the dreamer reports, without reservation of any kind, whatever thoughts come to mind. From these associations Freud attempted to reconstruct the "latent dream thoughts," the thoughts that have presumably played a part in the formation of the dream. These latent dream thoughts he called the "latent content" of the dream, which he distinguished carefully from the actual dream text, the "manifest con-

1. This chapter is adapted from a chapter on dreams and rational behavior in the author's *The Integration of Behavior*, Vol. 1: *Basic Postulates* (5).

35

tent" of the dream. By comparing latent content with manifest content, he tried to trace what has happened to the latent dream thoughts to transform them into the manifest dream content. This process of transformation he called the "dream work."

In the dream work the latent dream thoughts are treated with the utmost disregard for logic. Without regard for the sense of the latent dream thoughts, emphasis is often shifted along any available associative pathway, even the most superficial, such as a word or sound association. In this way the energy or affective interest belonging to two entirely different dream thoughts may be concentrated on a single middle term in a long chain of more or less irrelevant associations. Even diametrically opposite ideas are often condensed and represented in the manifest dream content by a single dream element.[2]

Freud concluded that the dream work exemplifies a mode of mental functioning that is characteristic of a special system of the mind, the system unconscious (usually abbreviated "ucs"). The mode of functioning of the system ucs Freud calls the "primary process." Its basic principle is free and massive displacement of energy from one psychic element to another along any available associative pathway, without regard for reality or logical relations. This massive displacement of energy is activated and guided by the need to avoid pain and to seek the pleasure of the moment ("pleasure principle"). Freud believed this to be the primary mode of mental functioning. He contrasted it sharply with logical thinking, which he called "the secondary process." In the secondary process the displacement of energy from one mental element to another is controlled by an end-goal or purpose and by recognition of real relationships and the rules of logic. Freud suggested that this is made possible by the fact that in the secondary process the mental apparatus operates with much smaller quantities of energy.

### Thesis that Dreams Have a Problem-solving Function

Another way of studying the dream work brings it into closer relation with the rational behavior of waking life. The motive, or, in Freud's words, the "motor," for the dream work is the need to find fulfilment for a wish. Dynamically the most significant part of the dream work is the part that leads directly from the motivat-

2. For a more complete description of the peculiarities of the dream work see Freud's own account (6).

ing wish to the manifest dream content. After a varying amount of elaboration, this wish encounters the dream censor. Yet the dream censor turns out to be not an impersonal system of the mind but a specific inhibitory motive, an appropriate reaction to this particular wish. Probably it is based in every case on the disturbing consequences of past attempts to fulfil a similar wish. Thus an intense dependent craving for love may arouse protest from the dreamer's pride; or a hostile impulse may give rise to a guilt reaction; or a sexual impulse in a man may stir up fear of the father; or the same sexual wish may lead to fear of rebuff from the mother-figure toward whom it is directed. When we study the dreamer's reaction to his conflict, we find that it is more than an attempt to give disguised expression to the disturbing wish. The inhibiting motive plays not only a censoring, but also a creative (1), role in shaping the fantasy activity that culminates in the manifest dream. The dreamer's pride, threatened by a dependent wish, may react with compensatory fantasies of independence and achievement or may try to conjure up a situation in which the dependent craving would not be too incompatible with self-respect. The dreamer whose guilt has been aroused by his hostile wishes may imagine himself unjustly treated, in order to justify his hostility; or his guilt may demand appeasement by a fantasy of being punished.

When we study this part of the dream work, we find that the mental apparatus is reacting, not to isolated fragments of a tangle of latent dream thoughts whose energy is being displaced along any available associative pathway, but rather to the situation created by conflict between the disturbing dream wish and the inhibiting motive. In every case we find the dream work struggling somehow to reconcile these two conflicting motives. This conflict constitutes a problem which the dream work must unceasingly struggle to solve. Thus we come to the conclusion that the dream work, like the thought-processes directing our ordinary waking activity, is dominated by the need to find a solution for a problem (3, 4).[3]

3. This method of studying the dream work is no innovation. It is the method that most psychoanalysts intuitively follow in the actual practice of dream analysis. They listen to the dream and to the dreamer's associations until the motivating dream wish finally dawns on them. Then they study the dreamer's reactions to this wish and try to understand the manifest dream content as an attempt to reconcile the conflicting wishes. If they succeed in understanding the dream and accompanying associations in these terms, they feel satisfied that they have grasped the meaning of the dream. The preceding discussion tries to make explicit what most psychoanalysts do in practice.

## Practical Grasp of Situations in Dreams
### and in Waking Life

If we examine the mode of mental functioning exemplified by the dream's way of dealing with the dream wish, we find that it resembles neither the logical thinking of Freud's secondary process nor the free displacement of energy of his primary process. In fact, it is not associative thinking at all, certainly not verbal associative thinking, but rather thinking in terms of a practical grasp of real situations: "If I act upon this wish, then I must expect such and such consequences. Shall I renounce the wish or suffer the consequences? Or is some compromise possible?" The dream's solution may not be very good from the point of view of waking life, but it is always intelligible, once we grasp the nature of the conflict.

As we follow the dream's way of dealing with its problem, we sense immediately to what it is comparable in our waking life. In most of our behavior in real life, too, we are guided not primarily by verbal reasoning, not by long chains of associations that have to be held in control according to the rules of logic, but by the same practical grasp of the situation that we recognize in the dream work's struggles with its problem. When we wish to get from one place to another, we study a map or picture the lay of the land and visualize our route accordingly. If we are putting together a mechanical device, we are guided similarly by a sense of the spatial and other relations involved, which we sometimes call "mechanical sense." In dealing with people, too, we size up the behavior of others, often without realizing exactly how, and guide our own behavior not by logical reasoning but by an intuitive sense of what others are likely to do. In dreams as in waking life, this is the primary mode of mental functioning. We begin to acquire our mechanical sense and our intuitive understanding of other people when we are babies, long before we know how to talk. It is only later that this direct and intimate knowledge is supplemented by what we learn through the medium of speech; and only still later do we acquire habits of logical thought.

Freud analyzed the dream work in terms of the associational psychology current at the time. However, he has several times stated (6, p. 489) that, for every superficial and illogical associative link in the unconscious elaboration of a train of thought, a corresponding "deep and logically significant associative link" can be found in the dream thoughts. This statement implies that superficial and illogical associations are not so meaningless and irrelevant as they seem to be. When we study the dream work in terms of our concept of the dreamer's practical grasp of his conflict situation, we discover that his attempts to find a solution[4] for his problem are handicapped by the fact that his capacity to understand his situation fluctuates during the course of the dream work. To adapt its understanding to the shrinking span of this capacity, the integrative mechanism must often form a highly condensed and oversimplified picture of the conflict situation by means of symbols and allusions (2, 3, 4). We suspect that the transformations resulting from such shrinkage of integrative span are closely related to the substitution of superficial and absurd associations for meaningful ones that Freud recognized, and that the impression of free displacement of energy without regard for reality or logic is an artifact, resulting from study of the dream work in terms of an associational psychology.

## BIBLIOGRAPHY

1. ALEXANDER, F. "About Dreams with Unpleasant Content," *Psychiat. Quart.*, 4:447–52, 1930.
2. FRENCH, T. M. "Reality and the Unconscious," *Psychoanalyt. Quart.*, 6:23–61, 1937.
3. FRENCH, T. M. "Reality Testing in Dreams," *Psychoanalyt. Quart.*, 4:62–67, 1937.
4. FRENCH, T. M. "Insight and Distortion in Dreams," *Internat. J. Psychoanalysis*, 20:287–98, 1939.
5. FRENCH, T. M. *The Integration of Behavior*, Vol. 1: *Basic Postulates* (Chicago: University of Chicago Press, 1952).
6. FREUD, S. *The Interpretaion of Dreams* (New York: Macmillan Co., 1933).
7. MAEDER, A. "Ueber die Funktion des Traumes," *Jahrb. f. psychoanalyt. u. psychopath. Forsch.*, 4:692–707, 1912.
8. MAEDER, A. "Ueber das Traumproblem," *Jahrb. f. psychoanalyt. u. psychopath. Forsch.*, 5:647–86, 1913.
9. MAEDER, A. "Zur Frage der teleologischen Traumfunktion," *Jahrb. f. psychoanalyt. u. psychopath. Forsch.*, 5:453–54, 1913.

4. The thesis that dreams have a "teleological" or problem-solving function was proposed and defended by Maeder (7, 8, 9) many years ago. Freud rejected this thesis of Maeder's (6, p. 533 n.). For more extended discussion of the relationship between the author's views and this controversy between Maeder and Freud see T. M. French (3).

# III

## HISTORY OF METAPSYCHOLOGICAL CONCEPTS

Edoardo Weiss, M.D.

BEFORE the work of Freud, the understanding of mental processes as dynamic phenomena was largely confined to works of philosophy and art. Many philosophers of the Western world, since the time of Aristotle and Plato, had formulated speculations regarding the human mind, and many great writers had accurately described various emotional manifestations and had intuitively sensed basic motivations.

### EARLY HISTORY

Schopenhauer recognized the force of unconscious will in its influence on all conscious thought and action, and Eduard von Hartmann further elaborated on Schopenhauer's conception of the unconscious. But for both these men the conception was metaphysical, and, as a consequence, many psychologists and other scholars were contemptuous of their assumptions. Nietzsche did not add to these conceptions, but, in his realization that conscious motives are rationalizations and that unconscious motives are the underlying forces, he recognized that the unconscious and the conscious are subject to different laws. Samuel Butler made a special contribution to the understanding of the unconscious in his theory of unconscious memory. William James explained mental processes as organic; that is, he considered that they were due to modifications in the brain and that the phenomena of instinct were explicable as an activity of the nervous system.

Because the early conceptions of the unconscious, as presented chiefly by Leibnitz and Herbart, were speculative, vague, and inaccessible to scientific scrutiny, classical psychology rejected them and explained mental phenomena by psychophysical and organic hypotheses. Coincident with the development of experimental and physiologic psychology and with the scientific approach to the study of neuroses, there arose an academic interest in unconscious mental processes.

Experimental psychology developed in Germany under the influence of Fechner and in France of Ribot, who recognized that a theory of the unconscious was necessary to explain mental phenomena. Ribot considered subconscious activity to be physiologic rather than psychologic, and he subdivided it into a "static" and a "dynamic" subconscious. With the stimulation of Ribot began the movement which brought forth the important clinical work of Charcot, Bernheim, and Janet.

Other experimental psychologists furthered the approach to the modern concepts of psychodynamics. In Fechner's presupposition of a "threshold of consciousness" lay the implication that there was something below the threshold. His principle of the tendency toward stability anticipated the psychoanalytic point of view concerning the phenomena of pain and pleasure which had already been studied by Hobbes and Helvetius. His observation of the dream state found confirmation in Freud's conception of the difference between dream activity and conscious mentation.

But, in spite of these isolated postulates, there was still no scientific dynamic approach to the problems involved in the understanding of mental processes or of mental disease. The etiology of psychotic and neurotic symptoms was considered to be organic— that is, to be the consequence of some disturbance in the brain. Charcot's work with hysterics laid the foundation for the scientific study of mental phenomena; and his experiments with hypnotized patients led to his discovery that morbid ideas produced hysteria and that these ideas, as well as the symptoms resulting from them, could be changed through hypnotism. Although he believed that there was an organic basis (deficiency in the brain) for hysteria, his approach to its study was psychologic, in that it included the production or elimination of symptoms by means of hypnotism. His investigations, therefore, mark the beginning of a genuinely scientific psychotherapy.

Bernheim, who carried further the research into the nature of hypnotism, discovered that when the human mind is in a certain state it accepts as truth, without proof and even against reason, statements made by an authoritative person. He thus interpreted hypnotism as suggestion and believed that the cause of hysteria lay in the individual's suggestibility and that, consequently, this tendency to be suggestible could be utilized in effecting a cure. His theory, therefore, was also psychologic.

Janet, too, used hypnotism as a method of investigation. Believing that mental life is a complete unit synthesized by psychic energy, he regarded neurosis as the consequence of a breakdown in the synthetic function of consciousness. He thought that the unconscious was merely split-off consciousness, and he gave no consideration to unconscious forces as a part of normal mental activity or as the cause of neurotic symptoms. He regarded the origin of neurosis as organic, on a hereditary or acquired basis.

The conceptions of these men gave no regard to unconscious dynamic motivation. That was for Freud to discover. Stimulated primarily by Charcot and Bernheim, less by Janet, Freud reached the conclusion that neuroses are due to conflicts within the mind in which one conflicting element is unconscious and therefore not accessible to introspection. Freud was thus the first to establish the unconscious as a field for scientic clinical investigation.

Freud's interest in neurology and neuroanatomy led him to Charcot's clinics, where he became acquainted with the views on hysteria held by Charcot and Bernheim. On his return to Vienna, where he practiced neurology, he began work with Breuer, who had discovered that the symptoms of hysterical patients depend upon forgotten but highly significant scenes or events in their lives. Breuer's therapy—a combination of hypnotism and catharsis—caused the patients to recall and reproduce these experiences under hypnosis. Breuer and Freud guided the patient's attention directly to the traumatic event in order to find the psychic conflict, so that the repressed affect might be freed.

The first work in psychoanalysis took place between the years of 1887 and 1895, when Freud and Breuer were trying intensively to understand and cure hysterical symptoms. With the publication (1893) of their paper on the psychological mechanisms of hysterical phenomena (4), the foundations of the structure of psychoanalysis were laid. The initiation of this investigation was due to Breuer's observation that some hysterical patients lost their symptoms if certain memories charged with emotions, of which the patient had not previously been aware, were brought to consciousness, whereby the emotional tensions were discharged. Thus the concept of "repression" was formulated, together with that of pent-up energy. To account for repression, the pain and pleasure principle was elaborated; this dynamic phenomenon led to the formulation by Breuer of the concept of a free-floating energy as distinguished from bound energy.

The disappearance from consciousness of mental content was thought to be the result of an act of repression because of the disagreeable nature of the material involved. Since the conscious individual cannot escape an inner unpleasant situation as he can an external danger, the inner situation is blocked from consciousness, and thus an emotional discharge is prevented. Through repression the mental content was not eliminated, but it maintained an affective existence unknown to the subject. In fact, the pent-up energy inherent in the repressed content was considered to break through into symptom formation, which always revealed a psychologic meaning when approached by the method of interpretation elaborated by Freud. The ensuing symptoms were sensed by the patient in the same way as symptoms of physical origin were. Recognizing that the process of repression is not always successful, Freud saw that symptoms are due to the failure of repression.

But Freud and Breuer disagreed on the explanation of the more intimate psychic mechanisms of hysteria, namely, on Freud's discovery of a sexual etiology for the neuroses. Very early Freud discovered that under the repressed memories and drives lay sexual conflicts. The sexual manifestations which revealed themselves through his methods of investigation were of such variety and so much related to the life of infancy and childhood that they aroused in patients and physicians alike a reluctance to investigate this field. Breuer clung to a physiologic theory. And so Freud continued alone. Freud found that the obstacle which had prevented his predecessors from admitting the existence of the unconscious was not only intellectual—what was not conscious could not be mental—but also emotional: by denying the existence of the unconscious, one denied also the repressed content.

Eventually, Freud abandoned hypnotism as a technique and adopted free association. Psychoanalysis proper, therefore, started with the rejection of hypnosis. When the patient failed to remember initiating traumas under hypnosis, the analytic work was blocked, and resistance was established which could not be broken down. Later it was recognized that only by proper changes within the ego could the resistances be overcome. These structural changes could not be obtained through hypnosis. The cathartic nonhypnotic method, which developed into psychoanalysis as it is known today, was built on the theories of repression and resistance and of infantile sexuality, on the phenomenon of the transference, and on the interpretation of dreams.

From these theories Freud developed certain abstractions: these concerned mental energy and its investment; repression and resistance and the associated concept of the topographic structure of the mind; the pattern of individual development from infancy to maturity. These concepts are, in no sense, dicta. They have grown and matured in the course of the years, with the clinical experience of Freud himself and with that of other scientific investigators. They still remain a challenge to further clinical investigation.

### MENTAL ENERGY AND ITS INVESTMENT

Psychoanalysis—an exquisitely dynamic approach to mental phenomena—deals with mental forces acting in the same, divergent, or opposite directions and with their resultants. The forces operating within the mind are subjected to what one could call the "integrative principle," which characterizes biologic processes— the organism and its structural parts form a coherent unity manifesting the tendency to preserve itself and to develop in determined ways. Thus the various needs and urges and impulses of the individual must be co-ordinated so as to lead to integrated conduct, which is necessary for his adaptation to the conditions of reality. Conflicts arise when two or more urges cannot be combined toward such behavior; and so emotional conflicts and their various consequences constitute the most important sources of knowledge of mental phenomena.

To account for the varying degrees of intensity inherent in any mental experience, one must postulate a "charge of energy" which is correlated to nervous excitation. The consciously perceived mental energy corresponds to what one usually calls "interest." It invests every mental process—corresponding to specific nervous tensions—and is discharged in feelings, affects, and emotions as well as in motor activity. Feelings, affects, and emotions result from the discharge of nervous tension in vasomotor, vasosecretory, and visceral processes, whereby the position of the individual as a whole remains unaltered in respect to the external world. Through motor activity the position of the individual in his environment is changed.

Following a general trend of biologic investigation, Freud approached the study of mental phenomena not only from a causal but also from a finalistic point of view. Everyone is directly aware of "aims" which he feels urged to pursue, though the source of the urge is not conscious. He is also aware that he must frequently achieve secondary aims in order to reach his conscious goal. An aim has an object. A simple example is the urge of hunger, the goal of which is to be satisfied and the object of which is food.

To describe a specific charge of mental energy, Freud devised the term *Besetzungsenergie. Besetzen* means "to occupy, to garrison." By the use of this term Freud compared a charge of mental energy derived from a specific source to a military occupational force which can be directed toward this or that position as the need arises. In the English translation the term *Besetzungsenergie* was rendered as "cathexis," and the illuminating analogy was lost. Since the cathexes are dynamic expressions of biologic needs and instinctive drives, Freud was concerned with the classification of the basic instincts and drives. This approach led to problematic and controversial formulations and also to a number of uncertainties which have required revision of many corollary concepts in the course of psychodynamic investigation.

In his first formulation of a dualistic concept of the basic drives, Freud distinguished the self-preservative or *ego drives* from the race-preservative or *sexual drives*. The former comprised all needs or urges concerning the preservation, growth, and development of the ego, which was conceived to be a person's own particular individuality but was not then considered in a structural sense; the latter included all interests in external objects in so far as they were not instrumental to self-preservative needs and the individual's developmental growth. In brief, in his earliest theory Freud included in the ego drives all self-interest, and he extended the concept of the sexual or erotic drives to comprise all interest in objects which did not serve the self-interest.

The dynamic force of the sexual drives in this broad sense was called "libido." The ego drives were considered to be empowered by a different energy which could not be transformed into libido, for the original objects and goals of which there could be no substitutes. All bodily pleasure not due to the satisfaction of the ego drives—thus not including such pleasures as those from satisfying hunger and thirst—was considered sexual or erotic, and the bodily zones susceptible to erotic stimulation were called "erogenous zones." Observation showed that libido could be displaced from one bodily zone to another and also that there could be substitutes for original objects and goals of the sexual drives.

But, as we have said, the drive consists of more than the dynamic element; it also includes an object and a goal. Thus the first difficulty encountered in distinguishing between ego drives and sexual drives arose from the obvious consideration that the individual himself derives erotic pleasure from his own body without the utilization of external objects. This was called "autoerotism," which is directed toward mouth, skin, excretory openings, and other erogenous zones. Moreover, the individual as a whole could become the object of erotic desires—a condition which was called "narcissism." In brief, it was realized that the sexual drives concerned both the ego and external objects, and, as a result, the distinction between ego drives and sexual drives could no longer be maintained.

While Jung admitted only one kind of mental energy, Freud, though altering his concept of the drives, remained faithful to his dualistic concept. It was in 1920, in *Beyond the Pleasure Principle* (18), that Freud dropped his former dualism, recognizing that the self-preservative and constructive developmental urges were empowered by the same force which characterized sexuality in the broadest sense of the word. But opposite to this kind of energy (libido), which includes all kinds of constructive drives, he postulated a destructive drive tending to dissolution and death. This dualism asserted that in the organism there normally arises not only a kind of energy which is discharged into pleasurable, constructive, and integrated activities but also another kind, the discharge of which determines disintegration and destruction—as it were, an "anabolic" and a "catabolic" energy. According to Freud, the two always appear mixed with each other.

Freud elaborated upon the manner in which the dynamic expression (libido) of the constructive life-drive, called "Eros," and that of the death drive, called "Thanatos," are supposed to be fused for the achievement of integrated goals. He also resorted to the "catabolic" cathexis to explain the so-called "negative" therapeutic reaction in some severe neuroses, that is, the worsening of the symptoms whenever an opportunity for improvement occurs. This sabotage by destructive energy is carried out by the guilty conscience, which demands punishment and destruction.

Whenever libido is fused with the fundamental destructive energy, Freud spoke of the "erotization" of this energy; the resulting aggression conveys pleasurable sensations. Sadism and masochism are examples of this fusion. Freud pointed out the complementary relationship between these two fundamental and antithetic cathexes toward external objects or toward the self. The greater the degree of extroversion, the less the introversive effect, and vice versa. Freud considered this circumstance responsible for the social phenomenon of war, which corresponds to a focusing of the destructive energy on the external world to protect one's self and one's allies from its deleterious effects.

Freud's stability principle is reflected in some recent theories based on fundamental biologic principles. Among these, Cannon's "homeostatic principle" (5), or "homeostasis," is the most important. According to this principle, the dynamic equilibrium in the living organism as a whole and in its component parts is re-established after every disturbance. Both Claude Bernard (3) and Fechner (6) formulated a "constancy principle," deriving various conclusions. The latter inferred from it the phenomena of pain and pleasure, stating that every increase in nervous tension above the constancy level must be felt as in disagreement with normal functioning and therefore as unpleasant and painful, and every decrease (discharge), with consequent return to dynamic equilibrium, as pleasurable. This theory does not account for all cases of pain and pleasure, since there are both pleasurable and unpleasurable increases of tensions above the constancy level. However, it does furnish a logical explanation for many sensations of pain and pleasure.

Federn (9, 10, 12) formulated a principle of the operation of the destructive energy which he calls "mortido." Its tension and discharge lead to suffering and to the avoidance of nonsuffering (pleasure); in antithesis to the *Lust-Unlust Prinzip*, according to which the erotic processes occur, he formulated the *Leid-Unleid Prinzip*, followed by the nonerotic, that is, destructive, processes. This view completes Fechner's economic explanation of the phenomena of pain and pleasure by adding to it a missing factor. According to Federn, will power and determination are due to the destructive component of the combined cathexes; they are, however, put at the service of a constructive goal. The distinction is that they are utilized in the mastery or the elimination of obstacles which stand in the way of the goal.

Some analysts resort to other explanations to account for aggression and destruction. They point out that, since these tendencies are biologically necessary for defense and for achieving security and satisfaction, they need not necessarily be derived from a hypothetical death instinct. French (15) points out that mobilization of energy to overcome obstacles is an essential part of all goal-directed activity. In rational purposive behavior, discharge of this mobilized energy is guided and controlled by a plan for achieving the end-goal. However, if obstacles prove insuperable, one loses hope of achieving the end-goal. When hope of achieving the end-goal is destroyed, the guiding influence of the plan for achieving this goal disappears; and the energy that has been mobilized, now released from restraint, tends to discharge massively in diffuse and violent motor activity. Thus frustration results in a kind of physiological disintegration of the pattern of a goal-directed effort.

The ultimate motive behind every urge and wish which determines human behavior is discharge of tension. But homeostasis alone cannot account for all biologic phenomena with which the mental drives are associated; it is responsible merely for the maintenance and re-establishment of the same conditions—the status quo—in the organism. No growth, no development, no expansion and propagation, can derive from homeostasis alone. These are due to another fundamental biologic phenomenon, namely, the endogenous production of excitation which continuously—and *selectively*—raises the organic tension above the equilibrium level. To characterize this phenomenon, Alexander (1, 2) introduced the "principle of surplus energy," and from it he derived certain biologic formulations and theories concerning erotism, growth, development, and propagation. He considered the production of endogenous excitation and the subsequent discharge from a quantitative, and not a qualitative, point of view. Through this approach no classification of drives can be formulated; a distinction is made merely between those tendencies which comply with homeostasis alone—maintenance and re-establishment of the status quo—and those which result from the surplus energy and its discharge in various activities. The latter Alexander calls "erotic drives." According to this theory, the discharge of all surplus energy, by which homeostasis is re-established, is pleasurable.

As mentioned before, the task of maintaining homeostatic equilibrium is complicated by the phenomenon of growth. According to Alexander's vector analysis, growth is based on the fact that more incorporated energy and substance is retained than is eliminated. When the limit of growth is reached by the mature organism, however, nothing can be added to it; the surplus, which during the process of growth could be added to the organism, is now expended in the form of propagation and care of the progeny. Propagation is accordingly considered as basically related to growth: it is growth beyond the limits of the individual.

The pregenital manifestations of sexuality also can be described as discharge of surplus excitation which is not utilized and integrated in the interest of self-preservation. According to Alexander, during early infancy many physiological functions are erotic in nature. The child playfully practices many of its physiological functions, such as sucking, anal activities, etc. The erotic component of these functions becomes lost when they are utilized secondarily in the interest of the total organism and are integrated into the total functioning that serves survival. Essentially, in this view, the sexual nature of a phenomenon rests on two criteria: (1) that it is a discharge of any psychological impulse which is in excess of the utilitarian needs of the organism and (2) that it is a discharge for its own sake (to get rid of surplus excitation) and is not utilized in the interest of survival as an integral part of the total functioning of the organism. In the framework of a similar conceptual system, French (15) subjected the principle of integration of psychic energy to a methodological study.

## Repression

Repression is the most important psychodynamic phenomenon which Freud discovered in his earliest studies of neuroses. The exploration of the consequences of this phenomenon led him to the formulation of unconscious, preconscious, and conscious states of mental activity; from these he later derived the topographic and the structural concept of the mind (19). The ego is the integrating organ which has access to the voluntary motor system and is endowed with other specific functions. When a drive or memory (mental representation of an experience) undergoes repression, it is excluded from the ego, is subjected to mental processes which are extraneous to the individual's conscious inner experiences, and, so long as it remains unconscious, it is inaccessible to introspection.

Since not all unconscious mental phenomena are excluded from the ego, only a very narrow span of mental phenomena can be conscious at any given moment. Most mental phenomena which the ego uses for thinking and, in general, for its integrative functioning are temporarily latent—unconscious—but can be awakened to consciousness according to need. These unconscious mental phenomena are called "preconscious." In this case the adjective "unconscious" is used in a descriptive sense. According to Freud, consciousness is not a necessary characteristic of mental phenomena. There are also mental phenomena which do not become conscious even when they are stimulated; they remain beyond the reach of the ego. These phenomena, unlike the preconscious ones, are unconscious in the systematic sense of the word. When Freud uses the term "unconscious" in this latter sense, namely, to indicate a certain category of mental phenomena, different from the preconscious, he adopts, in writing, the abbreviation "ucs"; analogously he uses "pcs" and "cs" for preconscious and conscious mental phenomena, respectively.

The confidence which a mentally sound person has in his capacity to act and behave coherently in his daily life, to express his thoughts, and to understand the speech and behavior of other persons is based principally on his feeling that he is making coherent use of the wealth of his preconscious memories and knowledge. Most contents of memories, of aims that one wants to reach, and of acquired ideas are, at any given moment, unconscious in a descriptive sense but become conscious at the proper time for thinking and acting: the preconscious is the integrative mental domain of the ego.

The phenomena of the "system preconscious" (pcs) are coordinated in time and according to concepts of space and causality. They are expressed mentally in words and are influenced by external contingencies. They do not differ from the conscious phenomena in any respect other than that they are not discharged in voluntary action.

Repression is one of the dynamic defenses against drives and memories which cannot be controlled by the ego and which thus jeopardize its integration. Repression and the ego defenses in general are closely related to the phenomenon of anxiety, which will soon be discussed. After undergoing repression, drives and memories, as well as connections between different mental data, do not participate in the preconscious system but are excluded from it. Therefore, they become subject to the patterns of mental functioning which characterize the "system unconscious," from which all drives and their pertinent cathexes derive. This system is also called the "id," the Latin neuter pronoun of the third person. This term expresses the impersonal nature of the system, namely, its independence of the ego. Freud pointed out that, in respect to the ego, the id is the inner (namely, mental) foreign country, just as the external environment constitutes the outer foreign country.

To comprehend the phenomenon of repression and its implications, one must study it from a dynamic as well as from a structural and topographic point of view. The first considers the forces employed by the ego to maintain the exclusion of a repressed drive from the ego and from consciousness in spite of its pressure from the id, where it may be strongly cathected; the latter concerns the localization of the process in the mental apparatus. It has been said that repression takes place between the system unconscious—the id—and the preconscious—the ego. These mental localities are not anatomically related to different portions of the brain, but are rather spatial symbols, that is, different patterns of mental functioning which maintain a constant reciprocal relationship. Only in this sense can mental structure and topography be understood.

### The Ego and the Id

A brief exposition of the functions of the ego and of the main characteristics of the id is indispensable for the clarification of the dynamic involvement of the ego in the process of repression. As was said above, the most important function of the ego is integration. It mediates between inner instinctive demands and the impositions of the outer world, making plans for obtaining gratification of its needs, properly timing the necessary intermediate goals, checking temporarily or permanently the discharge of such tensions as would interfere with the achievement of the end-goals, and eliminating contradictions between different urges. In brief, integration is a unifying function of the ego for coherent behavior and conduct. Special credit is due T. M. French (14, 15, 16, 17) for his thorough analysis of the integrative function of the ego.

The ego's function of intro- and extra-spection, namely, of perceiving inner mental data as well as, by means of the sense organs, the objects and events of the outer world, is indispensable for integration. But only through a dynamic understanding of the perceptive function can phenomena such as hallucinations and delusions be explained. These phenomena are "false perceptions"; that is, the ego mistakes mental stimuli for data of the external reality. In hallucinations the stimuli are perceived with sensory qualities. To account for the ego's ability to discriminate among the origins of perceived stimuli, whether they come from the outer or the inner world, Freud postulated an important function of the ego—"reality testing." He described the way in which this function operates as early as 1900, in his classical work, *The Interpretation of Dreams* (21).

In the beginning the infant utilizes a simple device to distinguish the origin of a stimulus: when through his movements the perceived stimulus disappears or changes position, it is recognized as deriving from the external world, while, if it remains unaltered by his movements, it is perceived as a stimulus from within. Subjectively, the external world is reality, the inner world is only imaginary. Upon the establishment of reality testing, the sensory characters of remembered or imagined data are suppressed, and only the situations which are recognized as real bring lasting satisfaction. This primitive device for testing reality becomes insufficient with the progressive development of the ego's orientation in the outer world. Motility alone is inadequate to convey a correct orientation to the real conditions and situations of the external world. In fact, the primitive "motoric" experimentation in testing reality is steadily augmented by the functions of thinking and reasoning. However, the complex nature of the mature function of reality testing does not always convey to the ego a feeling of certainty about external facts but may leave doubts and lead to varying degrees of uncertainty.

The earlier concept that delusions and hallucinations occurring in dreams and in psychosis are the result of a deficient reality testing does not account completely for these phenomena. It is true that these phenomena are due either to disintegrative processes of the ego or to its temporary weakening, as during sleep, but they are not caused directly by failures in reality testing. Federn speaks of a "sense of reality," as distinguished from reality testing. The acknowledgment of the reality of certain data is certainly based on reality testing; the individual may revise some of his formerly "recognized" realities, for example, upon obtaining proof to the contrary. But when a psychotic patient "senses" determined mental data as being real, that is, as corresponding to external facts, he does not "test" them, since reality testing for him has become useless.

On the one hand, it is well known that the paranoiac ego is highly logical in its thinking. On the other hand, repressed thoughts which break through from the unconscious into the ego may be sensed as external reality in defiance of any reality testing; they form the contents of the delusions. Therefore, the patient is confronted with the difficult task of bringing his delusions into agreement with the data of actual reality that he perceives and understands. This leads to what Freud called the "secondary elaboration," a process to which the contents of delusions are subjected. The manifest content of delusions (as in dreams) is a distorted product of repressed drives, and its latent meaning can be understood only through interpretation. But the ego's need for coherence is responsible for the elaboration of a meaningful appearance out of the images and thoughts which result from the alteration of repressed content in the unconscious; in other words, the concrete delusional ideas are so chosen as to present a logical façade, to appear consistent with the data of reality. In addition, the paranoiac patient finds artificial connections between different, or disconnected, perceived facts of reality, in order to substantiate the "reality" of his delusions; this is the mental activity of "mending." The latter, as well as the secondary elaboration of repressed thoughts, can be regarded as a kind of compensation for the omitted reality testing. Reality testing provides substantiation of consistent facts, as well as rectification of errors; secondary elaboration patches up a fictitious consistency between mental content, felt as external reality, and the actual reality, in order to safeguard the feeling of integration.

From the study of the behavior of the patient suffering from delusions as well as from the sensation of estrangement (unreality) from actually perceived outer objects, it becomes evident that reality testing does not fully explain the sense of reality. One of the important achievements of Federn's studies in ego psychology during the last thirty years is the clarification of the dynamic implications of the "sense of reality."

Only the main outline of Federn's theories can be presented here. They are based on an accurate description of the ego phenomenon as it is actually experienced by the subject. To account for the ego experience itself, Federn postulates an "ego cathexis," a form of excitation or "energy" which conveys this experience. It is a common realization that one's self-experience manifests fluctuating degrees of intensity: in certain states one feels numb; in others, more vivid. During dreamless sleep the ego cathexis is withdrawn. In the waking state one feels one's self (one's ego) introspectively as a coherent unity: all the bodily and mental elements which are included in any given ego experience are simultaneously invested by the ego cathexis, which thus exerts a unifying and integrating function. The ego investment of the cathexis, which includes the preconscious, necessarily has an extension, the periphery of which (in Federn's expression, the "ego boundary") is flexible; varying mental contents are included within and excluded from the ego at different times. In the ego boundary the sense organs are included and imbedded, like windows in a wall.

Only those mental stimuli which are intercepted and invested by the ego cathexis, thus being included and integrated in the ego unity, are felt to be mental (inner subjective experiences). They are recognized as "unreal" in so far as they do not belong to the facts existing in the external world. Certain disturbing drives, memories, or thoughts against which the ego mobilizes a dynamic barrier, called "countercathexis," do not obtain preconscious cathexis; thus they do not participate in the ego, nor do they come to consciousness even when they are strongly cathected from the id. Such mental data are repressed. The countercathexis constitutes the dynamic ego boundary toward the unconscious (the id). When the unconscious pressure of repressed drives challenges the efforts of the ego to maintain their repression, a state of anxiety ensues. When unconscious drives or thoughts, without investment by ego cathexis, break through into consciousness, they are sensed in the form of hallucinations and delusions as if they existed in reality.

These phenomena may be due either to a relative weakening of the ego resistance—the ego boundary—or to a relative increase of the drive cathexis. They are usually indicative of an ego weakness, temporary, as in states of exhaustion or sleep, or more lasting, as in psychosis. Ego weakness is understood to be a scarcity of ego cathexis, which may be innate or may be the economic consequence of too great investment of cathexis in such activities as repression. Whenever a mental structure enters the ego boundary from without, it is sensed as external reality; when it participates in the ego (is invested by the ego cathexis), it is recognized and felt as "inner mentality." In certain disturbances of the ego, the parts of the ego boundary in which the sense organs are imbedded are insufficiently cathected; in this case the perceptions of the actual external reality enter the sense organs but do not pass through the ego boundary. As a result, they are sensed as unreal and dream-like; this is the phenomenon of "estrangement."

In the present-day view, repression is of two types. In the first, material which has never been cathected by the ego but has remained in the id is kept repressed and never achieves consciousness (primary repression). In the second, material which was once conscious but which cannot be integrated in the present state of the ego is regarded as repression proper.

## The Unconscious

It is helpful to repeat that the preconscious and conscious mental phenomena are rooted in the unconscious system. Every drive and interest, every memory and representation of the "inner foreign country," originate in this system. Only upon acquiring the binding preconscious cathexis are they included in those coherent mental processes which can be reached by introspection. The binding or fixing character of the preconscious cathexis will be considered shortly.

The mental phenomena deprived of, or not obtaining, preconscious cathexis are subjected to processes which are characteristic for the system unconscious. They can be recognized through the analysis of their end-products as they are revealed in dreams and mental symptoms. These phenomena are very different from anything which can be perceived through introspection. In the system unconscious the cathexis is not fixed on the single representations but is "free-floating"; that is, the excitation of one representation can pass to other representations which are connected with it by associative links. Thus one stimulated representation can be substituted for another, irrespective of logical or rational motives. In fact, this phenomenon, called by Freud the "primary mental process," is not adjusted to reality. Some substitutions of unconscious representations by other images occur according to fixed inherited patterns, common to all human beings. Such archaic relations between many representations—of a man, of a woman, of children, of parents, and of persons in general, of death and birth, and especially of sexual organs and sexual functions— and the images determined by one's individual experience are called "symbolic." The symbols belong to the archaic traits of the system unconscious.

In this system no distinction between real and unreal is made.

The mental content which is cathected at any given moment is not related to external reality; no sense of reality or reality testing can function in the system unconscious. Nor can judgment, different degrees of certainty, doubts, or negation of mental content exist in this system. Its representations are not expressed in words as are those of the preconscious. Since, in Freud's opinion, there is no integration of the drives in the id, no incompatibility between contradictory drives can ensue; they may be aroused simultaneously, leading to a composite formation.

The primary process—the free displacement of mental excitation—does not lead to simple substitutions of one representation by another. Two or more representations can be simultaneously aroused. The cathexes of these representations may then be directed to still another representation, which thereby becomes strongly cathected (condensation of cathexes); or else a fusion of the stimulated representations may ensue (they may be "telescoped," to use a term introduced by French, into one representation). The primary process is checked by the intervention of the preconscious cathexis which concerns the representation of verbal expressions. Only when the id-cathected object representation (*Sach-Vorstellung*) is united with the preconscious verbal representation (*Wort-Vorstellung*) does the cathexis remain fixed on the representation, and displacement no longer occurs. Freud called this binding effect, resulting from the union of the id and the preconscious cathexes, the "secondary mental process" (23). It is the necessary presupposition for coherent and rational thinking.

Most dream images and neurotic symptoms appear meaningless and even absurd as long as they are not subjected to analysis. By this procedure the original unconscious content, which was altered by the primary process, can be detected. Repressed memories and drives, which are void of the preconscious cathexis, undergo the processes of the system unconscious just described. And only when, by the effect of the primary process, they become so disguised as to be unrecognizable by the ego can they reach the preconscious and consciousness.

## THE PHENOMENON OF ANXIETY

Freud's nondoctrinal approach to psychoanalytic problems is clearly illustrated by the evolution of his dynamic concept of the "phenomenon of anxiety" (24). In his earlier theory, anxiety was held to be the result of the inhibition (repression) of sexual excitation (libido), which thus built up tension to a level at which its emotional discharge, in the form of anxiety, was necessitated. He thought that libido was always transformed into anxiety when it was directly discharged from the unconscious. This theory was supported by a wealth of clinical experience. Patients developed neurotic anxiety when they repressed sexual desire or did not find adequate sexual satisfaction, especially when they were exposed for a certain length of time to excessive stimulation.

In 1926, in *The Problem of Anxiety* (24), Freud published his newer conceptions which had been modified from his earlier theory upon deeper consideration of many clinical manifestations. As a matter of fact, in his new concept, sexual tension maintained the role of a determining factor in the production of anxiety; but the dynamic formulation of the phenomenon of anxiety was revised in a decisive way, through connection with the economic concept of mental traumatization. Therefore, the more recent psychodynamic theory of the phenomenon of anxiety rests on the concept of trauma.

A traumatic condition ensues when the afflux of excitation into the mental apparatus can no longer be mastered; in other words, when the dynamic resources of the organism are insufficient to bind the impact of energies which cannot be discharged. Freud's German expression for countercathexis, *Gegenbesetzung* ("opposing stronghold"), conveys an excellent figurative picture of his dynamic concepts of defense and trauma. A physical trauma is a lesion of the external protective layer of the organism, the skin, which permits the entering of greater amounts of external stimulation than can be dealt with. Thereupon, the mental apparatus mobilizes defensive energies to check the invading stimuli. Freud called the external layer of the organism "stimulus protection" (*Reizschutz*).

Stimuli also enter the mental apparatus from within, from the id—the source of all needs, drives, and urges. It is the task of the ego to deal with the drive stimuli by binding and integrating them into a coherent behavior pattern. As has been explained, the ego uses the binding energy not only to fix the id cathexes on the single mental representation but also to keep them in check until the proper time for their discharge arrives, in accordance with its integrative plans for the achievement of the end-goals. French (16) points out that the ego's capacity to restrain subsidiary impulses from premature discharge is dependent on its confidence that it will be able to achieve the end-goal. When hope diminishes or fails, then the ego tends to lose its control.

The inner drive tensions can determine a traumatic condition in two ways. In the first place, the drive excitation may not find an outlet for its discharge, and its unchecked increase may prevent the re-establishment of psychic equilibrium. Second, the satisfaction of a given drive may be possible and, in itself, pleasurable, as is any drive satisfaction, but it may be dangerous by implication. In other words, its gratification may interfere with other important needs of the individual or may expose him to external traumatization, such as punishment, loss of love, or loss of esteem. One of the most important sources of danger, that is, of inner indomitable opposition, is the individual's conscience. This is a function of a third mental structure, the superego, the development and nature of which will be given due attention.

Anxiety is produced and experienced by the ego. Whenever the ego senses the threat of a traumatic condition, of an increase of tension beyond mastery, it reacts with what Freud called the "anxiety signal." This is a characteristic emotional state which stimulates the ego to mobilize all available dynamic resources to forestall the threatening trauma. When the threat is imminent and severe, the ego has to employ all its available energy to check the invasion of excess stimulation, so that its efficiency is more or less impaired. A fully developed anxiety state can even paralyze the ego, which then remains defenseless in the face of the oncoming danger. Freud considers the "danger," to which the ego reacts with anxiety, not as an objective situation but as a threat of a traumatic condition.

When the anxiety is due to the threat of an external danger, it is called "fear" (*Real-Angst*); when it is a reaction to an ungovernable drive stimulation, sexual or aggressive, it is called "anxiety" (*Trieb-Angst*), which is characteristic of neurotic anxiety states, especially for anxiety hysteria (phobia); when it is due to the tension resulting from the strictures of conscience, it is called "superego anxiety."

In Freud's opinion the physiological phenomena of anxiety, such as palpitation, shortness of breath, tremor, and increased bowel activity, represent a "hysterical fixation" to the first situation in which the individual helplessly experiences a tremendous increase of excitation which cannot be bound and discharged.

This was the situation when he was born. At every subsequent threat of a traumatic condition, those physiological phenomena which the individual experienced in that first traumatic situation are reactivated. It is understood, however, that these physiological anxiety symptoms are a constitutional reaction pattern and manifest themselves in every individual in a state of anxiety, irrespective of the severity of the traumatization which he himeslf experienced at his own birth. In Otto Rank's exaggerated generalization, all neuroses and psychoses were traced back to the "trauma of birth" (27).

The phenomenon of repression is induced by anxiety, as are all other defense measures of the ego. The countercathexes form the inner *Reizschutz*. As long as they keep the drives repressed in the system unconscious, anxiety is avoided. Every threat of the repressed drives to break through into consciousness arouses anxiety. The more repressions and other defenses the ego has to maintain, the less energy remains at its disposal in case of emergency. So it is evident that, with increased repression, the ego is impoverished, its integrative capacity is lowered, and it is more easily exposed to external traumatization.

The experience of an external trauma can provoke a traumatic neurosis in the individual. Such a person is unable, for a varying length of time after his withdrawal from the situation, to rid himself of the recurring impact of the traumatizing stimulation. The state of anxiety outlasts the traumatic situation because the individual was not successful in binding the afflux of excessive stimulation. And when he finds some relief in waking life through various diversions, the unmastered stimuli break through into the ego as soon as he falls asleep, provoking anxiety dreams in which the traumatic event is re-experienced over and over again. Eventually, the individual succeeds in binding such stimulations. The more unexpected the traumatic event, the more severe is its effect, for the anticipation of distress may mobilize in advance enough binding energy, in the form of anxiety, to prevent a lasting mental trauma. The development of anxiety in traumatized individuals during their mental re-experiencing of the traumatic event serves to bind the excess stimulation which remains uncontrolled.

## The Superego

"Identification" of one person with others is an important and complicated mental phenomenon. Sympathy, empathy, understanding of our fellow-men, pity, compassion, and conscience, which produces feelings of guilt, are based on various forms of identification.

The type of identification which leads to the formation of the mental structure called the "superego" can also be called the "internalization" of another individual. The latter is a more accurate term than Ferenczi's "introjection" (13), which found a general acceptance among psychoanalysts, since, as a matter of fact, nothing is introjected into one's own ego. Identification is the ego's adoption of traits and conduct in the likeness of another person; it is a kind of imitation whereby the ego feels itself to be, in the desired respects, like that person. Through this autoplastic duplication of another person, the latter becomes, as it were, internalized in one's own ego.

The innate tendency to assume the characteristics of the persons of one's environment and to learn to react as they do is manifested very early in the infant's life. No adequate development of behavior, social adjustment, and speech is possible without identification. It is still a controversial issue whether all features, achievements, and emotional reactions which derive from identification with other people, especially with the parents, participate in that mental structure which Freud called the "superego." While, according to Freud, the development of the superego begins at about the fifth year of life, in connection with the oedipus complex, Melanie Klein (26) and Ernest Jones (25) trace the beginning of its development back to earliest childhood, the first months of life. At any rate, no one doubts that the process of identification is already in effect at this early stage. Klein and Jones agree that the final superego structure is not completed until the fifth or sixth year.

Freud did not develop his conception of the main features of the superego, an inner institution which exerts the function of conscience, until the early twenties. Earlier (1914), in his paper on "Narcissism" (22), he described this function as derived from the individual's self-love. In order to satisfy his self-love, which is mortified by the discovery of his shortcomings as well as by numerous parental criticisms, reproaches, and punishment, the individual builds for himself an ideal image to which he wishes to conform. His self-love is thus displaced on this "ego ideal," which is built up according to the teaching and examples of the persons he admires, chiefly the parents. The inner institution which assumes the function of self-observation, and which is constituted by the internalized parents, was later called by Freud the "superego." In his earlier concept of conscience, however, he considered only the individual's narcissistic need to comply with the ego ideal. Gradually he came to consider conscience as only one function of the superego.

Although conscience is the most important regulating factor in human conduct because of its role in determining feelings of guilt and the need for punishment, the superego may also play a consoling, encouraging, supporting role, as Freud (20) pointed out in his article, "Humor," published in 1928. Indeed, when we consider that all parental attitudes are internalized, we realize that the superego must assume this supportive and comforting role as well as be critical and punitive. In undeserved suffering, the strength of endurance and the consolation that the individual is able to find within himself are derived from the superego. That it can also become a source of anxiety and of consequent repression was previously pointed out.

This chapter is intended to deal primarily with the history of metapsychological concepts, as they developed in the study of psychoanalysis. Elaboration of these concepts and further elucidation belong to the subsequent chapters in Part I, their application to the chapters in Part II.

## BIBLIOGRAPHY

1. ALEXANDER, F. *Fundamentals of Psychoanalysis* (New York: W. W. Norton & Co., Inc., 1948).
2. ALEXANDER, F. *Our Age of Unreason* (rev. ed.; Philadelphia: J. B. Lippincott Co., 1951).
3. BERNARD, C. *Leçons de physiologie expérimentale appliquée à la médecine* (Paris: J. B. Baillière, 1855).
4. BREUER, J., and FREUD, S. *Studies in Hysteria* (New York: Nervous and Mental Disease Publishing Co., 1936).
5. CANNON, W. B. *The Wisdom of the Body* (New York: W. W. Norton & Co., Inc., 1932).
6. FECHNER, G. T. *Einige Ideen zur Schöpfungs und Entwickelungsgeschichte der Organismen* (Leipzig: Druck und Verlag von Breitkopf & Haertel, 1873).
7. FEDERN, P. "Ego Feeling in Dreams," *Psychoanalyt. Quart.*, 1:511, 1932.
8. FEDERN, P. "Ichgrenzen, Ichstärke und Identifizierung" ("Ego Boundaries, Ego Strength, and Identification"), in *Almanach der Psychoanalyse* (Vienna: Internationaler psychoanalytischer Verlag, 1937).

9. FEDERN, P. "Narcissism in the Strucure of the Ego," *Internat. J. Psycho-Analysis*, 9:401, 1928.
10. FEDERN, P. "Zur Unterscheidung des gesunden und krankhaften Narzissmus" ("On Differentiation of Normal and Pathological Narcissism"), *Imago*, 22:5, 1936.
11. FEDERN, P. "Some Variations in Ego-Feeling," *Internat. J. Psycho-Analysis*, 7:434, 1926.
12. FEDERN, P. "Die Wirklichkeit des Todestriebes" ("The Reality of the Death Drive"), in *Almanach der Psychoanalyse* (Vienna: Internationaler psychoanalytischer Verlag, 1931).
13. FERENCZI, S. "Introjection and Transference," in *Sex in Psychoanalysis* (New York: Basic Books, 1950).
14. FRENCH, T. M. "Defense and Synthesis in the Function of the Ego," *Psychoanalyt. Quart.*, 7:537, 1938.
15. FRENCH, T. M. "Goal, Mechanism, and Integrative Field," *Psychosom. Med.*, 3:226, 1941.
16. FRENCH, T. M. "Integration of Social Behavior," *Psychoanalyt. Quart.*, 14:149, 1945.
17. FRENCH, T. M. "Reality and the Unconscious," *Psychoanalyt. Quart.*, 6:23, 1937.
18. FREUD, S. *Beyond the Pleasure Principle* (2d ed.; London: Hogarth Press, 1942).
19. FREUD, S. *The Ego and the Id* (London: Hogarth Press, 1947).
20. FREUD, S. "Humor," *Internat. J. Psycho-Analysis*, 9:1, 1928.
21. FREUD, S. *The Interpretation of Dreams*, in *The Basic Writings of Sigmund Freud* (New York: Random House, 1938).
22. FREUD, S. "On Narcissism: An Introduction," in *Collected Papers*, Vol. 4 (London: Hogarth Press, 1925).
23. FREUD, S. *An Outline of Psychoanalysis* (New York: W. W. Norton & Co., Inc., 1950), p. 45.
24. FREUD, S. *The Problem of Anxiety* (New York: W. W. Norton & & Co., Inc., 1936).
25. JONES, E. *Papers on Psycho-Analysis* (Baltimore: William Wood & Co., 1938).
26. KLEIN, M. "The Oedipus Complex in the Light of Early Anxieties," *Internat. J. Psycho-Analysis*, 26:11, 1945.
27. RANK, O. *The Trauma of Birth* (London: Kegan Paul, Trench, Trubner & Co., Ltd., 1929).
28. WEISS, EDOARDO. *Principles of Psychodynamics* (New York: Grune & Stratton, 1950).

# IV

## PERSONALITY DEVELOPMENT

### Therese Benedek, M.D.

THE psychoanalytic theory of personality consists of concepts concerning personality as an organization of the mental apparatus in general and of concepts concerning the processes which lead to differences specific for the particular individual.

In the infinite differentiations and integrations which make up the organization of the personality, it is useful to distinguish between the processes of maturation and those of development. "Maturation" refers to processes of growth which occur relatively independently of the environment; "development" refers to the interaction between maturational processes and environmental influences which lead to higher structuralization and to individual variations in the psychic apparatus. The development of the personality is the unfolding of an innate anlage—constitution—under the influence of the environment. Since the primary environment of the individual is created by the natural parents, who transmit to the child the patterns of the culture in which they live, genetic and environmental factors become closely interwoven, and "linked together they form"—as Freud put it—"an inseparable etiological unity."

The interaction between mother and child begins immediately at conception. We assume that the intra-uterine growth evolves through continuous gratification of basic needs, sheltered from external disturbances. However, not only the physiological processes of the mother favorable for the growth of the fetus are transmitted; more recent investigations indicate that fluctuations in the mother's physical and emotional well-being may also be registered by the fetus. Such influences, as well as the effects of obstetrical techniques, may modify the newborn child's adaptability to extra-uterine life.

Birth—the interruption of the fetal symbiosis—represents a trauma under any obstetrical condition. After a precarious pas-

sage through the birth canal, the newborn is subject to an overwhelming change in his physiology: he has to become active in
securing the basic needs for living; he has to breathe, suck, and
swallow. These vital functions are secured by reflexes co-ordinated during intra-uterine life. They are ready to function immediately after birth. Yet, since the network of the vegetative
nervous system is not yet quite organized, the first weeks of life
are characterized by vegetative instability. Irregular respiration,
sneezing, yawning, regurgitation, vomiting, fitful waking, startle
responses, give the impression that the newborn is not comfortable. It takes about four weeks—the "neonatal period"—for the
infant to advance in maturation to a level where smoother vegetative functioning occurs.

The activity pattern of the newborn reveals marked individual
differences. A stimulus intense enough to pass the threshold of a
"phlegmatic infant" may activate in another infant not only a
startle response but also a general excitation which provokes a
crying fit. Even more significant are the differences in the activity
and endurance in suckling, in the functioning of the digestive
system, in the rhythm of sleeping and waking. There are other,
less obvious differences in the sensory system of newborn infants:
their sensitivity to sound and tone, to tactile and taste stimulations,
shows marked variations.

According to Freud's hypothesis, the sleeping infant is in a
condition closely resembling that of intra-uterine life. Stimuli
from without and from within disturb this sleep. Hunger and pain
are the sensations which most often waken the infant crying. The
crying fit of the infant is a general motor discharge of excitement
caused by internal need. It is characteristic of the newborn that,
if the need reaches the threshold which activates crying, he continues with increasing intensity until the satisfaction of his need
is made available; then he grasps at the nipple and appears to
"work" with concentration until his hunger is stilled. If satisfaction fails to ensue, he may cry until his physical forces are exhausted.

The mother's genuine motherliness and her ability and desire
to protect the infant reduce the frequency of disturbing stimuli
and diminish the intensity of the crying fits. However, the
mother's behavior toward her infant is motivated not only by her
motherliness but also by the current customs of nursing care. In
our civilization these customs have changed during the last thirty

years, moving from one extreme to the other. Three decades ago, the nursing custom could be called "indulgent breast-feeding"; the infant was permitted to sleep close to the mother and be nursed any time the desire, not just imperative hunger, arose. As a reaction to the somatic effects of this indulgence, there followed the "strict regime" introduced by the German pediatric school (Czerny, Finkelstein). These pediatricians recommended keeping the infant isolated from the mother, and they established "feeding schedules," even at the cost of the infant's having to cry until exhaustion. It was later demonstrated that the all too routinized nursing care overlooked deprivations of various intensity and significance. Recently, a better balance between the child's needs and his gratifications has been recommended, thus allowing for individual differences rather than maintaining rigid regulations.

Normally, crying is a signal for the mother to take care of the baby. The rhythmically returning course of events is this: arising need—disturbance of sleep—crying—gratification—sleep again. As far as the newborn is concerned, this process evolves within the self, without the realization of an external environment. In this phase of extra-uterine symbiosis, the mother is part of the process of gratification. Sometimes one may observe intense sucking movements before the awakening of the infant. This phenomenon can be interpreted as repetition of the intra-uterine "practice" of the sucking reflex, which, in this early period of extra-uterine life, represents an attempt to continue the symbiosis and to preserve sleep. Naturally, the need remains unsatisfied and increases until it wakens the infant crying. The rhythmic alternation between need and gratification supplies the infant with the metabolic and emotional requirements for a smooth course of developmental events.

Feeding, especially at the mother's breast, not only satisfies hunger but also conveys to the infant the tactile and kinesthetic sensations of being protected; it preserves the security of the symbiosis. A biological communication between infant and mother is repeated with each nursing: the infant turns the head toward the mother's breast, incorporates it, retains it as part of the self, then separates himself from it, and by this, from the mother again.[1] The next step in growth is indicated when the

---

1. This process is supposed to represent the core (and the model) of the psychological process of identification, which is one of the basic patterns in personality development.

infant, after gratification of hunger—or after alleviation of discomfort and pain—does not fall asleep immediately but exercises "activities" already attained. He continues sucking playfully on the breast, enjoying the tactile sensations of lips and tongue, of fingers and cheeks, as they touch the breast; he learns to find his mouth in order to suck his fingers. While the infant enjoys the self-produced sensations, being awake enables him to perceive that the need originates within the self and the source of gratification—the mother—is outside.[2] We usually recognize this developmental step in the visual behavior of the infant: he follows the mother with his eyes.

The visual behavior of the infant is probably the first active manifestation of his need for communication with the environment, which, in the first place, is the mother. The infant's glance appears to greet the mother, his intent stare at her seems to grasp her and to hold onto her with his eyes before he can grasp her with his mouth. Soon after the visual co-ordination enables the infant to fix his gaze on an object, his mimical expressions become a rich means of communication. Not only the mother can interpret this body language; the trained observer also sees in it the content of the infant's primary relationship with his mother.

If the developmental process is undisturbed, the infant preserves the sense of security that all his needs are (and will be) satisfied. This sense of confident expectation from the mother is the content of the earliest affective relationship. Confidence is the intra-psychic correlate to the passive, receptive, dependent state of the infant; it plays an important role in his metabolic and psychic economy (9). Confidence sustains the mother-child unity and thus protects the infant from the intensity of external stimuli. Confidence acts as emotional shelter. It facilitates learning. The diminished instinctual tension enables the infant to give attention to the environment. The normal infant learns to understand the mother's facial expressions, just as the mother discerns in the infant's behavior the "signs and signals" of his needs as well as of his desires for activity. Through this preverbal communication, the child learns to accept the mother's reassurance in any new

2. Although a discussion of the maturation sequence is beyond the scope of this presentation, the author takes the growth processes and their observable psychologic manifestations more into consideration than is usual in psychoanalytic literature. It is in this sense that the author differs with Freud's concept that the newborn attributes all the pleasant sensations to the self and the unpleasant sensations to the environment.

step which his adjustment requires. The situation is different when the affect-position of primary confidence cannot develop. The conditions which lead to the disturbance of the primary relationship between mother and child keep the infant in a state of tension. Whether this is expressed in fitful sleep and crying fits and/or in feeding difficulties, the behavior of the infant reveals the disturbance of communication between infant and mother. Not trusting that his needs will be satisfied, his capacity for learning becomes inhibited, and in extreme cases (such as hospitalism), instead of learning, a reflex behavior develops. As the maturation proceeds, the healthy infant shows signs of recognition and a willingness to wait. The three-month-old infant recognizes the mother and the four-to-five-month-old follows attentively the preparations for his feeding.

By the time the infant turns his head toward the mother and smiles at her expectantly, the following developmental steps have been achieved: (1) differentiation between the self and the new environment, (2) perception of the mother as the "needed object" for relieving internal tensions, (3) experience of need as well as of satisfaction (pleasure of satiation within the self), (4) attention to animate and inanimate objects related to needs and gratification.

Since a psychic organization in which id is distinguished from ego emerges only gradually as a result of growth, from the point of view of personality organization the neonatal period represents an undifferentiated phase (32). The whole physiology of the newborn is in the service of survival alone. The maturation of the sensory and motor apparatus and certain emotional attitudes, such as the manifestation of the early relationship to the mother, are in the service of self-preservation and later will come under the control of the ego. The same growth processes produce a surplus of vital energies, which then become the source of pleasurable sensations and form a "reservoir of later differentiable psychic energies," which is the id (19).

With each step of the maturational processes of the motor and sensory organs, new needs for activity become manifest; it takes only a short while for the "practice" of these functions, that is, the functions themselves, to become a source of pleasure. For example, the unco-ordinated movements indicating discomfort, which one observes in the newborn when his blankets are removed, later become a push-and-pull game which reveals the infant's well-being. The pleasurable sensations come from all sources of vital energies and absorb the infant's attention immediately after the tension of the body is relieved. The relaxed infant either sleeps, or he is preoccupied with the pleasurable sensations of his body. These sensations, while originally representing only pleasurable excitation, may later become a need which demands gratification. Thus, at this stage of the development, one may differentiate between id and ego. The id generates impulses which may be supportive to, or in conflict with, the maturational and adaptive processes which form the tasks of the ego.

The libido theory was originally an anatomical concept. The organs which produce libido are the "erotogenic zones"; there the instinctual need is stimulated and is gratified. "Autoeroticism" is the gratification achieved by self-manipulation of the "zone" in which the need is perceived. The lips, the mouth, the skin, the anal mucous membrane, the penis, the clitoris, are considered erotogenic zones. In the center of the developmental organization is the erotogenic zone which is dominant at a specific age. In this sense, one speaks of "oral," "anal," and "genital" phases of development.

The first stage of libido organization is the "oral phase." The mouth is the erotogenic zone which experiences oral libido and its gratifications. The aim of oral libido is incorporation, and "the process is in the service of identification." This is, however, not an oral process exclusively. Olfactory, vestibular, and tactile sensations play a role in the feeding response of the newborn; some weeks later, auditory and visual sensations are also integrated into the feeding experience. Since all the sensory manifestations are in the service of the "receptive tendencies," these sensations as well as the feeding itself are a part of the process through which the infant evolves identification with the mother as well as a primary, affective relationship to her. The infant's capacity to adapt himself to his environment—the growth of his ego—goes hand in hand with the development of object relationship with the mother.

Not all the libidinal pleasure of the infant is autoerotic, generated by the self. The infant receives libidinal stimulation through the nursing care, through tactile, vocal, and tonal expressions of tenderness. Since the satisfaction of the physiological needs is fused with erotic, libidinous sensations generated by the mother, this continuation of gratification represents an urge strong enough to maintain object relationship. The interchange between auto-erotic and object-erotic gratifications is an important factor in successful infant care. The overstimulation of the loving mother, who does not let the waking infant be alone with his self-generated pleasures, actually frustrates the child; on the other hand, an excessive amount of autoerotic gratification at this age, similar to the extensive fantasy life of older children, turns the infant away from the object world and inhibits his efforts toward mastery of it.

Recent studies (41) of institutionalized children show that infants who did not develop object relationships or had to give them up because of neglect, withdrew from the environment and lived the life of preverbal fantasies which are expressed in the monotonous repetition of some form of autoerotic manipulation. Even if the condition is not extreme, overindulgence of the passive dependent needs can lead to an abundance of autoeroticism, since overindulgence deprives the child of the gains of his own expansiveness and inhibits his tendencies toward activity. There are many gradations between the compulsive, fixated autoeroticism of the withdrawn child and the happy, autoerotic pleasures of the well-developing infant. The former are diverted by hardly any substitute, while the latter turns his attention easily toward the mother and accepts her stimulation to external activities.

The primary process of mastery of the outer world repeats, to some degree, the process of incorporation. Grasping with the mouth is the first sign of not being afraid to incorporate (spoon, bottle, new food). Grasping with the hand and leading the object toward the mouth, putting it in the mouth and sucking on it, are the next steps in dealing with objects. (The child's own finger or toe is an external object in this respect.) The three-to-five-month-old baby grasps the bottle and holds onto it; the six-to-seven-month-old baby puts the objects which stimulate his interest into his mouth, in order to investigate them with his lips and tongue and thus to become acquainted with them. This is not a receptive, incorporative attitude alone; it is the manifestation of curiosity, through which the infant learns to recognize the objects of his surroundings. Learning is a receptive function later in life, too; what one really knows becomes a part of one's self. In infancy the receptive tendency appears manifest in oral activity—as if the baby has to be one with the object before he can learn to deal with it as a part of his external reality.

In deed, the receptive and incorporative tendencies and their psychic representation, oral libido, explain the psychodynamic processes of early infancy. The oral phase of development usually comprises the first year of life. Abraham (1) differentiated two levels within the oral phase: the *passive-receptive oral phase*, which lasts until the child becomes able to reach actively for objects; the *active-incorporative oral phase*, which is character-ized by attempts at mastery through incorporation (biting is such a manifestation).

Abraham's distinction between the two levels within the oral phase has more than descriptive significance. The term "active-incorporative oral phase" indicates that the receptive tendency is charged with aggressive impulses; these are usually directed toward the mother. Mothers cannot always provide infants with the requirement of undisturbed development. "Nervous" infants respond even to slight stimulation with uncomfortable tension. Since the infant has no other means than the crying fit of dis-charging his tension, nervous infants often respond with a veri-table "storm of excitation." It depends on the degree of maturity of the vegetative nervous system and the gastrointestinal tract whether the excitation becomes bound to definite parts of the gastrointestinal system. Since these systems are immature, colic, pylorospasm, diarrhea, or constipation may disturb the infant. Pain and tension increase the urge to gain relief and re-establish security by being close to the mother. The crying infant bites the nipple with force and suckles with greed. If the mother does not succeed in pacifying the infant, his physiological tension in-creases, and the need for incorporation becomes more and more charged with motor energy. This is called "hostile incorpo-ration"; although the psychic representation of hostility can hardly exist at that age, its model is formed. While the crying fit alienates the helpless mother, who feels rejected by her child, the child feels even more "annihilated" by the sense of frustration, which leads to his exhaustion. The manifestations of hostile, ag-gressive, incorporative tendencies thus indicate the developing interpersonal conflict between mother and child; they also repre-sent the origin of *ambivalence* in the infant and thereby the core of *intrapsychic conflict*.

The classical psychoanalytic theory of personality develop-ment was originally formulated by Freud and Abraham and con-sisted of the *libido theory*. Later, Freud developed the structural concept of the personality and defined its interacting functions as id, ego, and superego. Alexander (3, 4), considering that libido is produced by the positive balance (surplus) of the metabolic processes, defined psychic energy by the direction of its function rather than by the erotogenic zones (vector concept). These concepts are not contradictory; they complement each other.

This presentation of the developmental processes has traced the structuralization of the personality during the oral phase of the libido organization. Because of the physiology of the metabolic processes and the accompanying emotional needs, this phase can be described as the passive-receptive, dependent period of infancy. During this period, the differentiation of ego and id begins to evolve hand in hand with the development of primary object relationships. If the needs of the growing organism are not adequately met, insecurity, anxiety, and conflict develop.

Rado (39), Fenichel (18), and others pointed out that the first regulator of *self-esteem* (*Selbst-Gefühl:* a feeling of the self as a whole being) is the sense of security acquired by all the satisfactions connected with feeding; these analysts assume that the early disappointments and anxiety, which some infants experience in connection with feeding and digestion, may cause a sense of helplessness, inferiority, and worthlessness. If the positive, ego feeling is too often interrupted by its opposite, the ego development is impaired. (Fixation to the negative feelings within the self may become the core of psychosis or narcissistic neurosis.) The positive balance in the ego feeling, however, tends toward further differentiation for the sake of better adaptation.

The two principles of psychic processes—the *pleasure* and the *reality principles* (21)—are manifestations of the ego's adaptive function. The pleasure principle strives toward immediate gratification, and as such it serves the id; the reality principle tends to postpone immediate gratification in order to make later gratification secure by mastering the reality situation. Indeed, the infant learns soon to differentiate what causes pain and learns to avoid it; he learns also which of his actions bring the mother's—and other persons'—approval and expressions of love and which will bring about disapproval and withdrawal of love.

When the reality principle begins to take control of behavior, the child enters the second phase—the "anal-sadistic phase" of the development. This means that the anus becomes the leading erotogenic zone. Its double function—retention and elimination—becomes the center of interest and the source of pleasure. While the terms refer to the anal processes alone, actually urinary elimination and retention and the pleasure derived from them belong in the same developmental phase.

Toilet training is a crucial learning situation. In the authoritarian Western culture it was undertaken early. In recent years, with the increasing regard for the individual needs and expressions of the child, habit training is delayed to the second year. One assumes that compliance is easier when the child has achieved a degree of motor control. Walking is a good indicator of the change in the balance of the motor apparatus. When the child begins to walk, much of his attention is turned to this function. The increase in self-esteem which the child experiences with this achievement may easily be integrated with another achievement: sphincter control. At the same age the interpersonal relationships of the child have developed far enough so that he can understand the request of the adults and thus may "co-operate" in order to gain approval. The effectiveness of the parent's approval and disapproval as an instrument of habit training depends on several factors. One is the child's already established relationship to the parent; if this is ambivalent, the habit training becomes difficult. The other consideration is timing. There is an optimal time for habit training. This is when the stimulation of the urethral and anal passages is likely to create sensations intense enough to make the child aware of them and when the pleasurable quality of those sensations has not yet been enjoyed for too long a period. If the retentive and eliminative functions have already become an accustomed source of pleasure, the child will have difficulty in establishing control over them.

Toilet training is the ego's first conscious struggle for mastery over an id impulse. The process has several phases. It is usually the mother's task to influence the child—his ego—to exert himself against his tendency for soiling—against the id impulse. Actually, the child is offered a choice between various instinctual gratifications: the praise and love of the mother is one, and the satisfaction in soiling is the other. Thus the mother induces a conflict between rivalrous id impulses: an "instinctual conflict." With his compliance the child earns not only external approval but also internal satisfaction: a sense of mastery. When this sense of mastery becomes a goal in itself, the struggle reaches its next phase: the ego, stronger through gratification, tries to exert effort against the impulse without the help of the physical presence of the mother.

The request of the mother thus becomes incorporated, and the "sphincter morality" is gradually established. This represents a new structuralization within the self: the child becomes independent in so far as his ego can deal with the id impulse; but he also acquires the responsibility to do so—and this produces a new vulnerability. From this time on, anxiety signals danger when the id impulse is threatening to break through the controlling strength of the ego. Thus a "structural conflict" (8), i.e., a conflict between the incorporated prohibitions—primary superego—and the id impulse, is established and begins to control the behavior.

The method by which this result was achieved now pays its dividend. If the training was pursued with severity and punishment, the incorporated prohibitions appear to have such a strictly punitive quality that the child rebels against them and tries to turn the hostility back onto the mother. Defiance and hostile self-assertion during toilet training represent an attempt to externalize the conflict which has just been introduced within the self. The ambivalence—love and hate—thus expressed toward the mother creates a vicious circle: it increases not only the child's conflict with his environment but also the conflict within himself. It is more favorable for the further development of the child if at this time he is permitted and able to express his hostility toward the parent directly. If not, the defiance may be expressed by a failure in the rhythm of the sphincter functions: the child may eliminate when he should retain (lack of control: enuresis, diarrhea), or he may retain when he should eliminate (constipation). Under the confusing methods of toilet training, the excretory functions and their products become a highly appreciated value of exchange—an emotionally charged organ language—between the child and the environment.

Freud (27) described passive and active tendencies within the "anal-sadistic" libido organization. Abraham (1) attributed the passive anal-erotic tendencies to the first phase of that libido organization; he assumed that the first, the "passive-anal," phase coincides with the incorporation of and identification with the mother and with the development of ambivalence toward her. The second, the "active-anal phase," coincides, according to this theory, with the establishment of sphincter control and with the erotization of aggressive and self-assertive impulses. The child soon learns to transfer the active muscular impulses from his own body to others. The erotization of the aggressive impulses makes the term "anal-sadistic phase" appropriate for the second stage of pregenital development.

The psychic economy of the anal-sadistic phase is complex and precarious. The previously dominant passive-receptive tendencies, when the infant *was always given to*, changes to the awareness that he is also *taken from*. Retaining, of course, plays an important role not only in the physiological, but also in the emotional, metabolism. Receiving, retaining, eliminating—taking and giving—regulate the physiologic and psychic economy all through life. Actually, both physiologic and psychic economy have to remain in a positive balance in order to permit the active strivings of the organism to dominate over the passive receptive needs. If the balance of the economy is negative—this may be brought about by any serious deprivation or illness—a "regression" takes place; the active tendencies diminish or disappear, and the passive-receptive tendencies will dominate the behavior.

In the anal phase of development, when a "giving" attitude toward the environment is just at its beginning, the co-operation with the demands of the training may keep the child in a fearful tension, which repeats itself several times daily. Thus regression may occur repeatedly. This is the reason that infants, formerly happy and secure, sometimes become tense and negativistic and suffer from crying fits during a long-extended training period. After sphincter control is safely established, the conflict tension diminishes, and the child becomes free for the next step in his development. The greatest part of the infant's experiences, even those of the toilet-training period, occur mainly on the level of physiology and thus remain unconscious. But the experiences are not "organically" forgotten. The conditionings, during the oral as well as during the anal phase of development, and their psychic derivatives form a complex reaction pattern of somatic and psychic functioning.

It is in another area of maturation that the child learns to speak. This occurs usually during the second and third years of life. This complex process is considered to be the result of the progressing maturation of the speech apparatus and of intellectual accomplishments and is, therefore, not usually discussed in connection with the psychodynamic aspects of personality development. While the psychology of speech is beyond the scope of this presentation, we include some of its aspects which indicate the role of speech development in the structuralization of the mental apparatus.

When the infant coos and babbles in his crib, he uses his lips and tongue, also his vocal cords, not for communication, but for autoerotic pleasure. If his mother (or someone else whom he knows) enters his visual field and interest, the baby turns to his "dependable" means of communication: he smiles, he stretches his arms, grasps with his hands; he certainly makes his wishes understandable. When he is older and has already learned that movements of the lips and the tone accompanying them have importance for the mother, he babbles and coos back to her, trying to imitate her, though he is unable to co-ordinate the movements necessary for articulation. It has often been pointed out that the prevalence of oral gratification and the surplus excitation of the lips can be held responsible for the fact that, in every language, the word which means mother and the nursing person (and nursing implements) are formed by lip sounds: *ma—mom—mama; pa—ta—fa; ba—baba;* etc. These are the sounds which are first formed and are usually first noticed by the environment. But infants often repeat "unknowingly" some other sounds even earlier, sounds which accompany affects. Some infants inhale deeply when they are surprised or pleasantly amazed, and one can hear a definite syllable, like *hee, he, hei;* or they utter guttural tones, forming syllables when they are angry, like *ghroo, ghra,* or a combination of lip and hissing tones, such as *huppe, hppe.* Whether the infant "gets the idea" of speech by the experience that certain tones and sounds are forming the same way in his own mouth when he has certain feelings, one does not know. These affective utterances usually disappear after the child has learned to articulate in speech.

Each child learns to speak in his own way and at greatly varied times. Some children can speak one- to two-syllable words at nine months. Generally, children at first acquire a vocabulary which they use in single one- or two-syllable words, accompanied by gesturing. Some children, earlier than others but usually before the end of the second year, learn to speak a sequence of two to three words and then rudimentary sentences. In the third year they usually speak short sentences correctly and begin to speak of themselves in the first person.

Speech, phylogenetically the most recent acquirement, is abandoned quickly if the child is under the influence of affects. Not only in distress does the child cry rather than tell about his situation, but other emotions are also expressed by gesture rather than by word. The child jumps around with joy but does not say "I am glad," or he hides his face or himself altogether if embarrassed. Children in early years actually communicate by speech only when they are calm and their attention is directed. Under emotional influence, they revert to mimical expression. To this, we may add the body language of the urethral and anal functions to conclude that the language of emotions is primarily a body language; the verbal language, on the contrary, brings to the ego a means of communication beyond the purely physiological and emotional patterns of reaction.

The child learns to know many objects of his surroundings and to isolate them as functional units before he learns the word which designates the object itself. Since he hears the words, the names of things, he accumulates in his mind many word symbols before he can articulate enough to speak the words; and even more highly integrated must be the speech and the mental apparatus in order to express not only concrete things and needs but perceptions and feelings which are not directly connected with needs. Thus, when the child is able to speak the word "mama," he not only knows the mother as a person, different from others, but he has accumulated psychic experiences of identification with her, love, anger, and fear, and he also has stored in his mind symbols related to those experiences. These experiences, however, and the related symbols do not ever need to reach the level of verbalization. They form the content of the unconscious as the mental representation of physiological processes and/or as word and symbol representation of memory traces. The communication between these occurs through primary processes. In infancy and early childhood before the ego defenses interfere with the free flow of psychophysiologic energy, the demarcation between psychic and somatic processes is not so well defined as it is later in life. Therefore, only careful analysis of individual cases may reveal how much of the preverbal emotional processes occur purely on the level of physiology and how much reaches psychic elaboration which can be called "preverbal fantasy," how often and under what conditions they combine or change from one to another. All this needs to be investigated. Since the ego's control is not yet well developed, the child easily reverts to preverbal expressions. It is not words, therefore, but the child's activities, movements, and games, as well as his physiological regressions, which reveal the emotional processes which form his personality.

To take inventory of the psychosexual personality of the child

as he is about to outgrow the age of toilet training, we shall review
the various new differentiations within the psychic apparatus.

Since the prohibitions are introjected, the child has to protect
himself not only against the fear of the parent but against the
anxiety produced by the structural conflict. The primary superego manifests itself in the defense measures of the ego. The child
at this age level is capable of loathing and shame. Loathing and
shame are highly charged affects which used to be considered as
reaction formation of the ego against the instinctual impulse; but
they can also be defined as ego defenses, since they protect the ego
by making the id impulse undesirable. While shame and loathing
appear to be the manifestations of a strict superego, there are also
simpler defense reactions. Small children expose naïvely their impulse to undo the harm which is already done (soiling) or to deny
the blame. Undoing and denial are two typical ego defenses (19).
If the child's fear of the parent is too great and the ambivalence
conflict too intense, the developing ego defenses have a more serious character. Expression of the hostility against the parents or
against a sibling and/or discharge of hostility against animals or
turning the hostility toward the self are outcomes of the anal-
sadistic tendencies. Both the aggression directed toward objects
and the aggression turned toward the self play a significant role in
the fixation of the conflict constellation of the anal phase. The
sadistic, as well as the masochistic, tendencies and the structural
conflicts which they imply create the disposition for compulsion
neurosis as well as for paranoid reaction formations.

Normally, the simple ego defenses, together with the positive
identification with the mother-teacher, enable the child to withstand the pressure for immediate gratification of his instinctual
needs. While he postpones the gratification, the suspense presents
a new stimulation. Now the child is ready for substitute gratification of the diminished instinctual tensions. Masturbation may
begin through the suspense stimulation of the urethral and anal
zone; the stimulation may extend to the genitals, and thus genital
masturbation may channelize the urethral and anal excitation. The
child at this age, however, is able also to divert his attention from
direct, masturbatory gratification and can enjoy substitute gratifications in play with toys, with children and adults. The fantasy
gratifications of this age level are complex and serve not only the
gratification of the instinctual need but also the need of the ego for
mastery. Hand in hand with the expansion of the ego, the inter-

personal relationships of the child become manifold. He becomes aware of other people in his orbit besides the mother in the second half of his first year. In the second year these individuals begin to play distinct roles in his life. Innumerable identifications with the father bring him closer to the center of the child's psychosexual development. At the same time, the child explores the significance of siblings and responds to them day by day, to each one in a specific way. He may envy and hate one and admire another; he may feel that one is a source of security and reassurance or that he is a cause for competition, hostility, and ensuing guilt. The interpersonal relationships of the two-to-three-year-old are not based on the need for security alone; they are motivated by many other needs of the growing personality.

During the oral phase of development, there is hardly any difference in the emotional dynamics of the children of the two sexes. In the second year, during the anal phase, when self-assertion begins to play a role, marked differences are observed between boys and girls. The emotional security which results from the undisturbed relationship with the mother affects boys and girls differently. It gives the boy permission for self-assertion and courage that he may free himself from dependence on his mother and may start a development in which identification with his father becomes the leading motive. The girl's development takes a different course: the sense of security with her mother supplies her with the most effective impulses for identification with her mother. As long as the girl's identification with the mother is undisturbed, she learns from her easily. For example, it is well known to mothers that the toilet training of girls is usually achieved more easily than that of boys. Girls probably learn from the mother willingly and by identification, while boys learn from her only if and after their need for self-assertion has been satisfied.

Several behavior manifestations appear decidedly "masculine" or "feminine" even in two-year-old children. For the psychosexual integration, especially significant are the expressions of the child's interest in his body. During the anal phase the child learns a great deal about his body; he experiences some of its capacities and limitations. The ego gratification gained from good performance is abundantly enjoyed, but this pleasure is checked by disappointment and anger when the child fails to satisfy his ambitions. These reactions to failure are stronger in boys than in girls in general, and they become more obvious if the child compares himself with others. The roots of competitive behavior originate in the struggles for achievement of sphincter control. Jones (37) assumed that the competition in urinary behavior—the control and the power of the urine stream—is the model for all competitive behavior among men. Actually, it demonstrates the psychodynamics of competition in general: (1) the admiration for the successful competitor and the desire to be like him (identification); (2) anger toward the self because one is not like him and because the sense of frustration is not relieved; and (3) the projection of anger on the competitor who thus becomes responsible for one's failure.[3] During the anal and oedipal period the boy usually compares himself with his father; the effects of the comparison may contribute to passive reactions toward the father and to inferiority feelings. If the reactions of the child are too hostile to the father, the resulting fear may add to the developing castration complex. (Urinary competition with individuals of the same age is characteristic of the latency period.) The significance of urinary competition implies that the anus as an erotogenic zone is receding and that the penis is becoming the leading erotogenic zone: the boy enters the phallic phase of development. (The girl's responses to the experiences of her body at this age will be discussed later.)

The "phallic phase" is the third pregenital phase of development. In recent psychoanalytic literature it is more often referred to as the "oedipal phase," since the oedipus complex dominates its psychodynamic constellation. The term "phallic phase" originates in the concept that children of both sexes, at a certain age level, assume the existence of the same male genital in all persons. The term "oedipal phase" indicates that the child has arrived at that developmental level when his erotically colored demands are intensified and directed for gratification toward the parent of the opposite sex, i.e., the parent of the opposite sex becomes the object of the child's libido. Oedipus Rex (Sophocles) suffered blindness and exile as punishment for his unknowingly committed incest with his mother, Jocasta. The incestuous "crime" and the "punishment" for it represent the content of the oedipus complex. Several authors have attempted to be precise by intro-

---

3. "Projection of anger" sounds too severe a reaction in regard to the failure of the child. Yet we know how easily a child accepts the idea that a chair, a table, etc., is responsible for his hurting himself; he is relieved when he can "punish" it for its "misbehavior."

ducing the term "Electra complex" to define the conflict of the girl, caused by the heterosexual tendency directed toward her father. However, this seems to be cumbersome, and its use has not become general.

Boys begin to concentrate upon the genitals for gratification—in general—earlier than girls do. Boys' earlier awareness of the organ which produces pleasure is motivated by the anatomical differences in the sexual organs. The anatomy of the boy permits him to gratify his partial instincts freely. He can look at his penis and exhibit it; he can play with it while he urinates, and he may have sensations of fleeting erections. To this one may add the social evaluation of the male sex, the parents' pride in having a boy, and the pleasure of many fathers in stimulating sexual comparison in their sons and thus activating sexual preoccupation. The first manifestation of the awakening heterosexual interest is an intensified sexual curiosity which is normally directed toward the mother. She is the first object of her son's dependent love, and when he reaches another phase in his sexual maturation he holds onto the original object of his love. In this sense the male oedipus complex is simple.

The girls' development is more complex and somewhat slower. When the stimulation of the anal phase recedes, the sexual energy does not find an object for outlet through the body of the girl as easily as through the body of the boy. Thus, instead of concentrating on the genitals, the little girl's interest in and love for her body remains diffuse and is expressed mostly in pleasurable sensations of the skin and of motor co-ordination. The little girl's preoccupation with the mirror is not imitative; she is curious about her body, and she can look at it and enjoy its reflection. The diffuse narcissistic libido much later becomes directed toward the genital region.

There was, and still is, much discussion in psychoanalytic literature concerning the primary sexual development in woman. Freud's thesis (28) is that the genitals of the girl, except for the clitoris, remain undiscovered and without sensations until puberty; he assumed, therefore, that the first genital (i.e., phallic) response of the girl is curiosity regarding the genitals of the other sex, which she compares with her own. According to this concept, the first genital affect of the girl originates in the realization that she has no penis; the next may be the discovery of the clitoris as a substitute; the comparison results in a sense of inferiority which motivates the intense, biologically determined wish to have a penis. "Penis envy" is the center of the "female castration complex." Karen Horney (34) was the first in the ranks of the psychoanalysts who attacked this concept and pointed out that penis envy can be explained by the instinctually and socially preferred situation of the boy rather than by a biological inferiority of the girl.

The girl's oedipal development is not easy to explain. Her dependent needs satisfied by her mother, what motivates her in turning to her father for libidinal gratification? What mobilizes her heterosexual tendency? According to Freud's hypothesis, the penis envy mobilizes the tendency to incorporate the penis, to hold onto it, to possess it. This concept attributes a primary ambivalent motivation to the heterosexual tendency of the woman.

It seems that in the normal course of the maturational process, the feminine sexual anlage directs the libido toward the male sex. This threatens the girl with an instinctual conflict; her desire for her father's love represents a threat of losing the gratification of her dependent needs by the mother. This accounts for the prolongation of the pre-oedipal phase in the girl. Since she feels guilty because of her oedipal desires, any emotional upheaval in the little girl may be decided in favor of her dependent needs. The trial-and-error sort of fluctuation between heterosexual impulse and dependent needs has a significant role in the further development of sexuality.[4] When a regression to greater dependence occurs, the concurrent, diffuse erotization of the body may sustain the pregenital autoerotic behavior, or the libido may be steered to the genitals, stimulating masturbation and probably new conflicts. Through such repetitive processes, the girl finally develops the oedipus complex. This represents two conflicting instinctual tendencies: (1) the wish to be in the mother's place and to be loved by the father and (2) the wish to be the child and be loved by the mother. The first—the competition with the mother—carries with it the fear of punishment, the fear of losing the mother's love. This may be accepted by the girl as a stop signal, and she may turn back in her development to remain infantile but safe in her dependence. The other outcome of the oedipus complex may be that the girl, to be safe with the mother, strives for identification with the father or with a brother. Such an identification would make her safe against her heterosexual

4. This is usually repeated during adolescence, on another level of maturation.

wishes and would make her lovable to the mother as—she assumes—the father and/or brother are. Such a result of the oedipus complex intensifies the penis envy and, at the same time, fixates the development on an infantile level. The post-oedipal development of the girl continues in one of these two qualitatively different directions. The quantitative differences in the fixations account for the individual differences, namely, that the same process may lead to pathology in character formation in some individuals and to normal character development in others. Differentiation of these two main types is justified not only on the basis of the emotionally significant material but also on the basis of corresponding body-build and the evolving hormonal functions. Yet it would be a mistake to assume that these types are sharply delineated and definitely fixed. "Developmental processes" mean the struggle to overcome the factor which may interfere with an integration of the personality in which all factors are balanced.

The boy's oedipal development is more direct, less hesitating, than that of the girl. Yet the oedipus complex holds the crucial conflict of the male child also. The boy who was encouraged and stimulated to grow through identification with his father feels, at this step in his development, the urge to compete with his father and to take his place with the mother. Although his phallic tendencies cannot be consummated, the boy's sense of guilt for his sexual striving becomes concentrated upon the penis. He expects retaliation to be directed toward the organ from which he receives pleasure. The fear of castration—mutilation—develops, in varying intensity, even if a threat of physical punishment was never uttered. The castration fear impels the repression of the sexual tendencies toward the mother and sets in motion the most significant structuralization of the personality.

Castration fear changes the boy's relationship to his father; it brings out the mutual ambivalence. Even if the father has not been punitive and his attitudes have not intensified the son's hostility, the internal conflict alone is sufficient to bring out the guilty feelings of the boy. He hates and fears the rival father, whom he loves and appreciates as his protector outside the conflict area. Under the pressure of guilty feelings, the boy will tend to intensify his dependence on the father; he will try to please him, and, by identifying with him in other than sexual matters, he tends to idealize his father. As the child imagines that the parents do not exercise sexuality, which they forbid, he introjects an asexual image of the parent, and thus the sexual prohibition becomes internalized. By the strength of the internalized prohibition, the boy attains the capacity to respond to the moral code of the environment, not out of fear of retaliation, but because the parents' prohibition has become a part of his own personality: in this way, the superego is established. This is such an important structuralization within the ego that Freud (21) attributed to it the quality of an inner psychic institution which controls and regulates instinctual impulses. It would be a mistake, however, to assume that the superego is a topically defined entity, functioning from above, mastering the id impulses and policing the ego. The superego represents the sum of those differentiations within the ego which develop through internalization of prohibitive influences. We have discussed one of its earlier manifestations in the adaptation to sphincter control. While the repression of the oedipus complex is a thrust for the stabilization of the superego, it does not represent its final organization. It takes many years through the process of mastery of castration fear and resolution of the oedipus complex before the mature superego becomes an integrated part of the personality.

What are the sexual manifestations of the third pregenital organization, the oedipal phase? Infantile sexuality is essentially autoerotic and is expressed in diffuse manifestations of partial instincts. The oedipal phase represents the first or primary concentration of erotic strivings upon the genitals. Yet the manifestations of this infantile genital organization naturally remain autoerotic, albeit the instinctual need has an "object" outside the self, in the parent of the opposite sex. But the father and/or the mother have "normally" a nonaccepting attitude toward the erotic impulses of the child. The rejection (nonacceptance) of the heterosexual parent, on the one hand, and the fear of the parent of the same sex, on the other, keep the oedipal tendencies of the child in check; the genital tendencies may turn toward substitute objects and are often acted out with siblings and playmates; they also supply the libidinal excitation for genital and substitute masturbation.

Besides the direct manifestation of sexual impulses, there are psychosexual activities, characteristic of this period, which reveal not only the sexual tendencies but also the ego's defenses against them. They indicate the psychodynamic processes by which the oedipus complex is finally repressed and resolved.

1. *Sexual curiosity.*[5]—The desire to gain knowledge about the sexual apparatus and its functioning is an attempt at mastery by intellectualization. In the guise of objective inquiry, the child is allowed partial gratification; in talking about it, the child expresses his sexual tension and conveys it in a limited measure to the parent toward whom it is directed. Since the answers, whether they are objectively informative or evasive, cannot lead to gratification, the child's questioning may become a compulsive preoccupation. Factual information may coexist in the child's mind with sexual theories of his own creation.

2. *Infantile sexual theories.*—Such theories are characteristic attempts at solving the riddle of one or the other aspects of the propagative functions. Usually a child has a "theory" for only one phase of sexual functioning. For example, one child is more preoccupied with the idea that impregnation occurs through the mouth; another with the theory that birth occurs through the anus; etc. Although aware of the genitals and able to perceive sensations from them, the child cannot imagine their functions or accept them emotionally. In his own "sexual theory," the child admits that the body of the adult actively participates in the act of procreation, but he attributes the process to organs the functions of which he has experienced and, in some sense, understands. In his sexual theories the child seems to charge the organs —gastrointestinal tract, mouth, anus—with new libidinal interest at a time when he is about to overcome the libidinal organization centering around them. This fluctuation between the libidinal charges actually helps to *deny* the significance of the genitals.

3. *Denial.*—Denial is an ego defense which represents a step toward the repression of an ego-alien impulse. The child, convinced that "that cannot be which should not be" in his effort to desexualize the parents, tries to believe: "My parents would not do that." And even later, when the child knows about the "facts of life," he may still cling to the idea with a slight modification and often believes that the parents have had intercourse only as many times as they have conceived children. Such denial of the parents' sexuality is the result of the incorporated taboo of sexuality. Measured by such an idealized image of the parent, his own

5. Freud (25, 29) considered sexual curiosity to be the root of all intellectual curiosity, since its instinctual energy can be transferred to other areas of knowledge: if sexual curiosity is inhibited by fear and its energy repressed, intellectual curiosity may also become inhibited.

sexual impulses appear unacceptable to the child; thus they cause guilty feelings and fear of punishment.

The repression of the knowledge about the parents' sexuality is caused not only by the anxiety implicit in the oedipal conflict but even more, or probably primarily, by the discomforting tension which the unintelligible sexual excitation activates in the child. The auditory and visual perception of the parents' sexual intercourse represents the "primal scene."[6] The concomitant sexual excitement of the child and the anxiety aroused by it may represent a trauma of pathological intensity. Its affective charge may be reactivated again and again until it has been slowly mastered through fantasies, through symptom formations, and, finally, through the developmental processes which were set in motion by the oedipal conflict. While it is easy to understand the significance of the primal scene for those who have witnessed it, it is interesting that the psychic elaboration of the parents' sexuality also plays a role in the fantasy life of those children who have never been exposed to this experience. This indicates that, if sexual impulses mobilize the ego's struggle against them, the child draws into the area of sexuality previous experiences of non-genital nature. He may elaborate all sorts of prohibitions as sexual prohibitions, all kinds of tenderness as sexual seductiveness, and all gentleness between the parents as "primal scene." Thus he may sustain fantasies which are necessary for the intra-psychic "working-through" of the oedipal conflict. We may assume, however, that the repression of the sexual impulses and with it the desexualization and idealization of the parents evolve more smoothly if the child is not exposed to overwhelming sexual stimuli. If the child is unable to repress the affects caused by witnessing the primal scene, he is impelled to rationalize his anxiety caused by sexual tension. This leads usually to the following process.

4. *A sadistic concept of sexuality.*—The anxiety-producing idea that sexual intercourse is an extremely brutal activity which endangers the life of a parent (usually the mother) changes the meaning of sexuality. Instead of love, the child attributes to it aggressive tendencies of threatening intensity. This necessarily intensifies the fear of his own sexual impulses. The increased conflict tension often leads to massive inhibition of the sexual

6. Freud referred to this also as "primal fantasy" (24).

impulses, or it may seek solution in identification with the opposite sex.

5. *The identification with the opposite sex.*—Such identification is a defense against intense castration fear and/or wish. The loss of the penis is not inconceivable to the little boy. He is "prepared" for it by previous experiences which he might have interpreted as a loss of a part of his body. Thus impressions, like the loss of the nipple from the mouth, the loss of the feces from the anus, might reinforce the fear of losing the penis (2). The fleeting tumescence of his penis, which comes and goes beyond his control, may be frightening. When the boy discovers the female genital region (his mother's or some little girl's), the danger of losing his penis may be corroborated; he realizes that there are human beings not so endowed. To the boy who, by anlage or by experience (or both), has developed intense castration fear, this discovery may be a traumatic experience. To him the female genitals appear as a devouring organ, which may incorporate his penis and keep it. To avoid this catastrophe, the identification with the dangerous individual appears to be the efficient defense. Through the identification with the mother, the boy develops a "negative oedipus complex": instead of identifying himself with the father in order to have heterosexual feelings toward the mother, he offers himself, so to speak, as a passive love object to the father and wants to replace the mother. Thus the negative oedipus complex diminishes not only the fear of the vagina but the boy's fear of the strong father (who would punish him for his sexual feelings toward the mother). During such a negative oedipal phase, the boy may hate the mother, whom he considers an intruder between him and the father, but he may also regress and intensify his passive dependent attachment to the mother, or he may try to avoid the father, especially if the father is not sympathetic toward the son's passive tendencies. Escape into femininity is not a socially acceptable solution. Soon the passive tendencies are in conflict with the need for self-assertion and masculinity. After new attempts at identification with the father, the normal positive oedipus complex may finally be achieved.

The retarding effect of the identification with the male sex on the girl's oedipal development has been pointed out before (see p. 81). Referring to this, however, we usually do not speak of a negative oedipus complex. When the girl recoils from her heterosexual tendencies and turns to the mother for love, she repeats the pattern of her dependence on the mother. Yet, if the girl's fear of the feminine sexual function becomes intensified by the sadistic concept of sexuality, the resulting "female castration complex" may interfere with the further oedipal and sexual development: the fear of the male (father's penis) impels the intensification of the girl's incorporative tendencies, the goal of which is, in this instance, the *identification with the aggressor*. The little girl's fascination with the penis and the ensuing active curiosity are manifestations of her heterosexual tendency, but its goal is the possession of the penis. Some girls, obsessed by this need, become very aggressive toward little boys in the oedipal age; other girls, more passively, try to imitate the boy's behavior. In all these instances, penis envy, as a defense against the female sexual tendencies, dominates the outcome of the oedipal conflict.

The various phases of the oedipus complex may occur not only in time sequence but also side by side in the same individual. The active heterosexual tendency and the fear of its punishment, as well as traces of identification with the opposite sex, are present in every individual. The psychodynamic significance of these factors and their interaction depend upon the tendency to bisexuality.

Bisexuality is a primary quality of the biological anlage. Its manifestations may be discerned in the variations of the child's tendencies for identification. But it takes the struggle of the oedipal phase to reveal the quantitative differences between masculine and feminine tendencies; between readiness to take the risks of heterosexual development or recoil from it because of the strength of the opposing tendencies. In the *Studies on Hysteria* Freud (15) developed the concept that the unresolved bisexual component of the oedipus complex is responsible for the fixation of libido which tends toward discharge in *conversion hysteria*. Hysteria is generally considered as a neurosis referable to the oedipal conflict, since the psychic energy maintaining its symptoms originates in the unresolved conflicts of that developmental phase.

Since the structuralization of the personality progresses, the conflicts of the oedipal period can be more clearly differentiated than those of the anal period as: (1) instinctual conflicts, arising between the various instinctual tendencies; (2) structural conflicts, arising between the instinctual tendencies and the already introjected prohibitions: superego. The ego—as an organ of adaptation—seems now to have developed far enough to undertake the function of mediation between (1) instinctual needs and their prohibitions (superego), (2) instinctual needs and external reality, and (3) internal (structural) conflict and reality. At this stage of development, the ego can best safeguard its functioning by repressing the sexual tendencies. Freed from the tensions and disturbances caused by immature sexual impulses, the personality is prepared for the next developmental phase: *the latency period.*

In our culture the beginning of the school age (six years) usually, or ideally, coincides with the emerging latency period. The desexualization of the child's interest enables him to comply with environmental requirements and thus to expand in mental and social growth. The latency period is considered, generally, as the age of character formation.

The early psychoanalytic concepts considered character traits as transformations of and reaction formations to the originally libido-charged, instinctual tendencies. Abraham (1), with a brilliant comprehension of psychic connections, ascribed specific character traits to the transformation of specific libido organizations. Thus he described oral, anal, and genital sources of character trends. According to our present concepts, character trends represent well-defined structuralizations within the ego. The previous discussion of developmental processes, such as learning of sphincter control, desexualization and idealization of the parents in establishing the superego, may serve as examples of the differentiation of psychic energies through which the integration of character trends within the personality may take place.

The primary biological tendencies of giving and taking, of retaining and eliminating, appear as habits of the ego function during the latency period. The continuation of the oral receptive pleasure is manifest in the desire to receive material as well as spiritual gifts. The need to receive may express the normal degree of dependence, or it may increase to insatiable demandingness. Some children at this age show a willingness to give and to share, while others are unable to separate themselves from possessions; others again seem always to be afraid of losing something. The tendencies for aggressive incorporation appear in manifestations of envy, jealousy, and maliciousness. The intensity of these emotions may lead to stealing. Stealing at this age does not necessarily indicate a lasting trend toward delinquency. It is considered rather the "acting-out" of an emotional tension resulting from the child's struggle with several concomitant frustrations. After the child has renounced gratification of sexual impulses, he may experience intensification of the receptive-incorporative tendencies. This may cause, for example, an irresistible desire for sweets or to own things which do not belong to him; it may also increase the child's desire to resist the authority of prohibitions set up by adults. Thus stealing, while it satisfies the child's incorporative urge, also expresses his need for self-assertion. Children resort to stealing usually when they feel helplessly abandoned to several inconsistent prohibitions. Stealing is an emergency reaction of the ego; it indicates how narrow the margin is between what we expect as normal and what we call abnormal behavior at this age. The reason for this is in the "brittleness" of the newly formed superego reactions. At first, the internalized prohibition tends to be overrigid and strict. If the frustrations are not relieved or if they are too severe, inhibiting several areas of the personality, the superego may yield, and "acting-out" or other regressions occur.

Even more complex are the character trends related to the anal retentive and eliminative tendencies.[7] The latency period is the age in which the child's attitude toward orderliness appears "characteristic." Some children cannot be taught orderliness; they lose their possessions, scatter them, forget about them. Other children are meticulous. Some children who were orderly before become rebelliously disorderly and unclean during "latency." The dynamics of this reaction is similar to stealing. Restriction in one or many areas of the personality may demand regressive behavior in another area, especially if this area was highly charged in the previous developmental phase. For example, children who were toilet trained early may become quite unclean as far as their general habits are concerned.

The retentive tendency may become manifest in the *passion for collecting* and in the desire to systematize the collection. The cherished objects may change often, since renouncing interest in previously valued objects, discarding them, or forgetting about them have their developmental significance, too. Since the objects have symbolic value, toying with them represents substitution for and/or stimulation of sexual fantasies. It is well known that the difference in the emotional makeup of boys and girls is

7. This enumeration of "character trends" is incomplete and serves only as examples of the organizational processes within the ego.

revealed in the objects they collect. Every age has its characteristic fad. Young boys usually collect stones, pieces of string, keys, mechanical tidbits—objects which represent masculine occupation. Some years later they change to stamps, to work models, to bugs and butterflies, etc. Little girls usually collect boxes, ribbons, and beads, all sorts of materials useful for dolls. When somewhat older, they collect pictures and picture cards, cutouts, and things to "trade with." If boys show interest in the objects usually cherished by girls, or vice versa, this fact is considered a sign of bisexuality. However, the interest may take definite turns. The developmental changes in the psychodynamic tendencies are responsible for the lability of emotional value (object cathexis) represented by the collected material. For some children, possession in itself remains significant even after the collective urge has diminished; for others, the possessions become a means for developing interpersonal relationships. Some children feel the need to "overpay" for friendship; they give away what they value (whether it belongs to them or to someone else) in order to gain prestige and love; others, again, develop skilful acquisitiveness by turning their interest from valued objects to objective values. None of these characteristic attitudes, although they are referable to the primary biological tendencies, can be considered simply as sublimation of, or reaction formation to, any one tendency alone. Any new attainment has to fit into the already established patterns of functioning, in order to safeguard the positive balance within the systems of the personality necessary for undisturbed development. If this cannot be achieved, the arising conflict tension motivates new attempts for solution.

Fantasy is an intra-psychic safety valve which yields relief from tension and at the same time provides intermediary steps in development. Fantasy is a form of primitive thinking which, in contradiction to logical and realistic thinking, permits the wishes and desires—the psychic representations of the instinctual needs— to appear attainable or even fulfilled. The fantasies most crucial for the personality development have been discussed in relation to the oedipus complex. The biological urge which motivates those fantasies is the impulse to grow and become like the parent. But the struggle for the repression of the oedipal fantasies and the "threat" which they imply indicate that identification with the parent in order to be safe must be achieved by small steps. Characteristic of the latency period are fantasies which, either through imagination alone or through games, repeat and channelize the developmental conflicts, paving the way for their resolution. The universal inclination of girls to play with dolls is an example. These games give the girl opportunity to express (1) dependence on the mother: "I love my doll as I want to be loved by Mother"; (2) hostile conflict with the mother: "I treat my doll badly, I hate her, as my mother hates me and treats me badly"; (3) conflict within the self: "I hate my doll because she is like me, a girl," or "I love my doll because she is like me, a girl," or "I love my doll because she is what I can be"; etc. There are innumerable variations of fantasy games played by boys and girls which prepare them for mastering situations and for satisfying their ambitions.

Since it affords autistic gratification, fantasy tends to make the child independent of the environment (in the area of the needs gratified by the imagination). Fantasy yields pleasure and brings consolation for pain. Since it reduces action to endopsychic function, it diminishes the conflict with the environment and thus serves as protection against fear. If the child feels unable to cope with a situation, the protective use of the fantasy may grow out of hand; the rampant imagination may bind an unduly great part of the child's psychic energies and thus interfere with his adjustment to reality. Not all fantasy yields protection. Some fantasies create conflicts with the superego and produce anxiety. One fantasy may even counteract the psychodynamic effect of another. Fantasies may absorb the psychic energy of conflicting tendencies and thus become the focus of developmental disturbance.

The concept of "latency period" implies that, after the psychodynamic tendencies of the oedipus complex have been repressed, the child becomes free from sexual impulses and, protected by his ego defenses, lives in a quasi-asexual environment. He has repressed his need to expose and express erotic tendencies and with it his wish to hear, to see, and to know about sexuality altogether. Yet observations reveal that sexual impulses can easily be stimulated in the child by external as well as by internal experiences, even if an asexual period has been achieved. In a great percentage of children, a complete latency period does not develop at all. Even if the content of the oedipus complex is repressed, the pregenital sexual tendencies, fixated by infantile eroticism, persist and stimulate sexual activities of various extent and significance. Whereas desexualized pregenital tendencies can be integrated in the ego as character trends and mitigated libidinous tendencies can be dealt with in ego-permissible fantasies, sexual impulses of greater intensity cannot be mastered in any way but by discharging them in sexual activity. Sexual behavior and its accompanying fantasies—disturbances of the latency period —often determine the ways and practices by which the individual will attain sexual gratification throughout his life.

The concept of latency period as a biologically determined phase of human development has provoked criticism and has caused a great deal of controversy. Objections are based mainly on anthropological data. Children of many primitive societies do not develop a latency period because the moral code of their environment does not imply sexual prohibitions like those of the Western cultures. Incest is taboo in primitive civilizations, as well as in ours, but the structure of the family organization in most primitive cultures permits a dispersion of the child's psychosexual energies among many persons, without provoking such exclusively significant focus as the father and mother are in the patriarchal family of Western civilization (38). However, individuals of the primitive cultures described in this connection do not develop such differentiation of the psychic apparatus which our superego represents.[8] Superego is the "intra-psychic institution" by which, in our civilization, the family achieves its cultural function and "carries the cultural demands from generation to generation." This educational process is the result of a continuous two-way communication between the child and his parents.

In discussing the developmental processes from early infancy thus far, we have referred repeatedly to the processes of introjection and identification; they represent basic adaptive responses of the child to the parents. We have not mentioned, however, the parents as individuals, as persons with specific wishes and ambitions, with problems of their own personality and experience. Yet the parents in their everyday living express in a way perceivable to the child their expectations and gratifications, the hopes, fears, and frustrations related to their parenthood. Parental behavior is rooted in the personality development of each of the parents; it is modified by the parents' relationship to each other,

8. In comparison with the individualistic superego in our culture, the superego in primitive societies is collective.

and it unfolds toward the child in innumerable manifestations of love, care, tenderness, as well as of impatience, anger, and punitiveness. Through countless processes of mutual identifications and projections, the relationship between the parents and the child forms an intrinsic psychodynamic unity—*the family triangle:* father-mother-child. The culmination of the complex interactions within the family triangle is reached in the superego.

Freud arrived at his concept of the superego and its function for the individual as well as for society by studying individuals reared in patriarchal families. The psychodynamic processes within the family triangle appear to have been simple in the traditional patriarchal family as compared with "individualistic" families. In the patriarchal family, the role of the parents was well defined: the father, strong, infallible, the threatening representative of the moral code; the mother, the main (or only) source of tenderness, herself abiding by the authority of the husband. The parents, supported in their function by religious and secular authority, pursuing their educational goal with unwavering but simple principles, were well suited for idealization and for becoming the core of a strict and prohibitive superego. But even in the patriarchal family the child introjects not only the aims and wishes of his parents but also their inconsistencies and shortcomings.

In our present individualistic civilization the dynamic forces of the family triangle tend to become more involved. The parents, eager to maintain and to emphasize their own individuality in relationship to each other, are inclined to minimize the differences in the role of the father and that of the mother in regard to the child. In the attempt to convey to the child the meaning of his own individuality, they often diminish the distance between themselves and the child. Thus modern individualistic parents renounce, often too early and too much, their rights and responsibilities for guiding the child. By leaving him to his own "decisions," they confuse the child about his powers and his limitations. The ambiguities of such parent-child relationship become even more apparent if the sexual education is too permissive or seductive. Thus, while the child is not compelled to repress his impulses, he is exposed to several internal conflicts without being able to resolve them after a pattern set by the parents. Such parents often interfere with the goal which they are anxious to achieve. Instead of furthering the individualization of the child, they do not afford the conditions in which a stable superego can be established. Too many children incorporate the doubts and conflicts of their parents in such a way that in specific areas of their personalities they do not learn to distinguish right from wrong. Thus a deformed character develops.[9]

Compulsion neurosis is a condition caused by the strictness of the superego. It develops when rebellion and hostility toward authority has to be repressed early and under the pressure of great fear. Indeed, the authoritarian regime of the traditional patriarchal family is conducive to the development of compulsion neurosis. It should not be overlooked, however, that personality development is motivated by too many factors to be pressed into relatively simple equations. It happens often that in families where the father is lenient and "understanding" the children may develop compulsion neurosis. Their superego responds to an unconscious guilt in proportion to the lenience of the father and sets up a rigid internal regulation of behavior.

Generally, the superego is strict and rigid during the latency period as a protection against ego-alien impulses which the father did not sufficiently control. Therefore, children in these years often suffer from compulsive neurotic symptoms. Many of the games are but compulsive activities or magic ceremonies that serve the purpose of overcoming superego demands. If the family triangle is responsible for the development of a superego which encompasses many conflicting tendencies, the intra-psychic struggle may lead to depressive or to delinquent personalities. In the former "autoplastic solution," the punishment is doled out to the self before it can become guilty in action; in the latter "alloplastic solution," the ego—too weak to stand the internal pressure of the conflicts—"acts them out" to invite the punishment of the environment.

The next developmental phase is introduced by the physiological maturation of the sexual apparatus. From the first manifestations of the secondary sex characteristics until the completion of functional maturity, several years pass. The term "puberty" indicates the time of physiological maturation; the term "adolescence" refers to the complex interaction between the physiological and psychological processes involved in the developmen-

---

9. Several studies of the development of delinquency demonstrate such disturbances in the ego development (Szurek, 42; Johnson, 36; Bettelheim and Sylvester, 14; Emch, 17.

tal task of this period. *Adolescence* can be considered as a new chance for the reorganization of the personality. The disquieting manifestations of adolescence cannot be attributed alone to the physiologic upheaval of puberty. Since no developmental phase is entirely overcome and since each new developmental achievement, or its failure, possesses the characteristics derived from the earlier history of the personality, it is to be expected that puberty will bring to the fore the conflicts which were latent. Adolescence, indeed, puts the ego to a hard task; the ego, using the newly upsurging psychosexual energy (which is at the same time a source of uneasiness), must master the old conflicts and integrate them into the functions of the adult personality. It is no wonder that this process, strongly overdetermined by sociological and cultural factors, is circuitous and takes a longer time for reaching its goal than does the physiologic maturation itself.

The early signs of physiologic maturation are noticeable in many instances—in boys and girls alike—as early as the age of nine, but, on the average, the physiologic changes of puberty take place gradually between the ages of ten to fourteen. The psychology of the *prepubertal period* is largely that of the latency period, which, once established, only slowly gives way under the influences of the physiologic growth. Helene Deutsch in her study, *The Psychology of Women* (16), discusses the manifestations of the girl's "last defense" against the oncoming sexual maturation. Shyness and shame because of the growth of the breasts may trouble some girls; others may be concerned about expected menstruation. Normally, these emotions are reactions to the libidinous feelings caused by the physiologic processes and may soon give place to *positive narcissism:* a normal libidinal cathexis of the body. If, however, the *bisexual* tendency is dominant, the onset of feminization of the body may activate anger and hostility toward the self, which may be expressed in various indirect manifestations of self-destructive tendencies, for example, in overeating. In these instances, we may speak of "negative narcissism."

The boys' reaction to physiologic changes of prepuberty are normally free from denial and shyness. Since the center of his body narcissism is the penis, the boy accepts the growth of his genitals and the other signs of the beginning sexual maturation with a sense of gratification and pride. Thus the male puberty is characterized by a more or less free expression of autoeroticism.

Yet (and this is the perplexing problem of male adolescence in our culture) boys go through a complex developmental process which leads from the *early genital phase* to the *final genital phase*. The latter implies, as Abraham (1) stated, that the boy has "attained a point in his object relation where he no longer has an ambivalent attitude toward the genital organ of his heterosexual object, but he recognizes it as a part of that object whom he loves as an entire person."

Not only the male but the female also has to overcome the remnants of the castration complex in order to become able to reconcile with love the existence and function of her own sexual organ and that of the heterosexual love object. In the case of male development, the oedipal phase ended with the desexualization of the mother and the depreciation of sexuality. The rejection and loathing of the female sexual organ is an integrating part of sexual repression; the result of it is the fear of the "castrating" female sexual organ. At puberty, the arising sexual needs again mobilize the earlier castration fear with increased intensity. Psychodynamically similar are the effects of the female castration complex. At the time of puberty, the fear of the (envied) male organ is mobilized again. This recharges the defenses against the male and causes the flight from the feminine sexual role. As the sexual maturation proceeds, the libido tension finally succeeds in overcoming the fear of being hurt, and by this the sexual act becomes possible.

The hormonal function of the maturing sexual apparatus together with other processes of growth produces "surplus energy" (3, 6), which charges the body with a sense of well-being. "Primary narcissism" is the libidinal energy which originates in the positive metabolic balance. The primary narcissistic libido is channelized in activities which satisfy the ego's sexual needs as well as the needs for mastery in nonsexual areas. Through the accomplishments of ego-syntonic and ego-elating activities, the ego becomes charged with a sense of the value of its functioning. "Secondary narcissism" is the term for the libidinal charge of the ego which, originating in the satisfaction with one's self, serves as a defense against disappointments in one's self. The adolescent struggle for intra-psychic equilibrium may be described in terms of exchange between primary and secondary narcissism.

Adolescents, boys and girls alike, when they perceive sexual impulses after the latency period, attempt to master them by repeating the effort which was successful at the oedipal phase: namely, repression. As the struggle against sexuality proceeds, all the available resources of sublimation are mobilized, and expansion of interests and achievements is generated. The fascination for abstract problems, the tendency to project one's subjective problems into the realm of the absolute or into the culturally significant, and other feats of creative imagination can be considered—from one point of view—as ego defenses of the adolescent. Since they afford ego gratification on a high level, they reassure the youth of his individual merit at a time when internal turmoil threatens his equilibrium.

For the repression of the primary narcissism and its sexual manifestations, the youth is rewarded by the augmentation of his secondary narcissism. Yet the ego, even though its power is enhanced by secondary narcissism, cannot withstand for long the pressure of the instinctual impulses; the defenses yield and the instinctual tension is released. Since the span between the ego's aspirations and the sexual impulses is great, however, the sexual gratification is soon followed by remorse. This again reactivates the ascetic attitude and its gratifications, but only to fail and to yield again to the instinctual demands. Thus develops the "polarization of affects" which Anna Freud (19) finds characteristic of adolescence. It is obvious that the effect of the vicious circle between asceticism and indulgence may drive the adolescent farther away from adjustment to reality.

The normal adolescent, however, can hardly enjoy his isolation. His need to withdraw is disturbed by the internal stimulation of the sexual need, as well as by his need to conform with external reality. He is too aware that insecurity is the root of his need for isolation. Hence the shyness, awkwardness, and hypersensitivity lest others will notice what he wants to hide; hence the rebellious pride that he displays in defending his new values, which he has acquired to satisfy a new ego ideal and which he appraises as different from the old one, formed after the father and/or the mother. Thus old, hidden ambivalence conflicts become buoyant and are easily provoked into some sort of discharge by incidents which would seem insignificant at any other time. The defiant, often exasperating, behavior of the adolescent may be considered as a symptom, and, in some instances, it may actually reach a pathological, asocial degree; yet generally it is a manifestation of the resolutions of the original conflict with the parents. Through many repetitions of the rebellious, hostile behavior, the adolescent "fights it out," the boy more with the father, the girl with the mother. The emotional upheavals brought about by such hostile episodes reach deep into the unconscious and lead finally to a shift in the structure of the superego. In "The Passing of the Oedipus Complex" (26) Freud formulated one of his fundamental concepts. There he points out the dynamics of the processes by which, through many repetitions, the ambivalence conflict embodied in the superego finally reaches its resolution. Its aggressive (destructive) energy discharged, the superego loses its rigidity; it becomes more pliable than before, since it is independent of the past (parents).

In interaction with such structural changes in the personality the sexual drive reaches its integration step by step. Usually this process involves the overcoming of the auto- and homoerotic tendencies. Conflicts between these and the heterosexual impulses and between them and the inhibiting factors of the personality motivate the inferiority feelings and induce the moodiness which seems to justify the assumption that adolescents suffer from narcissistic neurosis. Through tribulations and depressions, the adolescent boy relives his early unconscious identification with his mother. The conscious manifestation of this is his conviction that he "understands" women—usually one woman whom he does not need to fear and may therefore begin to love. This phase of adolescence is governed by different dynamics in the girl's development. The bisexuality of the girl is already intensified in prepuberty and may persist with various oscillations for a long time. As the sexual maturation proceeds, the emotional manifestations of the feminine, passive-receptive tendencies diminish the effect of masculine identification and prepare the girl to find a heterosexual love object.

The resolution of the adolescent conflict does not mean merely that the adolescent has achieved the capacity for genital gratification—the male, sexual potency; the female, sexual receptiveness. Heterosexual love is not a function of sexual physiology alone. It is an achievement of the total personality which, through the *adolescent process*, reaches a new level of integration.

No doubt there are many adolescents who do not achieve maturation through the sequence described here. There are many who seem to reach the goal by passing through all phases in a relatively short time; some experience one or more phases only in dreams and fantasies; others may pass through one of the stages quickly and then may be caught in another for a long delay and struggle. In many instances the process seems to repeat itself, for regression may occur after disappointments of any kind. Therefore, many of the experts are inclined to speak of this torturous process as the "normal psychopathology" of adolescence.

The most significant difference from the process described above is presented by those individuals who do not develop a latency period. In their adolescence they do not need to "discover" the genitals of the other sex, since they "knew" of their existence all the time; they do not "learn" to accept the genitals as part of the beloved person because they reverse the process of "falling in love." Instead of expanding the love to include the genitals of the beloved, they transfer their more or less persevering ambivalent interest in the genitals to include the person whom they "love." The reason for this attitude lies in the denial of the castration fear which is a characteristic outcome of the oedipal conflict of these individuals. Since they have not succeeded in repressing the fear of the castrating effect of the female genitals (respectively for girls, the fear of the damaging effect of the male organ), through the sexual practices of a latency period, they try to prove their lack of fear. The sexual curiosity and activity of the latency period is then more a demonstration of lack of fear than a manifestation of emotional need. The adolescent process can only rarely overcome such "habit-forming" fixations; thus sexuality usually remains in these cases, even after physiological maturation, an act of self-assertion and overcompensation. This explains the cynical attitude of such individuals toward the sexual object who is sought out in order to repeat compulsively a fixated sexual pattern. Such persons avoid the painful experiences of adolescent suspense and delay of gratification, but for this "convenience" they pay with a limitation of personality development. The heterosexual affect repressed, there is no drive to set in motion the process through which a new equilibrium of the personality can be achieved. This accounts for the puerile behavior which remains characteristic of such individuals for a lifetime. Measured by the requirement of our culture, these individuals do not achieve the developmental goal.

"Sexual maturity" means that the individual learns to find gratification for his instinctual needs in the framework of his conscience. This includes not only the organization of the ego for acceptance of the sexual drive but also the adjustment of sexual gratification to the requirements of external, sociological realities. This brings about the motivation for further development. As in the earlier phases of development, each new achievement serves as an urge for the next one, so in adolescence the sexual maturation itself supplies the motivation for the next phase, which is achieved in marriage and through parenthood. In simpler societies this goal can be achieved with more safety and probably in shorter time than in ours. Here the individual himself is responsible for the choice of his love object, and sexual activities outside marriage are considered to be against society rather than a part of it; yet, since the economic basis of marriage is difficult to achieve, this often forces the man to postpone marriage. Thus the two aspects of development—sexual and social—often oppose each other and delay or even arrest maturation. In primitive societies and even in the majority of societies with strict patriarchal organization where the society takes care of and assumes the responsibility for the sexual activities of the adolescent, his place in the community is determined by the social order. Thus the co-ordination of the sexual and social aspects of maturation evolves in sequence and reaches its goal— although without that degree of individuation required by our culture—with fewer remissions and with less delay.

The maturation of the sexual function and the development of the personality are, indeed, intricately interwoven. The integration of the *sexual drive* from its pregenital sources to the *genital primacy* and to functional maturity is the axis around which the organization of the personality takes place. From the point of view of personality development, the process of interaction is the same in both sexes. Men and women alike reach their psychosexual maturity through the reconciliation of the sexual drive with the superego and through the adjustment of sexuality to all other functions of the personality. Regarding the integration of the sexual drive from the point of view of its goal—procreation— the difference between the sexes is obvious. *The sexual drive is organized differently in man and in woman, in order to serve specific functions in procreation.*

The woman's life, more markedly than the man's, is divided into periods defined by her reproductive function. "Menarche," the first menstruation, definitely indicates her puberty. Menstruation is frequently considered a traumatic event in the girl's life, since it represents an offense against the integrity of the body. Yet the anticipation of menstruation, as well as the conscious response to it, are influenced by cultural factors. In our present civilization, education and hygiene prepare the girl for menstruation in a sympathetic way and diminish her manifest rebellion against it. But the bleeding and discomfort, which often may increase to the point of pain, may stir up her latent anxiety. These sensations impel her to realize that women have to adapt themselves to sexuality, not only to its pleasurable function, but also to its discomfort.

The female sexual functions are under highly complicated hormonal controls which result in the cyclic functioning of the ovaries. The ovary has the dual function of forming the female sex cells—the ova—and of producing two kinds of hormones: (1) the estrogen, produced by the ripening follicle, and (2) the progestin, which prepares the uterus for the nidation of the fertilized ovum. From menarche to menopause, in cyclic intervals, the woman prepares for conception which, if it fails to occur, is followed by menstruation, after which the new cycle promptly begins.

The periodicity of the gonadal functions and their influence upon the behavior related to reproduction are well established in mammals. In the human the direct manifestations of the sexual drive are modified by the developmental processes which establish patterns of sexual expression and conditions for its gratification. In spite of this—in a series of investigations in which the state of the ovarian function was determined by vaginal smears and the course of affect-manifestations was followed by psychoanalytic observations, it was found that the emotional manifestations of the sexual drive, like the reproductive function itself, are under hormonal influence and, therefore, in correlation with the gonadal cycle—an emotional cycle evolves (13). The term "sexual cycle" includes both the hormonal and the emotional aspects of the process.

To summarize: the sexual cycle begins with the ripening of the follicle. The estrogen secreted by the follicle mobilizes the manifestations of active, heterosexual tendencies; these are expressed by conscious or by disguised heterosexual desires and by increased alertness in all kinds of extroverted activities. Parallel with the increasing estrogen production, the heterosexual need increases[10] and reaches its height at the time of *ovulation*. About the time of ovulation, the hormonal state is that of maximum estrogen and of incipient progestin production. The emotional state of the woman accords with the biological readiness for conception; her body flooded with libidinous feelings, she is receptive to her sexual partner. After ovulation, the direction of the sexual drive appears to change; the libido is turned toward her person, especially toward its gratifying, pleasurable care. In correlation with the increasing progestin production, the passive-receptive and retentive tendencies motivate the emotions which are expressed in wishes and desires concerning pregnancy and the love and care for a child—or in the defenses against pregnancy and in conflicts about childbearing and child care. If conception does not occur, the hormone production declines, and the woman's emotional reactions reveal her inner perception of the "moderate degree of ovarian deficiency" (35) which the premenstrual-menstrual phase represents. Her behavior often changes; the woman feels and acts less composed; she is more irritable and aggressive, or more dependent and moody than she was at the height of the same cycle. Generally, the woman reaches the most complete psychosexual integration of which she is capable at the height of the hormonal cycle. In correlation with the decline of the hormone production, the psychosexual integration regresses from the genital level to the pregenital, anal-sadistic and/or the oral-dependent level. The analysis of the sexual cycle reveals that, corresponding to the gonadal cycle, the emotional cycle represents a condensed repetition of the processes of the psychosexual integration of the woman's personality development.

The study of the sexual cycle permits significant conclusions in regard to the basic organization of the female sexual drive and its psychic representations. Helene Deutsch in her extensive study, *Psychology of Women* (16), on the basis of general psychoanalytic observation, came to the conclusion that a deep passivity and a specific tendency toward introversion are char-

10. In evaluating the intensity of the heterosexual need, one has to consider the changes in affects occurring with gratification or from frustration; in the same way, one has to consider the variety and affect-content of the defenses in order to use them as indicators for the hormone production.

acteristic qualities of the female psyche. The study of the sexual cycle confirms this assumption, since it demonstrates that these propensities of the female psyche are repeated in cylic intervals in correspondence with the dominance of the specifically female gonadal hormone, progestin, the function of which is to prepare for and help maintain pregnancy. On this basis, we assume that the emotional manifestations of the specific passive-receptive and narcissistic retentive tendencies represent the psychodynamic correlates of the biological need for motherhood.

The psychology of pregnancy belongs to the scope of this presentation only as it indicates the role which childbearing plays in the evolution of the woman's personality. The psychodynamic processes accompanying pregnancy can easily be understood in the light of the progestin phase of the sexual cycle. As the woman, through the monthly repetition of the physiologic processes, prepares somatically for pregnancy, so does the corresponding emotional state prepare her for that introversion of psychic energies which motivates the emotional attitudes during pregnancy. The enhanced hormonal and general metabolic processes necessary to maintain normal pregnancy intensify the receptive tendencies of the woman. Whether they are expressed orally in overeating and/or in a general increase of the receptive dependent needs, they are manifestations of the biological process of growth which they serve. The "surplus energy" produced by the active metabolic balance replenishes the reservoir of primary narcissistic libido which is concentrated on the self, on the pregnancy and its content, the child-to-be. Thus the psychic energy which supplies the placid, vegetative calmness and well-being of the pregnant woman becomes the source of her motherliness. Her general behavior during pregnancy may appear withdrawn and regressive in comparison with her usual level of ego integration; yet the condition which seems to indicate regression of the ego actually represents a growth of the integrative span of the personality on a biological level: motherhood encompasses the child in the psychodynamic processes of the woman.

The trauma of birth interrupts the symbiosis of pregnancy, leaving the mother with a varying degree of physiological and emotional readiness for the complex, emotionally charged functions of motherhood. After parturition, the organism of the mother is preparing for the next function of motherhood—lactation. The hormonal control, related to the production of prolactin, stimulates milk secretion and, with it, usually suppresses the gonadal production. Thus it induces an emotional attitude which is similar to the progestin phase of the sexual cycle. The trend toward motherliness in now, as then, expressed, actively or passively, by receptive tendencies. During lactation, both the active (giving) and the passive receptive tendencies gain in intensity; they become the axis around which the activities of motherliness center. The mother's desire to nurse the baby, to be in close bodily contact with it, represents the continuation of the symbiosis, not only for the infant, but for the mother as well (12). While the infant incorporates the breast, the mother feels united with her baby. The identification with the baby permits the mother to enjoy her "regression" and to repeat and satisfy her own receptive, dependent needs. The emotional experience of lactation and of the sundry activities of nursing care, through the processes of mutual identification, lead step by step to the integration of motherliness.

Motherhood, through the libidinally charged processes of pregnancy and motherliness, sets in motion a reorganization in the mother's personality. To be a good mother and love the child —to be able to respond to the child's needs in the most constructive manner—is the ego ideal of every normal mother; if she fails, she feels punished by the child as much as, or even more than, she ever felt punished by her parents. Thus the child, through his unceasing needs, becomes a strict superego of the conscientious mother. As the child becomes older, the mother's identification with him becomes more complex. While the mother consciously strives to make the child's needs and goals a part of her own ego aspirations, unconsciously she may project onto him her own expectations, hopes, and frustrations. One mother may burden the child with the hope that he will satisfy her aspirations; another may reject the child because of her own frustrations, assuming that her child, being like herself, cannot or will not be able to undo her own failures. Thus the mother, reliving with her child, and with each child in an individually significant way, those emotional experiences which determined her own development, is a conveyor of the past and a participant in the future at the same time.

Motherhood, indeed, plays a significant role in the woman's personality. Physiologically, it completes maturation; psychologically, it channelizes motherliness. The specific qualities of

motherliness originate in the primarily introverted narcissistic
tendencies; their sublimated expression becomes a part of the
woman's personality even if physiological motherhood does not
replenish its primary sources. Sympathy, responsiveness, the desire to care for others, and other sublimated manifestations of
motherliness develop in every woman through similar, if not
such intensive, processes of empathy and identification which
govern the mother's feeling toward her children. Thus motherliness, in its sublimated manifestations, widens the span of the
personality.

The organization of the sexual drive in the male is simpler
than in the female. The propagative function of the male, under
the control of one group of gonadal hormones—androgens—is
discharged in a single act. There seems to be a coincidence between gonadal hormone production and the urgency of the
sexual impulses. However, there is no regularly returning cycle
of recessions and reintegrations of the psychosexual pattern directly comparable with the sexual cycle in women. Men are not
prepared for parenthood by cyclical repetitions of emotional
expressions originating in the reproductive need. Yet there are
emotional, originally instinctual, trends which, together with
cultural trends, complement those which find expression in
motherhood.

Under conditions which impede the reproductive function,
such as sterility of either of the marital partners, or enforced
separation, such as occurs during war, man's instinct for survival
in his offspring becomes accessible to study. If man's survival is
threatened—directly, as in war, or symbolically in the many
ways which may destroy his self-esteem—his anxiety activates
dependent needs. But, in the process of growing up, man's dependent needs have fused with the aspirations of his virility. In
gratifying his sexual need, man reassures himself of his virility,
especially in the hope that he may create a representation of
himself in his child. The analysis of such cases reveals that the
instinct of propagation is but a special form of the instinct of
self-preservation in adults. The psychology of fatherhood can
best be understood as the manifestation of two tendencies of
man's biological urge for growth. One is the urge to conquer
his own dependent needs through heterosexual love and the other
is to fulfil his desire to become like his father or even to surpass
him. These ambitions take many turns during his development,

until they triumph when he himself becomes a father: his self survives as once his father did, in his child. In man, as well as in woman, the instinctual need for parenthood originates in the narcissistic reservoir of "surplus energy." When this is discharged in the germ cells, it surpasses the boundaries of the self and creates a continuation of the self.

Since the father's biological function is completed in one act, the psychodynamic processes of fatherhood are strongly influenced by cultural requirements. In societies where the organization of the family affords the development of a family triangle, the adaptation to fatherhood is psychodynamically similar to that of motherhood. The father, like the mother, tends to identify himself with his child; he, too, repeats unconsciously through identifications and projections the steps of his own aspirations and hopes, in order to achieve completion through the child. While fatherhood channelizes man's narcissism, it also puts harsh requirements upon him and acts as would a severe and relentless superego. The responsibilities to which the father is pledged by our society become the axis around which the organization of his further development takes place.

The mother normally achieves identification with her infant through libidinally charged processes which permit her to become a child with her child again. This is not so for the father. He is impelled to renounce and repress his receptive dependent needs when they arise—as they may—in identification with his offspring. He has to become the provider. Alexander (5) has discussed the psychodynamics of this complex developmental task which requires that the man, who once needed a mother for the gratification of his dependent needs, should become the father-provider for his wife and children. Although men are prepared by previous identifications with their own fathers for the task which is taken for granted in our culture, they may often fail, or they may pay for fulfilment with various types of mental or psychosomatic suffering. Overcompensation of their dependent needs in demanding, domineering, or even despotic behavior is one, regression to direct gratification of oral needs in overeating and alcoholism is another, expression of the repressed passive-dependent needs. More complex and more disguised psychosomatic symptoms may ensue if the father overdraws his libidinal resources in the effort of being a provider.

Against the restrictions and renunciations of id gratifications on the other side of the ledger, adult man has his gratifications in and through his work. From childhood, achievement, in whatever form and level it occurs, is absorbed in the personality, enlarging its span. Mastery, through its affective gratifications of secondary narcissism, delineates the psychodynamic role which work plays in the emotional household of men in our civilization. In youth the instinctual needs are more compelling; in adulthood, especially after the father has incorporated the gratifications and restrictions which his family represents, work and its satisfactions gain emphasis in the psychodynamic processes. Fortunate is the man whose primary emotional gratifications keep balance with the spending of psychic and physical energies in work. Even the gratifications of secondary narcissism may become a steady drain upon the psychic resources, leaving but little libido for primary emotional gratification. Such a process may lead to rigidity of the ego and finally exhaust the adaptive capacity of the individual. Since work, through sublimation as well as by its material gratification, plays an integrative part in the expansion of man's personality, the renunciation of work often represents a trauma; it necessitates a readjustment of the total emotional economy. If the individual can look back upon a successful career and can give up work by his own decision, the adjustment may be smooth, although it is not always so. If, on account of social and economic circumstances or because of age and disability, the man is compelled to give up work, his ego may collapse. New attempts at success or his sense of guilt because of his failure may exhaust his psychic resources. The mental health of the adult male is best guaranteed by a smoothly functioning interchange between primary libidinal gratifications (provided by his interpersonal relationships within his family and community) and the satisfactions of his secondary narcissism, which he achieves by work.

The decline of the reproductive period in man and woman approaches slowly. Normally, it evolves as a process of maturation through continuous adaptation to the internal and external requirements of living. The term "climacterium" is often applied to the period of abating reproductive function in both sexes. Climacterium, however, according to the different organization of the reproductive function, is a dynamically different process in man and woman.

The woman experiences fluctuations in gonadal hormones

from puberty on; her organism adapts itself to the psychosomatic reactions which accompany the monthly hormonal decline. Thus, when the gonadal stimulation definitely subsides, the healthy woman's emotional economy is not severely harmed by the loss of hormonal stimulation. The integration of the personality once established, the woman appears independent of gonadal stimulation for maintaining the sublimations of the reproductive period.

Many women suffer from neurotic, psychotic, or psychosomatic manifestations which, because they occur about or after the menopause, are usually attributed to the stresses of climacterium. The psychoanalytic study of such cases reveals that the symptoms, which appear aggravated during this period, have already existed before. Even if they were not manifest, they have been pre-formed under the influence of the precarious balance of the personality. Those women who were unable to adapt to the premenstrual hormone decline and suffered from premenstrual depressions and/or dysmenorrhea usually suffer again from the vegetative discomforts of the climacterium. The study of the personality structure and life-experience of women who manifest severe emotional disturbances at climacterium reveals that in these cases (1) the bisexual component played a dominant and obviously disturbing role; (2) the psychic economy was dominated by the strivings of secondary narcissism rather than by primary emotional gratification of motherliness.

Climacterium is different for those women whose psychic economy has not been exhausted by previous neurotic conflicts. When menopause indicates the cessation of the propagative functions, these women often respond to the desexualization of their emotional needs with an influx of extroverted energy; their still flexible personalities seek and find new aims for psychic energy. As in early childhood, when repression of the sexual impulses led to superego formation and socialization, so in climacterium the cessation of the reproductive function releases a new impetus for socialization and learning. The manifold interests and productivities of women after the climacterium, as well as their improvement in general physical and emotional health, serve as evidence that woman's climacterium may be regarded in a psychological sense as a "developmental phase" (10).

In man the reproductive period lasts longer than in woman; his procreative capacity is expected to last as long as orgastic potency remains. Both the sexual urge and the reproductive capacity may be rekindled, even if they appear to be extinguished. Thus man has no definitely marked cessation of his reproductive capacities, which would justify the concept of a "male climacterium" on the basis of hormonal physiology alone. Such a concept, however, has a broader biosociological implication.

Men in our society respond sensitively to the signs of aging, and they may relate any functional decline to it, for aging is considered a menace, which they watchfully expect and detect in the oscillations of sexual potency, in work or sport achievements, in general health. Aging is a source of insecurity for the modern man. In patriarchal society the social significance of old age was different. Whatever the oscillations of his sexual potency were, man did not need to feel threatened, since marriages were stable and, socially, the man's prestige increased rather than decreased with age. In our culture, men are not protected by such tradition. They feel compelled to compensate for their lessening capacity by increasing competitive productivity. While this may enhance man's self-reliance, it may increase his intrapsychic tension: success and mastery dominate his activity at the cost of primary emotional gratification. Slowly or suddenly, as, for example, in a traumatic failure in sexual potency, the aging man's psychosexual economy becomes similar to that of the adolescent. Just as in adolescence, sexual potency and mastery in achievement have acted as opponents, now again the insecurity in regard to sexual potency enhances the narcissistic significance of each sexual act and every other activity as well. Thus the "polarization of affects" may be repeated. Any failure may appear as an irreparable damage to the personality and may activate the ever latent castration fear; this mobilizes the specific conflicts of the individual, and these, in turn, may determine the specific symptoms which, occurring at this age, make the assumption of "male climacterium" justifiable. However, "male climacterium" is motivated mainly by the multiple psychosomatic effects of man's struggle in a competitive society. If the adaptive task which men have to meet is not motivated by factors other than that of the physiology of the declining sexual function, "climacterium" does not develop, for man's aging is a continuous, not a pathological, process.

Chronological age has a different significance for the individual as well as for his community, depending upon many cultural factors. It is common knowledge that, in spite of its stresses and discomforts, civilization has extended man's life-expectancy. Even more significant is it that modern man can look forward to a much longer period of productive enjoyment in life than the average man ever could before.

The psychodynamic process of growing old is characterized by a change in the vector of the psychic and somatic processes. The giving, expansive attitudes, needed for the functions of the reproductive period, slowly become outweighed by the retentive, self-centered tendencies characteristic of old age. Since the redistribution of the vital resources induces an introversion (retention) of psychic energy, both men and women obtain manifold gratifications of a narcissistic nature. Whether the aged individual applies what he has learned in a lifetime and surveys his world in broad philosophical concepts or just cares for the grandchildren, the pleasure which "warms his heart" is the gratification of being able to think, to do, to feel, to be aware of the self in special activity and achievement. There is no doubt about the enhanced narcissism of the old, which, since it cannot draw on the resources of newly produced surplus energy, enlarges the gains of their available resources by identification with the young and by rekindling the memories of past achievement and gratification.

In the obviously self-centered phase of senescence, the receptive dependent needs dominate the aged individual's relationship to his environment, often causing great irritation in the younger generation, who complain about the egotism of the old. The gratification of the dependent needs, however, serves more than the mere maintenance of life. In old people as in children, the gratifications of the dependent needs are taken for manifestations of love; being loved increases the sense of security and enhances the value of the personality. The senescent individual, aware of the failing of his own capacities, becomes hypersensitive in regard to the fulfilment of his dependent needs, which are often expressed as a need for prestige and recognition. While the old person is dissatisfied with himself, he demands from those who love him the impossible, namely, that they shall make him unaware of his weakness. Thus the regression within the personality structure of the senescent often manifests itself in a paranoid conflict with the environment.

As the exhaustion of the vital energies proceeds, the restriction of the emotional household becomes more and more manifest. Expenditure has been limited long before; at that late stage, also, the receptive needs diminish because abundance can no longer be enjoyed. When life has no more strength than to maintain itself at a low metabolic rate, mental functioning is reduced to a minimum, and one can no longer speak of the structuralization of the personality.

In this chapter, we have discussed the processes through which biological and cultural forces become organized and form the personality. "Personality" is the capacity of the total organism to function as a whole—a unique, discernible self, distinguished from other members of the species and from other members of the same social group. In the most general psychodynamic terms, one may define personality as the product of the various ways of dealing with psychic tensions which, in turn, produce recognizable trends and predictable behavior. Personality is a continuous function, resulting from infinite interactions between the individual and his society. "Emotional maturity" is a term often used to describe a personality which has fully developed its potentiality for reconciling internal, instinctual needs with the external requirements of society. "Emotional maturity" in this sense does not mean a consciously applied philosophy; it indicates rather an unconsciously functioning psychic economy which operates with a positive balance. This implies that the organization of the personality allows for an easy mobilization of psychic energies whenever a new adaptive task requires it. Thus emotional maturity is a relative concept. It can be evaluated only in reference to the question: "Mature—for what?"

The key to the understanding of all pathological processes is the evaluation of the adaptive task in respect to the total psychic economy. Preventive psychiatry has as its purpose the diminution of the gap between the requirements of the adaptive task and the individual's capacity to master it. This aim, however, is beyond the scope of any single discipline. When all cultural and economic forces of a society bend their efforts together in behalf of the individual, then we may secure that stability and security which will reduce the risks involved in the complete individuation of the personality.

BIBLIOGRAPHY

1. ABRAHAM, K. *Selected Papers* (London: Hogarth Press, 1927).
2. ALEXANDER, F. "Concerning the Genesis of the Castration Complex," *Psychoanalyt. Rev.*, 22:49, 1935.
3. ALEXANDER, F. *Fundamentals of Psychoanalysis* (New York: W. W. Norton & Co., Inc., 1948).
4. ALEXANDER, F. "The Logic of Emotions and Its Dynamic Background," *Internat. J. Psycho-Analysis*, 16:406, 1935.
5. ALEXANDER, F. "A Note on Falstaff," *Psychoanalyt. Quart.*, 2:592, 1933.
6. ALEXANDER, F. *Our Age of Unreason* (rev. ed.; Philadelphia: J. B. Lippincott Co., 1951).
7. ALEXANDER, F. *Psychosomatic Medicine* (New York: W. W. Norton & Co., Inc., 1950).
8. ALEXANDER, F. "The Relation of Structural and Instinctual Conflicts," *Psychoanalyt. Quart.*, 2:181, 1933.
9. BENEDEK, THERESE. "Adaptation to Reality in Early Infancy," *Psychoanalyt. Quart.*, 7:200, 1938.
10. BENEDEK, THERESE. "Climacterium: A Developmental Phase," *Psychoanalyt. Quart.*, 19:1, 1950.
11. BENEDEK, THERESE. *Insight and Personality Adjustment* (New York: Ronald Press Co., 1946).
12. BENEDEK, THERESE. "The Psychosomatic Implications of the Primary Unit: Mother-Child," *Am. J. Orthopsychiat.*, 19:642, 1949.
13. BENEDEK, THERESE, and RUBENSTEIN, B. B. *Psychosexual Functions in Women* (New York: Ronald Press Co., 1952).
14. BETTELHEIM, B., and SYLVESTER, E. "Delinquency and Morality," in *The Psychoanalytic Study of the Child*, Vol. 5 (New York: International Universities Press, 1950).
15. BREUER, J., and FREUD, S. *Studies in Hysteria* (New York: Nervous and Mental Disease Publishing Co., 1936).
16. DEUTSCH, H. *The Psychology of Women*, Vols. 1 and 2 (New York: Grune & Stratton, 1944–45).
17. EMCH, MINNA. "On 'the Need To Know' as Related to Identification and Acting Out," *Internat. J. Psycho-Analysis*, 25:14, 1944.
18. FENICHEL, O. "Frühe Entwicklungsstadien des Ichs," *Imago*, 23:243, 1937.
19. FREUD, A. *The Ego and the Mechanisms of Defence* (London: Hogarth Press, 1937).
20. FREUD, S. *Collected Papers*, Vols. 1–5 (London: Hogarth Press, 1924–50).
21. FREUD, S. *The Ego and the Id* (London: Hogarth Press, 1927).
22. FREUD, S. "Female Sexuality," *Internat. J. Psycho-Analysis*, 13:281, 1932.
23. FREUD, S. "Formulations Regarding the Two Principles in Mental Functioning," in *Collected Papers*, 4 (London: Hogarth Press, 1925), 13.

24. Freud, S. *A General Introduction to Psychoanalysis* (New York: Boni & Liveright, 1920).
25. Freud, S. *Leonardo da Vinci: A Study in Psychosexuality* (New York: Random House, 1947).
26. Freud, S. "The Passing of the Oedipus Complex," in *Collected Papers*, Vol. 2 (London: Hogarth Press, 1924).
27. Freud, S. "The Predisposition to 'Obsessional Neurosis,' " in *Collected Papers*, 2 (London: Hogarth Press, 1924), 122.
28. Freud, S. "The Psychology of Women," in *New Introductory Lectures on Psycho-Analysis* (New York: W. W. Norton & Co., 1933).
29. Freud, S. *Three Contributions to the Theory of Sex* (New York: Nervous and Mental Disease Publishing Co., 1930).
30. Gesell, A., et al. *The First Five Years of Life* (New York: Harper & Bros., 1940).
31. Hartmann, H., and Kris, E. "The Genetic Approach in Psychoanalysis," in *The Psychoanalytic Study of the Child*, 1 (New York: International Universities Press, 1945), 11–30.
32. Hartmann, H.; Kris, E.; and Loewenstein, R. M. "Comments on the Formation of Psychic Structure," in *The Psychoanalytic Study of the Child*, 2 (New York: International Universities Press, 1947), 11–37.
33. Hartnik, Jeno. "The Various Developments Undergone by Narcissism in Men and Women," *Internat. J. Psycho-Analysis*, 5:66, 1924.
34. Horney, K. "On the Genesis of the Castration Complex in Women," *Internat. J. Psycho-Analysis*, 5:59, 1924.
35. Hoskins, R. G. *Endocrinology* (New York: W. W. Norton & Co., 1941).
36. Johnson, A. M. "Sanctions for Superego Lacunae of Adolescents," in *Searchlights on Delinquency* (New York: International Universities Press, 1949), p. 225.
37. Jones, E. "Urethralerotik und Ehrgeiz," *Internat. Ztsch. f. Psychoanal.*, 3:156, 1915.
38. Mead, M. *From the South Seas* (New York: Wm. Morrow & Co., 1939).
39. Rado, S. "The Problem of Melancholia," *Internat. J. Psycho-Analysis*, 9:4:20, 1928.
40. Reich, W. *Character-Analysis* (3d enl. ed.; New York: Orgone Institute Press, 1949).
41. Spitz, R. "Hospitalism: An Inquiry into the Genesis of Psychiatric Conditions in Early Childhood," in *The Psychoanalytic Study of the Child*, 1 (New York: International Universities Press, 1945), 53–74.
42. Szurek, S. "Notes on the Genesis of Psychopathic Personality Trends," *Psychiatry*, 5:1, 1942.

# PART II
# CLINICAL PSYCHIATRY

# V

## NEUROSES, BEHAVIOR DISORDERS, AND PERVERSIONS

### FRANZ ALEXANDER, M.D., AND LOUIS B. SHAPIRO, M.D.

#### NEUROSIS DEFINED

FREUD defined neurotic symptoms as substitute gratifications in fantasy for co-ordinated action, adequate to satisfy impelling subjective needs. Because fantasy gratification can never completely relieve the pressure of unsatisfied needs, neurosis is always connected with frustration. Neurosis is, then, an inadequate, unsuccessful attempt to restore the emotional equilibrium disturbed by the presence of unsatisfied or poorly satisfied subjective urges.

The adequate satisfaction of subjective needs is the function of the ego. Every neurosis can be understood in final analysis as a disturbance of ego functions. In this respect, neurosis can be compared with any other disease. Disease is a result of inadequate functioning of an organ system. In the case of neurosis, the failing organ is the co-ordinating center; it fails in its biological task of gratifying subjective needs in harmonious co-ordination with one another and in congruity with existing external conditions upon which the gratification of the subjective needs depends.

Any or all of the four fundamental functions of the ego may be disturbed: (1) internal perception of subjective needs, (2) correct external appraisal of the environmental situation, (3) integration of the data of internal and external perception with each other, and (4) the executive function based on the ego's control over voluntary behavior (see chap. iii). In most neuroses all four functions are to some degree disturbed. For example, in hysteria, the internal perception is primarily disturbed by repression, whereas in behavior disorders chiefly the executive function of the ego is impaired.

As discussed before (chap. iv), the ego acquires its functional efficiency during postnatal development by a gradual learning process. The first requirement for integrated and goal-directed behavior is an adequate capacity for controlling one's impulses, a capacity which is only gradually acquired. The child's capacity for conscious control—renunciation or postponement of impulses —is weak; and, in order to maintain the integrity of the ego, he can only resort to the process of excluding from consciousness all impulses that the ego cannot control and harmonize, those impulses which would otherwise give rise to anxiety, guilt, and shame. This process is called "repression." Repressed impulses represent quantities of energy which have either to be held constantly in check or to be drained off in some other manner not threatening to the ego. Many of the psychodynamic phenomena in the field of psychopathology (chap. i) are auxiliary methods which support repression or represent substitutive vents for repressed psychological forces.

Repression is essentially denial. In a sense the ego denies the existence of an internal impulse or an external event that might lead to a painful consequence. Ideas—the carriers of instinctual strivings—must become conscious in order to gain motor expression. In repression the ego excludes from consciousness any pain-producing idea or impulse by refusing it entrance to its domain. Repressed impulses are therefore not permitted any modification through the learning process. The more the infantile ego has to make use of the drastic measure of repression, the less it can fulfil its function of gratification of the subjective needs by modifying them and adapting them to one another and to external conditions. Excessive repression has a twofold result: (1) the ego's supply of energy will be impoverished, since the dynamic forces over which the ego rules are excluded from its territory; (2) a great deal of the ego's energy will have to be utilized for defense against the pressure of repressed tendencies. Having once repressed an objectionable impulse, the ego's task is not finished. Energy is constantly required to maintain the repression. This may be manifested clinically in the neurotic's complaint of fatigue and lack of energy adequate to meet the daily problems of living. In many cases the ego's task of dealing with a dangerous or unpleasant impulse by repression proves to be unsuccessful, and the ego is therefore forced to take recourse to auxiliary defenses.

Although neurotic symptoms represent inadequate gratification, still they contain a component of gratification which they both seek and deny. This is the basis of the "neurotic conflict." This conflict, which exists in the mind and yet is unknown to the person, is a struggle between two sides of the total personality. It can be demonstrated when one attempts to cure a patient of his symptoms. When the therapist applies the analytic technique of unraveling the symptom, the patient unknowingly and unwittingly opposes this effort with strong resistance. This becomes apparent when the therapist is about to make conscious to the patient some unconscious material related to the symptom and at the same time particularly painful to the patient. It becomes obvious that the patient prefers to retain his unwelcome symptom rather than to become conscious of the particularly painful association. The symptom is a substitute for the latter, which remains in the unconscious. This struggle of the patient to obtain relief from his symptoms and yet to avoid making conscious the unconscious processes underlying his symptoms is the core of every neurosis. All symptoms can be understood as results of the conflict between repressed and repressing forces.

Neurotic disturbances can be classified according to the type of defenses which the ego employs or according to the nature of the repressed impulses. In the actual clinical classification of neuroses, as a rule, a combination of both criteria is utilized. Freud suggested that there may be an intimate connection between special forms of defense and a particular neurosis, as, for example, between repression and hysteria. He also called attention to the relation between aggressive and sadistic impulses and reaction formations in the ego, such as overcleanliness, exaggerated scrupulousness, meticulousness, and defensive techniques employed in obsessional neurosis. Helene Deutsch (2) has noted that possibly each defense mechanism arises at first to master some special instinctual impulse during infantile development. Anna Freud (3) has suggested that repression is used against sexual impulses, while other mechanisms are employed against aggressive impulses.

The fact that repression is generally the chief technique used by the ego in hysteria is probably due to the attitude in our culture toward sexual impulses. Adults often behave as though sex were nonexistent. In hysteria we see the same attitude adopted; that is, the unacceptable impulse is viewed as if it simply did not exist. In other words, the cultural attitude toward the instinctual impulses supplies the tool that the ego uses in dealing with sexual impulses. Aggressive impulses, on the other hand, although acknowledged as existing, are stamped by our culture as bad, and the ego is called upon to exercise various techniques, such as "overcompensation" or "undoing," to counteract this force. This explains the presence of overcompensatory techniques in those neurotic pictures characterized by aggressive instinctual drives, as, for example, in obsessive-compulsive neurosis.

Neurotic disturbances can be divided into two large categories —chronic and acute. Emotions of excessive intensity, such as anxiety, rage, and frustration, may temporarily impair both the integrative and the executive functions of the ego. Anxiety, if excessive, may have a paralyzing influence. The same is true for rage. An enraged person is likely to concentrate on one single aim—that of vengeance—and leave out of consideration everything else. In all excessive emotional states the primary objective of the organism is to find immediate relief from the tension. This urgency interferes with a comprehensive handling of all external and internal factors.

Common examples of acute neuroses are the so-called "traumatic neuroses" (see chap. vi). In the traumatic situation the ego is incapable of carrying out its co-ordinating and adaptive functions. This failure may precipitate not only a regressive evasion of the traumatic situation but also a strong regressive movement toward a more dependent, helpless state of infancy. Loss of consciousness, of the faculty of locomotion or of speech, or of the co-ordinated use of the extremities may be the result. Acute conditions may easily develop into chronic neurotic states, and therefore it is important that acute conditions should be treated early. In the early phases supportive measures frequently suffice to prevent the development of chronic neurotic states as a result of an acute neurosis. The emotional support may serve as encouragement for the ego to make new attempts to regain its mastery, which was only temporarily disturbed under the influence of the excessive stimulation of the trauma.

The chronic failures of the ego functions usually can be traced back to disturbed interpersonal relationships in childhood. Sometimes traumatic interpersonal relationships are of later origin. Accordingly, there is a continuum between acute, subacute, and chronic states. In the development of a chronic neurosis the following phases in general can be distinguished:

1. Circumstances that precipitate the actual situation with which the patient cannot cope.

2. Failure in solution of the actual problem after some unsuccessful attempts.

3. Replacement of realistic adaptive measures by regressive fantasies or behavior.

4. Reactivation of the old conflicts which in the past induced the ego to give up the old adaptive patterns in the course of maturation.

5. Efforts of the ego to resolve the infantile conflict revived through the evasion of the actual life-situation. As has been said, the differentiation between the several forms of neurosis is based to a great extent on the type of defensive measure employed to resolve the anxiety, guilt, and inferiority feelings resulting from the reactivated original neurotic conflict.

6. Secondary results of the chronic neurotic state. The symptoms, which are the ego's attempt to resolve the conflict, absorb the patient's energy and make him even less effective in dealing with the real problems of his life. This secondary conflict necessitates further regression and produces new symptoms which, in turn, decrease the ego's efficiency by absorbing more energy. This is the neurotic vicious circle which results as the end-effect of the chronic neurotic state.

## TYPES OF NEUROTIC CONDITIONS

In the following discussion the main criterion used for classification of the several forms of neurosis is the differentiation of defenses used by the ego to resolve the neurotic conflict. Only secondary consideration is given to the nature of the ego-alien impulses against which the ego has to defend itself. According to the authors, classification based on "instinct-qualities" is much less reliable. In fact, the validity of some customary generalizations concerning the nature of ego-alien impulses and the degree of regression postulated in the different conditions is questioned by the authors.

### HYSTERICAL CONDITIONS

Three clinically well-defined conditions belong in this group: (*a*) anxiety neurosis, (*b*) phobia, and (*c*) conversion hysteria. Although these three neurotic states outwardly appear as quite different, the one common feature which justifies classifying them together is that the principal defense employed in all three is repression. In anxiety neurosis, repression is not supported by any other defense mechanism; in the phobias, repression is supported by displacement; and in conversion hysteria, the symbolic use of body innervations serves as a substitute expression of ego-alien tendencies. The validity of the statement common in psychoanalytic literature that in hysteria the repressed impulses are mainly of genital-sexual nature is not fully convincing. The presence of pregenital tendencies, particularly oral and sadistic, are commonly observed both in anxiety and in conversion hysterias. The argument that these pregenital impulses are regressive retreats from genital impulses is true in all forms of neurosis. There may be a preponderance of genital-sexual impulses in this group, but this generalization still requires further confirmation.

*a) Anxiety neurosis.*—Some form of anxiety is a well-nigh universal concomitant in all forms of neurosis, and it is also a common reaction in healthy individuals. Anxiety is the ego's reaction to the internal danger represented by the pressure of impulses, the gratification of which would involve the person in conflict with external or internal standards. In anxiety neurosis, anxiety is the central symptom, a constant or regularly recurring condition which has a paralyzing effect upon behavior. It appears without conscious motivation—it is "free-floating," without being firmly attached to any ideational content.

Free-floating anxiety, as a rule, is a reaction to repressed hostile impulses and represents a fear of retaliation. The hostile impulses are mostly aroused by sexual competitive drives, no matter how deeply these drives may be repressed. The unconscious content of anxiety in man, accordingly, is castration fear or masochistic homosexual fantasies; in women it is typical masochistic fantasies resulting both from guilt toward the mother and from hostile (castrative) fantasies toward the man.

Free-floating anxiety, seldom a chronic state, is the introduction to the development of some other more stable neurotic condition. Since neurotic mechanisms serve to allay anxiety aroused by the central conflict, anxiety neurosis can be considered as an initial phase, which exists before the ego forms adequate defenses against the anxiety. Nevertheless, free-floating anxiety may persist occasionally for a long period of time or may flare up periodically under conditions which mobilize the patient's conflict. The central mechanism is repression without any of the auxiliary defenses which are utilized in other neuroses to circumvent anxiety. Accordingly, anxiety neurosis can be considered the simplest form of neurosis, and the other neurotic conditions can be understood as different methods by which the central core of neurosis —neurotic anxiety—is handled by the ego.

The following case illustrates the dynamics and clinical picture seen in anxiety neurosis. It particularly high-lights the etiology and demonstrates how the anxiety neurosis can be the initial phase of a breakdown in ego functioning and then lead into the development of a clinical picture characterized by phobic and depressive features as the ego's defenses become operative.

A 34-year-old married white woman, following a serious quarrel with her mother-in-law, developed an acute attack of anxiety. Her free-floating anxiety, obviously a reaction to repressed hostile impulses, became manifest in tachycardia, palpitation, loss of appetite, and weakness and tremulousness of both upper and lower extremities. The anxiety soon became attached to the idea that she had heart trouble and that she was going to die. This phobia persisted for several months and finally led to hospitalization and cardiac study. After six weeks she returned home to her husband and three children, relieved of the thought that she had heart trouble. However, the unconscious hostility toward her mother-in-law and marriage now became displaced by obsessive thoughts that her husband and children would die or that he would divorce her. By the time she was referred to the psychiatrist, she was deeply depressed and full of remorse and self-accusations.

*b) Phobias.*—In the phobias, in place of generalized anxiety as seen in anxiety neurosis, the fear is focused on certain highly specific situations, such as being in the dark, in crowds, in inclosed places (claustrophobia), in wide-open spaces (agoraphobia), or high places (acrophobia). It is not our purpose to give an exhaustive description of the great variety of specific forms which phobic anxiety may take. In all instances the patient reverts to some early childhood fears, which are common and normal in infancy, such as fear of strange people, of darkness, of falling, of being alone in a crowded street. The etiological question is to establish the cause of the regressive reactivation of childhood fears.

The phobic fear reveals itself as a substitute for an actual fear of the problems of life which the patient cannot meet. The most common among these problems which the patient tries to evade are those connected with mature sexuality, the responsibilities of marriage, having children, and occupational tasks requiring independent decisions, competition, and all those complex interpersonal relations which are a part of adult existence.

A common example is the street phobia of women, who displace their anxiety because of prostitution fantasies (street-walking) to the fear of crowded streets. In acrophobia, the fear of ambition, responsibility, and leadership is symbolized by being "high up"; and the wish to accept a more humble position—in men, often a female position—is frequently replaced by the fear of falling.

Phobic anxiety has a tendency to spread, making the patient avoid more and more of the trivial situations of everyday life. In severe cases the patient retires completely from independent activity and indulges in a vegetative existence within the four walls of his home. This end-phase demonstrates clearly the unconscious trend toward infantile dependence—an escape from all the risks and efforts of adult existence.

The following case illustrates the clinical picture of a phobia:

A 31-year-old single white woman, in addition to vague complaints of chronic indigestion, suffered from a street phobia. This became particularly manifest when she was about to cross a street. She usually waited until others came along and then surreptitiously joined them as they went to the other side of the street. Her fear was that she would fall or faint. The street phobia in this woman was not only a displacement of her anxiety of unconscious prostitution fantasies but also a fear of her intense ambition and masculine strivings. Her feminine sexual strivings, repressed by her masculine protest, found discharge in the rich prostitution fantasy that led to one part of her street phobia. Her masculine protest led to a professional life, bringing her into a competitive relationship with men. However, strong unconscious trends toward infantile dependence became activated whenever she made important advances in her professional career and moved into positions calling for greater responsibility and leadership. Following such an advancement in position, her fear of falling became so acute that she felt giddy and dizzy even when walking on the sidewalk along the buildings. Her gastrointestinal distress also became more acute. In short, her unconscious infantile longings to be nursed and cared for became so intensified that the fear of ambition and the wish for a more humble position was replaced by the fear of falling.

A second example of a phobia is the case of a young lawyer who had a morbid fear that he would someday contract rabies. Not only was he fearful of being bitten by a dog, but he was afraid even to be near or touch anyone who owned, petted, or had been near a dog (example of the tendency of phobic anxiety to spread). As a youth he was exposed to the frequent quarrels of his parents, and often heard his mother refer to his father as a "baser Hund" ("mad-dog"). In fantasy the young lawyer often pictured himself as the rescuer of his mother and the avenging destroyer of his father. It is clear that his fear of rabies is a displacement and reaction to both his hostile wishes as well as his passive submissive trends toward his father.

The phobic anxiety in the latter case is similar to that of "little Hans" and the "Wolf man" from Freud's clinical studies (4, 6). In little Hans the fear of the falling, kicking horse was a displacement of the fear of the father who little Hans wished would fall over dead, while the Wolf man's fear of being bitten was a reaction to his unconscious passive feminine strivings toward his father.

*c*) *Conversion hysteria.*—The underlying mechanisms in conversion hysteria are essentially the same as in the common expressive innervations of the body, such as weeping, laughter, and blushing. Conversion symptoms express and relieve emotional tension through bodily changes, which have no other function but to relieve emotional tension. The differences between normal bodily expression and hysterical conversion symptoms is that the latter are individual uncommon innervations and the underlying emotional content is completely repressed into the unconscious. On the other hand, the normal channels of emotional expression may also be utilized for the drainage of unconscious ego-alien impulses, in which cases we deal with hysterical uncontrollable weeping or laughter. These patients are unable to say why they are laughing or weeping. A woman patient reported repeated instances of uncontrollable laughter at funerals and condolence visits. In her case unconscious malicious pleasure about the tragedy which befell persons against whom she had ambivalent feelings was the unconscious motivating force.

The forms which conversion symptoms may take are extremely variegated and are determined by the traumatic experiences of the individual. Contracture and paralysis of the limbs are the most common conversion symptoms in the field of the voluntary muscles. The contracture or paralysis has a symbolic meaning, which, at the same time, expresses both the gratification and the denial of the unconscious content. A contracted leg may symbolize the castrated male organ and thus express both the unconscious castrative wish as well as the punishment for it. In the great hysterical attack described in the older textbooks of psychiatry, several details of sexual intercourse are represented, such as the rhythmic movements, episthotonus, forced respiration, etc. What is missing is the experience of sexual gratification.

Hysterical conversion symptoms may appear not only in the voluntary muscles but in all sensory systems, producing an immense variety of paresthesias, anesthesias, pain, blindness, deafness, etc. The unconscious meaning is the denial of some ego-alien gratification connected with the affected sense organ.

The functions of some smooth muscles under the control of the autonomic nervous system may be the seat of hysterical conversion. The most common example is hysterical vomiting, the unconscious meaning of which is the rejection of some oral fantasy (fellatio, oral impregnation, biting, etc.). Such symptoms are not contradictory to the statement that conversion hysteria is restricted to the field of the sensorium and voluntary movements, because swallowing is a part of a complete co-ordinated physiological function, the first phase of which is the voluntary act of eating.

The excretory functions, also, are controlled by a combination of voluntary and automatic innervations. Accordingly, a combination of hysterical conversion mechanisms with those of vegetative neurosis is a common occurrence in the gastrointestinal tract.

It is a widely held view that hysterical conversion symptoms are utilized primarily for the expression of genital impulses, in contrast to depressions and compulsive obsessional states, in which pregenital (oral and anal) impulses are prevalent. The detailed study of conversion symptoms, however, seems to indicate that all kinds of instinctual tensions may find expression in conversion symptoms.

The prevalence of genital impulses holds more true in what is often called the "hysterical personality." These patients are inclined to go through the motions of feeling without actually experiencing the very emotions to which they often give an extremely dramatic expression. The feelings which the hysterical patients so desperately try to capture and which they are unable to experience are, as a rule, those characteristic of mature sexuality. This emotional shallowness is particularly frequent in connection with the sexual act itself and is the basis of the widespread phenomenon: sexual frigidity. Many frigid women go through the external motions of sexual gratification without being capable of experiencing it. Play-acting in place of actual experience, however, usually spreads out to all interpersonal relationships.

In connection with conversion hysteria, a phenomenon described very early by Freud deserves special mention. The patient identifies himself with another person but restricts the identification to assuming the sufferings of the chosen person. He imitates the disease symptoms (such as coughing or pains and aches of all kinds) of the one whom he both loves and hates. In the identification the patient gives unconscious gratification to his wish to be in the other person's position—for example, to have the same lover—and at the same time he gratifies the need for punishment by sharing the suffering of the envied person.

The following case is an illustration of conversion hysteria:

A woman of 32 developed a hysterical paralysis of her right arm and hand after her husband lost his job and developed a gradually increasing degree of impotency. The frustration she experienced as a result of his inadequacies led to the generation of strong unconscious hostile impulses. These, as well as substitutive sexual expressions, were repressed, but found expression in her conversion symptom of paresis. This occurred through the process of displacement and symbolization.

A dream reported during the second week of analysis reveals her unconscious hostile castrative impulse toward her husband as well as the masturbatory strivings. She dreamed that she returned home with a bag of groceries. She put her hand into the bag and took out an onion. She looked at it and said: "It has gone to seed, it is rotten." The hand, which is innervated by the hostile as well as the masturbatory impulse, is punitively immobilized. The onion that has gone to seed is an obvious reference to her husband's atrophied testicle.

In this case the conversion symptom has a symbolic meaning which, at the same time, expresses both the gratification and the denial of the unconscious impulses. The hand paralyzed is a symbol of punishment and gratification for the hostile castrative wish against the husband's genitals, as well as punishment and gratification for the infantile masturbatory impulses.

### OBSESSIVE-COMPULSIVE STATES

Full-blown cases of obsessive-compulsive states present a dynamic equilibrium in which obsessive preoccupation with ego-alien fantasies (incestuous, coprophilic, sadistic-homicidal ideas) are precariously balanced by rituals representing an exaggeration of social standards, such as cleanliness, punctuality, consideration for others. The obsessive ideas are mostly asocial in nature, whereas the compulsive rituals are caricatures of morality. The dynamic formula is similar to bookkeeping, in which on the one side of the ledger are the asocial tendencies which the patient tries to balance precisely on the other side with moralistic and social attitudes. The 50-50 ratio is characteristic of these patients and explains their central characteristic: doubt, indecision, and ambivalence. Every asocial move must be undone by an opposing one. Many of the complicated touching and washing rituals can be explained by this peculiar polarity in the emotional household. The endless hand-washing is a response to coprophilic tendencies. Touching is a symbolic substitute for hurting; the left hand must undo the sin committed by the right hand.

Psychodynamically, the compulsive-obsessional states differ from the hysterical conditions primarily in respect to the defense mechanisms. In the hysterias the principal defense is repression. In the compulsive-obsessive states the repression is not successful —the ego-alien ideas appear in consciousness sometimes without any distortion whatsoever. The defense consists in allaying anxiety and resolving the conflict by compensating measures (overly moralistic rituals), by which the asocial tendencies are undone, and by isolation of the ego-alien tendencies from the rest of the mental content. The objectionable ideas are de-emotionalized; they appear disconnected and almost as abstractions, like foreign bodies for which the patient does not feel responsible. Displacement, too, may play an important part in obsessive-compulsive symptomatology. This could be demonstrated in a 65-year-old patient who developed a mild, lifelong counting compulsion which suddenly became aggravated to an almost psychotic degree a week after his sixty-fifth birthday. Formerly a wealthy man, the patient was then forced to realize the precariousness of his financial situation. Instead of facing the hard financial facts and his future economic problems, which required some calculation, he began to count everything in his environment and was unable to free himself from this compulsion for even a few minutes during his waking hours. Meaningless counting of any countable objects substituted for his facing the highly disturbing numerical facts of his future economic existence. Counting objects is one of the most primitive forms of mastery—bringing some order into the chaotic world. A regression to this form of mastery when all other methods of controlling one's life-situation fail is a not uncommon form of neurotic evasion.

The preponderance of anal-sadistic impulses is well established in compulsive states. The defensive measures employed are particularly suited for dealing with the conflicts aroused by hostility.

The following is an illustrative case of obsessive-compulsive neurosis, showing the presence in consciousness of incestuous, coprophilic, and sadistic fantasies, as well as the ego's constant preoccupation with making restitution, isolating, or undoing the above-mentioned ego-alien impulses. This clinical example also demonstrates the psychodynamic difference in the defense mechanisms of the obsessive-compulsive state as contrasted with the hysterias.

A 31-year-old married white woman who had always been a compulsive and scrupulously clean housewife was forced by financial reverses to seek her father's help. He lived with two older sisters of the patient, one married and childless, the other single. The patient consciously resented the relationship of the father to the older sisters and frequently referred to them angrily as her father's "wives." Conscious hatred was felt for her father and the two sisters. The patient felt guilty about these hateful emotions but did not admit into consciousness any of her hostile death wishes. Instead, they appeared in consciousness in the form of acute anxiety or panic states whenever any disaster occurred. She was unable to read the newspaper headlines or listen to the radio for fear she would hear of some recent disaster. If this happened, she was then plagued with doubt that she had not performed her compulsive mental rituals correctly. If the disaster was a fire, then she wondered if she had not said "long life" the last time she saw the word "fire." If she had been talking to someone or looking at someone, she felt she must go over and over in her mind certain ritual phrases that were designed to deny the presence of any hostile wish that someone should drop dead, or burn to death, or come down with some dread and crippling disease. For example, she would repeat such phrases as "I mean she should not get sick" or "there should be no fire" or "I mean there should be no war." Frequently, doubt would arise in her mind as to whether she had got the phrase right, thus indicating quite clearly the breaking-through of the hostile wish.

Sometimes this tendency to undo or negate was directed against anal-sadistic impulses. For example, thinking about a man or being in his presence might force her to mumble to herself, "I don't mean kiss my behind." Further evidence of her anal-erotic fixation is indicated by her sexual responses to her husband's advances. She was unable to enjoy sexual activity with him unless she guiltily indulged in fantasies about spanking. In these, some other woman was always being spanked. It is interesting to note that the patient's father, a surgeon, was frequently plagued with a compulsive doubt regarding his preparation for the sterility of the surgical field, or he wondered if he had made all his sutures tight enough.

Being forced to return to her father's home for help threw the patient back into the unsolved oedipal conflict of her childhood. Her mother had died when she was six, and she and the two older sisters were reared by this father with the aid of housekeepers. At the time of the mother's death the child developed some kind of rectal trouble requiring frequent enemas. There was some regressive soiling at that time, with frequent punishment by her father.

It is not difficult to see that this patient resented her father's "wives" and wished them dead; but fear that her magical death wishes might cause their deaths, just like the real mother's, aroused intense anxiety and led to the displacement and spreading of the hostility to cosmic proportions. The compulsive cleanliness and anal-sadistic fantasies are obviously a regression to a previously overstimulated erotic zone that was accidentally fixated by the constant enemas and spankings.

### DEPRESSIONS

In depressions, also, ego-alien impulses—in this case, hostile tendencies—can no longer be excluded from consciousness by repression, and the ego has to use other modes of defense against them. The principal method is to turn the hostile impulses originally directed against other persons against one's own self. The melancholic patient indulges in an orgy of self-accusation which substitutes for destructive wishes toward others. The original target of hostility is always an ambivalently loved and hated person. Because of the love component, the hostility cannot be vented freely and must be turned back against the hating person himself. This is a suitable defense, because to hate a person whom one also loves is the source of the most intense sense of guilt. Attacking one's self—a kind of self-punishment—not only drains off the aggressive impulse but also serves at the same time as an atonement for wanting to destroy the beloved person.

The picture is further complicated by another important dynamism, which is of specific significance in depressions—identification. The love relationships of the depressive are tenuous and easily regress under frustration to a precursor of mature object love, that is, to identification. The lost object is reconstituted within the ego by the process of identification. The ambivalent conflict originally entertained toward the object now continues intra-psychically toward the person introjected. The process of identification thus favors the retroflection of the hostile impulses toward the self.

The quality of the impulses which participate in this dynamism are primarily of oral-aggressive nature. The tendency to incorporate the object as a part of the ego corresponds to that early period of development in which the interpersonal relations are of oral-dependent and oral-aggressive nature. According to Freud (5) and Abraham (1), the depressive patient has a fixation to the early oral phase of development and regresses to it whenever his tenuous object relationships in later life are disturbed. The dynamics of the depressive reaction are identical with those of mourning. In a depression the ambivalent character of object relationships is more pronounced, and the whole process is more intensive and prolonged. Because there is ambivalence in every object relationship, mourning is a universal phenomenon.

The following is an illustrative case of depression:

A 26-year-old white man developed a severe depression following the death of his wife. His depression was typically accompanied by feelings of guilt and ideas of a self-accusatory nature. He hated himself for not being kinder and blamed himself for her death because she had died in childbirth. During his depression that lasted about nine months, he suffered from frequent bouts of nausea and was unable to eat anything but baby foods. Analysis revealed that their $3\frac{1}{2}$ years of married life had not been very congenial. His wife had wanted a baby soon after marriage, but he claimed it was not wise because of financial reasons. There were frequent quarrels between them because he did not care to go out with her socially except to visit his mother's home. He also fussed about his wife's failure to develop into as good a cook as his mother. When she finally did become pregnant, he was openly neglectful and frequently left her alone to visit his mother or to be with the "boys."

The oral fixation and the ambivalent attitude to the wife are obvious in this case. The depression lasting nine months and his nausea and vomiting are indicative of an oral incorporation of the dead pregnant wife. By this process of identification, the hostility that he felt for his wife was turned upon the introjected object. In this case it can be clearly seen how the principal defense of depression, namely, a turning of the hostile impulses originally directed against his wife against his own self, is made possible by the process of oral incorporation and identification. It is interesting to note that as a child he suffered from a severe eating problem and had to be placed in a boarding house for several months.

### HYPOCHONDRIASIS

Only because it so frequently occupies the central place in different forms of neurotic conditions does this syndrome deserve discussion under a special heading.

Anxious preoccupation with one's own body and fearful expectation of a disease are always manifestations of a deep-seated need for suffering which derives from unconscious guilt feelings. A further important factor is that the preoccupation with a supposedly diseased part of the body can serve as a particularly suitable excuse for withdrawal of interest from the external world and for concentration of all love and attention to one's own self. The fact that this excuse consists in suffering allays guilt feelings, which a mature adult feels because of an excessive degree of self-concern.

A third factor is that the preoccupation with a concrete disease symptom allows the patient to displace a more intensive form of anxiety (such as castration fear or its feminine equivalent), as in the phobias, to one circumscribed area. The important role which narcissistic withdrawal and guilt play in these cases explains why the hypochondriasis syndrome is usually either the substitute for or a component of a depressive state.

## BEHAVIOR DISTURBANCES

Behavior disturbances are "neurotic character," "fate-neurosis," "psychopathic personality," and "impulse-ridden character." The outstanding feature of these conditions is that ego-alien impulses find outlet in actual behavior rather than in neurotic symptoms. As we have shown, neurotic symptoms are symbolic substitutions in fantasy for co-ordinated activity. Neurotic characters, however, are not satisfied with such tenuous gratification; they "act out" these impulses. Their life, in contrast to the neurotic, who suffers from typical symptoms, is dramatic; it is not just a private affair of the patient, it involves the environment. Because the ego-alien impulses are often of an aggressively antisocial nature, these patients often get into conflict with the law and form the major portion of the delinquents. Other neurotic characters express their unconscious impulses in eccentric behavior. Many famous adventurers, collectors, mountain climbers, and daredevils belong to this category. Neurotic acting-out of an impulse is the equivalent of a neurotic symptom. The difference lies in its alloplasticity.[1]

---

1. Ferenczi differentiated between autoplastic and alloplastic adaptations at the disposal of the organism: (1) changes within the organism (for example, development of heavy fur in the Arctic regions); (2) changes in the environment (for example, building fire or homes as protection against cold). Neurotic symptoms exemplify the first category because subjective needs are satisfied merely by internal processes, such as fantasy. Neurotic characters, on the other hand, gratify their alien drives by full-fledged activity which directly influences the environment, such as delinquent or unconventional behavior.

However, like neurotic symptoms, such symptomatic behavior is still only a substitute for realistic gratification of the repressed tendency, which is only rarely acted out in unadulterated form by severely disturbed psychotics.

This group of behavior disorders has long baffled psychiatrists, and the diagnosis "psychopathic personality" has come to be considered a wastebasket diagnosis. From the psychodynamic point of view, however, this diagnosis is not more difficult to make than any other diagnosis of a neurosis. The differential criterion is "neurotic acting-out" versus neurotic symptoms. The presence of an unconscious neurotic conflict can easily be recognized. It manifests itself by the following phenomena:

*a*) Irrationality of behavior, which is ill-motivated so far as conscious awareness of motives is concerned.

*b*) Stereotyped repetitive acting-out of unconscious motive forces which are not accessible to the modifying influence of conscious inhibition. This explains why, for example, neurotic delinquents repeatedly decide to start a new life and end their irrational behavior, only to fail again and again in their determination to reform. The opinion of most people, including many psychiatrists, that this inconsistency is a deception leads to the faulty view that these patients lack a superego and are fundamentally—indeed, constitutionally—asocial. There is no evidence that constitution is of greater significance in these patients than in those suffering from any form of neurosis.

*c*) Marked self-destructive tendencies which express the neurotic conflict. Neurotic delinquents always manage to be caught, as a result of a strong need for punishment, an outcome of guilt feelings, which themselves arise from the asocial impulses.

*d*) The actual neurotic behavior is a distorted substitute for unconscious fantasies. The actual crime, for example, is often a substitute for incestuous or patricidal impulses. The criminal who is acting from a guilty conscience, as described by Freud (7), attempts by a more or less trivial delinquency to express his crime, and in this way he appeases his unconscious guilt and makes a bargain. He suffers consciously for a smaller crime, while in his unconscious he secures substitutive outlet for his deeply repressed asocial tendencies, for which he would be punished much more severely. In fact, he exchanges the unconsciously dreaded castration as the expected punishment for his oedipal guilt with a more trivial form of suffering, such as imprisonment or, at most, hard labor.

The following case is illustrative of the acting-out neurotic character and demonstrates the features so typical of this condition, namely, the acting-out of ego-alien impulses, suffering being experienced by those in the environment because of the aggressive, antisocial nature of the impulses.

This is the case of a 27-year-old white male who is the youngest of three children. Both the older brother and sister are now hospitalized for schizophrenia in a state institution. His father, a very aggressive and successful business promoter, who was somewhat unscrupulous and inclined to alcoholism, died several years ago. The patient was attached to his mother, who was an indulgent and weak-willed woman who failed to exercise any discipline. The father was a bully, so that the patient was thrown between the spoiling of the mother and the bullying of the father. Although his intellectual capacity was adequate, he did poorly in school because of his truancy and defiance of male schoolteachers. He quit after two years of high school and then showed an even poorer work record. He was inclined to get into frequent quarrels with others and would then show traits that were imitative of his father. He would talk in a "big" and grandiose manner, scold, and act in a physically threatening manner. He most often associated with people of questionable character, because he felt ill at ease with those of his own set. He was easily affected by small amounts of alcohol and would evince the picture of pathological intoxication at times, approaching a confusional state. These periods lasted from only a few days to three weeks. Twice during such periods he became married to scheming women who had to be paid off and the marriage annulled. From one of these women he contracted syphilis.

This case reveals the unconscious competition and identification with the powerful and bullying father and the guilt about his incestuous attachment to his indulgent mother. But the neurotic conflict, instead of being discharged autoplastically, is drained off alloplastically in acting out the role of the superior and bully toward his inferiors and in choosing the indulgent prostitute as both a denial and a gratification of his incestuous attachment.

## ALCOHOLISM AND DRUG ADDICTION

These conditions deserve special classification for practical reasons because of the combination of the physiological effect of the drug with an unconscious emotional need.

The essential factor is that, by means of their narcotic effect, both alcohol and the different forms of drugs favor the possibility of regressively escaping conflictful life-situations. Through the narcotic effect, alcohol and drugs give physiological support to the regressive tendency to re-establish the carefree, passive state of Nirvana, of early infancy, when the child's needs are satisfied at the mother's breast. On the other hand, the initial stimulating effect of the drugs, which sooner or later is followed by the sedative effect, permits the patient to overcome his psychological inhibitions. The latter factor is particularly important in alcoholism. Alcoholics are often recruited from neurotics who are particularly inhibited in their human relationships and suffer from intense feelings of insecurity. The physiological effect of alcohol allows these patients to express themselves more freely and to feel effective and superior.

In the second phase of the intoxication the effect of alcohol dulls the pains of self-depreciation and insecurity. In other words, narcotics are pain-killers not only in the physical but also in the psychological sense.

The fact that indulgence in alcohol is socially sanctioned and that it offers pleasant, although temporary, relief from emotional stress explains its widespread use and partially explains the difficulties of therapy. In fact, alcoholism—both in theory and in therapy—is one of the most puzzling problems of present-day psychiatry. The question is: What makes certain persons become victims of this drug, from which other people derive only temporary relaxation from the tribulations of everyday existence? Some hidden allergic sensitivity of the organism has often been postulated, but no objective findings have been presented for the support of this hypothesis. On the other hand, there is indication that a psychological susceptibility, a basic weakness of ego control, might be the crucial factor.

### SEXUAL PERVERSIONS

One of Freud's early formulations was that a neurosis is the negative of a perversion (8). In other words, what a neurotic person represses and can gratify only symbolically by symptoms, the pervert expresses directly in his sexual behavior. Little can be added to this formulation, but the factors which are responsible for one person's developing a sexual perversion and another a psychoneurosis are still largely unknown.

In perversions either the quality of the sexual strivings or the object of the sexual striving is abnormal. In sadism, masochism, exhibitionism, voyeurism, and transvestitism the nature of the sexual striving is disturbed. In homosexuality, pedophilia, and zoöphilia the normal object is replaced by an unnatural one. In fetishism the object of the sexual striving as well as its quality is abnormal.

Etiologically, it is of primary significance that perversions show fixation to early pregenital forms of gratification. Regression to points of fixation is often manifest, but usually the perversion can be traced back as a continuous inclination of the patient from early childhood. There may be exacerbations and remissions, and occasionally there may be a long interval between fixating childhood experiences and the manifestation of the perversion in later adult life.

Because of the significance of the fixating childhood experiences, one should consider perversions as manifestations of an interrupted sexual development rather than as a disintegration of mature sexuality into its pregenital components. Although disintegration may play a certain role, in pronounced cases sexual maturity has never been firmly established. This fact might be responsible for the unusual difficulties which these patients offer to any form of treatment.

In sadism, inflicting of pain is the main content of the sexual urge. This aggressive impulse is completely dissociated from any utilitarian goal, such as the elimination of an enemy or an obstacle. Inflicting pain is an aim in itself and the source of sensual gratification. The same is true of masochism. Here the suffering of pain is the content of the sexual sensation. Voluntary endurance of pain is an important component of rational adaptive behavior. In order to achieve a cherished goal, a person may often willingly subject himself to all kinds of suffering. This, however, is not masochism. In masochism the endurance of pain is not subordinated to any goal but is a pleasurable aim in itself.

In exhibitionism, the showing-off becomes an isolated aim and the source of sensual gratification. Voyeurism can be described as the sexualized form of curiosity. Curiosity, too, is an integral component of purposeful behavior. When curiosity becomes a goal in itself, it assumes an erotic quality.

These forms of perversions, in which the quality of the instinctual strivings retain their pregenital form, substantiate the thesis that sexual gratification does not depend upon the quality of the instinctual urge but upon the mode of discharge. Every emotional tension, such as aggression and endurance of pain, curiosity, or vanity, can be expressed in sexual and nonsexual form. What is characteristic of the sexual expression is that here the emotional tendency is not subordinated to a self-preservative function but is an aim in itself. Object love also can be expressed in a nonsexual and in a sexual form, as is demonstrated by the double meaning of the word "love."

In the group of perversions in which only the object of the sexual tendency is disturbed—homosexuality, pedophilia, and zoöphilia—the sexual maturation is more advanced than in the group mentioned above. Here the influence of the oedipal conflict manifests itself in the replacement of an incestuous object by another one. Accordingly, homosexuality is often a defense against an intensive mother- or father-fixation. Another common mechanism in male homosexuality consists in identification with the original forbidden object of the sexual striving, for example, with the mother. At the same time, the person's own role is projected onto the homosexual partner. The sexual relationship re-establishes the mother-son relationship in which the patient plays the role of the mother and enjoys vicariously the pleasures of the partner who has the role of the son. The same mechanism is equally common in cases of female homosexuality.

In fetishism the main function of the perversion is to bind intensive castration fear. This is borne out by the fact that fetishism is restricted to the male sex. The fetish, usually a part of the female body or some article of female apparel (for example, shoes), represents the male genital, which the fetishist insists on attributing also to the female sex. By this he denies the existence of a castrated being (a body lacking a penis), which would arouse his own castration fear to an unbearable degree.

It is not intended to give illustrations and clinical examples of all the various perversions. However, the following case of homosexuality in a male is cited to illustrate some of the salient factors noted above. Analytic study of this case revealed that the perversion had been expressed by the patient from early childhood and at no time had been completely absent. This case also demonstrates the fact that perversions are a manifestation of partial interruption in the sexual development, partial because some degree of heterosexual development took place. This patient also shows that his homosexuality was not only a direct expression of libidinous striving of that nature but that this avenue of discharge was also used to drain off frustrated emotional striving arising from other sources.

This is the case of a 31-year-old married white male who came for treatment only after he had been picked up by a plain-clothes policeman for attempting a sexually perverse act. He is a well-built and handsome man but has a somewhat effeminate appearance. His mother is a very dominating and domineering woman, who came from a wealthy family. The patient's father, a soft-spoken, passive, timid creature, who was always browbeaten by his wife, worked in the father-in-law's business. A younger brother had to be hospitalized in a state institution for the feeble-minded.

This patient's homosexual experiences go back to the age of eight, when he seduced a colored man servant into fellatio and mutual masturbation. From then to his present age he has actively sought homosexual partners. He usually tries to find large muscular men, with whom he engages in mutual embracing or fellatio. When he was fifteen, his parents were quite conscious of his difficulty, sought help, and sent him to a military school. The behavior of the patient's mother in regard to sex was traumatic to him. The patient remembers awakening to find his mother examining and handling his genitals.

It is interesting to note that his libidinal organization influenced his vocational choice. He became interested in women's hairdressing and is now engaged in a thriving business. Although the idea of heterosexuality nauseated him, about two years ago he married a soft-spoken, mild sort of a woman, who can, however, be hard and firm upon occasion. This was shown by her ability to stand up to his dominating mother (her mother-in-law). The patient has always been contemptuous of his father but has been fearful of his mother.

When he came into therapy he revealed a boyish and infantile sort of orientation. He was still "mother's boy" and often spoke petulantly of his wife's ill-treatment of him. Sexual relations with her were only a matter of form. His desires often led him to such places as men's lavatories in hotels. This tendency on many occasions increased under any kind of stress. Quarrels with his wife, troubles in business, or difficulties with his mother often led to homosexual release. In his fantasies he often pictured himself being hugged and made love to. It was understandable that this man's trouble was greatly aggravated when his child was born and that he got into particular difficulty with the child's nurse.

This case of male homosexuality is illustrative of intense "mother-fixation," with the solution being a regression from the oedipal conflict because of fear of incest to a passive, oral position. Fear of the tyrannical mother made him turn to men for his passive oral gratification. He then sought for male lovers who would love him as he wanted and feared to be loved by his mother. Unconsciously, he established a love relationship with these men and played the role of the young child, giving the mother role to his male partners. A female creature was unthinkable because of his disgust and fear of the tyrannical mother. His feminine identification was further enhanced by his intense longing for the strong father whom he had never had in childhood.

## BIBLIOGRAPHY

1. ABRAHAM, K. "Manic-depressive States and the Pre-genital Levels of the Libido," in *Selected Papers* (London: Hogarth Press, 1927).
2. DEUTSCH, H. *Psychoanalysis of the Neuroses* (London: Hogarth Press, 1932).
3. FREUD, A. *The Ego and the Mechanisms of Defence* (London: Hogarth Press, 1937).
4. FREUD, S. "Analysis of a Phobia in a Five-Year-Old Boy," in *Collected Papers*, Vol. 3 (London: Hogarth Press, 1924).
5. FREUD, S. "Mourning and Melancholia," in *Collected Papers*, Vol. 4 (London: Hogarth Press, 1924).
6. FREUD, S. "Notes upon a Case of Obsessional Neurosis," in *Collected Papers*, Vol. 3 (London: Hogarth Press, 1924).
7. FREUD, S. "Some Character Types Met with in Psychoanalytic Work," in *Collected Papers*, Vol. 4 (London: Hogarth Press, 1924).
8. FREUD, S. *Three Contributions to the Theory of Sex*, in *The Basic Writings of Sigmund Freud* (New York: Modern Library, 1938).

# VI

## ACUTE NEUROTIC REACTIONS

### Leon J. Saul, M.D., and John W. Lyons, M.D.

U NUSUAL external stresses may elicit acute reactions. These stand in contrast with those chronic neuroses which are reactions to long-standing difficulties and are, by comparison, more independent of the external life-situation.

If a number of people are exposed to the same stress, only certain ones develop neurotic reactions. Earlier psychiatrists attributed this to constitutional weakness, while others stressed the reactivation of repressed infantile experiences by the trauma. More recent formulations (12, 28), born of the experience of World War II, utilize the concept of "specific emotional vulnerability" —how and when *any* individual will succumb depends, in the main, on the violence, duration, and nature of the stresses bearing on the specifically vulnerable parts of his personality. An individual's vulnerability is determined in part by constitutional factors, of which little is known, and in part by his emotional development, of which considerable is known.[*]

[*] These relations have been schematized in the following formula (28):

$$V_s \times S_s \propto \frac{A\,d}{F} \times \frac{R}{P} \propto \frac{T}{E} \propto N \,,$$

where

$V_s$ = Specific emotional vulnerability;
$S_s$ = External stresses, especially in relation to specific emotional vulnerability;
$A_d$ = Difficulty of adjustment, internal and external;
$F$ = Flexibility, adaptability, including capacity for temporary and partial regression;
$R$ = Regressive forces, including fixation (toward childish dependence or infantile attitudes or reactions);
$P$ = Progressive forces (toward independence, responsibility, productivity, maturity);
$T$ = Emotional tension;
$E$ = Ego strength (especially control and integrative capacity);
$N$ = Degree of neurosis.

Since war, with its unusual physical and emotional hardships, is probably the most fertile source of the acute reactive neuroses, most of the literature deals with reactions to the stresses of war, and this chapter is based chiefly on the study of war neuroses.

Freud considered the central feature of traumatic neurosis to be a psychic fixation to the moment of trauma (9). The neurosis then becomes a reproduction or a repetition of the situation, because the task of mastering and digesting it is still to be accomplished. Freud stated that constitution and infantile experiences are complementary and that minor traumata might reactivate infantile responses in a predisposed individual. This observation helps to explain the wide range of breaking points in various people to specific traumata.

In 1921 Freud (11) wrote that, if previous research had not substantiated the sexual theory in war neurosis, neither had anyone shown it to be incorrect. Freud, of course, used the term "sexual" in a broad way to mean (1) "sensual" and (2) "love" in its widest sense. The experience of World War II bore this out, in showing that prolonged frustration of emotional needs was a central factor in many cases of war neurosis.

Freud felt that the intra-psychic representative of reality may consist not only of genuine superego (that is, roughly, "conscience"—the internalization of parental ideals and standards) acquired in childhood but also of later and more superficial identifications with various other authorities. War, with its rigorous training and living conditions so dissimilar to peacetime, may create a "war superego" which permits the expression of forbidden impulses and tempts the ego with demands intolerable to the real superego. Freud felt that in many of the war neurotics a "peace ego" arises in defense against the "war superego." This view was confirmed by Abraham, Ferenczi, and Jones (11). Freud wrote (9) that the individual is impelled by a self-seeking, egoistic motive, and his quest for protection and self-interest maintains the conflict, once the symptoms occur. This aims at protecting the ego from a repetition of the trauma and persists until the danger is no longer present or until some compensation has been received.

Ferenczi (11) believed that not only love of others (mature love, "genital attitude," "object interest") but its precursor, love of self (narcissism), was affected by war. The symptoms of terror, depression, instability, etc., arose from increased ego sensitivity as a result of the withdrawal of libido from the object into the ego, in other words, from a retreat from the usual mature interests in others to preoccupation with one's self. This is the tendency under stress—to abandon other considerations and take care of one's self. Thus those predisposed by a high degree of self-centeredness (narcissism) will be susceptible to traumatic neuroses. Because of the universality of the narcissistic stage, no one is immune. Children only gradually outgrow their self-centeredness and become capable of adult parental responsibility and sacrifice.

Abraham (11) agreed that men who developed war neuroses were predisposed before the trauma. Since their previous adjustment was dependent on self-interest (narcissistic concessions), they were ill-prepared for the selfless sacrifices demanded by war.

Jones (18) wrote that the conflict was between fear and the adaptation to war. Conflicts over killing, dirt, and discipline, combined with fear of being maimed or killed, tend to overwhelm the ego.

In the traumatic neurosis the dream life continually goes back to the disaster situation, indicating a "fixation" to the trauma. Freud felt that, if the wish-fulfilment theory of dreams were to be maintained, then dreaming suffers a dislocation along with other functions and is sidetracked from its usual purpose. He postulated a "repetition compulsion" for powerful experience that goes beyond the "pleasure principle" (8). According to this hypothesis, the dreams represent a regression to a more primitive mode of mastery. Through repeated reliving of the trauma, control may be slowly regained by the gradual discharge of energy and relief of tension. Recent work (29), without contradicting this hypothesis, indicates that some, if not all, catastrophic nightmares of the traumatic neuroses fit perfectly into Freud's well-established theory of dreams.

Freud believed that the ego developed in part at least for the purpose of avoiding traumatic states by its ability to anticipate expected trauma and prepare the individual so that the effects are softened. Economically (quantitatively), such preparation consists in making ready amounts of "countercathexis" (countercharge of emotion) to bind the expected excitation. To be forewarned is to be forearmed. Unexpected traumata are experienced more forcefully. Pathological and archaic attempts at mastery may be utilized to stem the painful incoming stimuli. An incident may have a traumatic effect in direct relationship to its unexpectedness.

Simmel (32) stated that there were no appreciable differences between the neuroses of World War I and those of World War II. He felt that the dynamic conflict lies within the ego itself, in its attempt to mediate between instinctual demands and external reality. The ego in its struggle for survival is undermined by the prospect of annihilation from the external world. The symptomatology results from the ego's use of the mental mechanisms of defense in transforming real anxiety (fear of death) into neurotic anxiety.

A nation at war, as an external representative of the parents, permits a return of the repressed aggressive impulses and sanctions them if used against the enemy. However, if relations to the parents were bad, then there is a tendency to be hostile against all authority. Soldiers indoctrinated in a military unit are joined libidinally and are collectively identified with a leader, who becomes the externalized superego (10). Thus the soldier is in the old child-father relationship and feels secure and even immune to death as long as the relationship with the superior is good. However, discrimination, poor leadership, and disappointments tend to isolate the individual and render the authority unsuitable as an externalized superego. Since he feels released from the group, the man's original conscience and standards function again. The ability of the ego to withstand trauma now depends on the strength and normality of the soldier's peacetime superego.

War symbolizes the ambivalent conflict with the father in a specific manner. Where the self-esteem is hurt by authority, the authority becomes the hated father. The aggressive destructive tendencies previously aimed at the authorities are turned inward and tend to augment the strictness of the inner superego. This guilt may then paralyze the personality by phobic reactions and may cause overt aggression or pathological heroism. In other words, repressed hostility to superiors can reach such intensity and cause such guilt as to generate neurotic symptoms. To the predisposed, war can also represent the original oedipal situation in the form of the enemy symbolizing the father and the home country the mother.

As Simmel saw it, the symptoms of war neurosis are mechanisms of escape from an unbearable situation, as in psychosis. These mechanisms turn into neurotic symptoms through the interference of the superego, which is able to turn the external danger into an internal, instinctive danger. Thus the symptoms are not converted erotic longings but destructive impulses. That is, they are powered not by sensual feelings but by anger, hate, and hostility. By forming symptoms, the ego avoids a complete psychotic break with reality and brings about a release of the tensions toward the superego. By protecting himself against the danger of his own hostile aggressiveness, the person maintains his stability.

In treatment Simmel stated that, if the war neurotic can turn anxiety into rage and aggressive action, the ego will find its way back to reality. Consequently, he introduced and encouraged the venting of rage on dummies and recommended the assumption of a benevolent superego (kindly, tolerant, permissive) attitude on the part of the therapist.

Kardiner (19) finds that there is no specific neurosis created exclusively by war conditions but that war offers an opportunity for the development of neuroses in greater concentration and frequency. He discusses inhibition as the major force, operating broadly and disordering the various mechanisms of adaptation. The neurosis becomes the organism's attempt to adapt itself under the circumstances of vastly reduced resources. The continuous conflict necessitates constant control and inhibition. This tends to change the individual's conception of himself and the outer world. It produces a feeling of helplessness and a tendency to give up and to be parasitic (regression). His altered conception of the outer world as a threatening place inhibits vital psychological functions, in part as a defense against further traumata. His regression to infantile helplessness in the face of the threatening world engenders further fear and hostility. Catastrophic dreams then occur because of the feared retaliation for his own hostility. Though his regression may give him some inner security, it may also tend to perpetuate the neurosis.

A sudden loss of control over the situation causes lasting damage to the adaptive capacity. Rado (24) postulates an emergency control mechanism which tends to remove the individual from dangerous situations. The basic pattern is described as being a conflict between military duty and self-preservation, with an ensuing flight into illness, fixation on the trauma, and a secondary gain from the illness. The emergency control mechanism, spurring toward flight or blind attack, is in conflict with the sense of duty, which requires calmness and rational thinking. The traumatic period becomes the last straw, and the man finds relief from tension in a flight into illness, especially if it can last for the duration of the war.

In the post-traumatic period the anxiety perpetuates itself by creating the illusion that he is still in battle. There are sporadic resurgences of rage and anxiety as the personality relaxes its subjugation to the emergency control mechanism. As time goes on, the process gradually subsides. If, however, the traumatic phobic factor is too strong, the fear of recurrence becomes dominant, and the patient regresses to dependency and unconscious appeals for support. The sexual function is vulnerable because of its susceptibility to anxiety since childhood (castration fears).

Grinker and Spiegel (12, 13) find the nuclear problem of war-induced neuroses to be anxiety, much of which results from the stresses of war bearing upon the integrative functions of the ego. War, equated with potential injury or death, stimulates every emergency biological mechanism for flight. The conflict between the desire for flight and the fear of punishment from officers floods the ego with emotion. Further sources of anxiety are the individual's feeling of helplessness and the unusual situation of actually having approval for hostile and destructive behavior. Anxiety springs also from the liberation of primitive reflexes and its associated energy, such as the noise, sight, and smell of battle. Thus the ego is flooded with anxieties from external reality, from the man's own instinctual drives, and from the reactions of the superego. On the other hand, the ego is protected from anxiety by a number of factors: the individual's ability to identify with a group, approval of war aims, sense of invulnerability, and ability to express hostility outwardly.

Ego-exhausting factors, such as fatigue, hunger, pain, sensory overstimulation, traumatic identification, guilt, and expected injury and death, tend to undermine the ego from without. At the same time, previous neurotic trends and traumata bore from within. As the pressure on the ego continues, its inhibitory and intellectual functions weaken. Signs of free-floating anxiety, confusion, and poor concentration result. The process may go on to complete disintegration, as in fugues, stupors, or schizoid dissociated states. This loss of ego function appears to be a biological regression to more primitive levels of adaptation. Anxiety may subside also by being bound to conversion symptoms, leaving the rest of the ego to function normally.

In a later publication (2) Grinker states that "in the interval before returning to the U.S. war neurosis seems to undergo a change of pattern; the newer reactions are engulfed by old patterns and the total picture stands out sharply, showing the reactions to war to be a repetition of old reactions to previous conflicts."

Saul (28) proposed a theory of acute neurotic reactions to cover the highly individual factors as well as the general causes. He combined the concept of "specific emotional vulnerability" with the concept of emergency physiologic mobilization for fight or flight. The specific vulnerabilities, in addition to the various general factors discussed above, such as superego conflicts and ego depletion, account for the individual variations in symptomatology; the psychophysiologic "fight-flight" reaction accounts for the similarity of the syndromes.

## INCIDENCE

Acute neurotic reactions are seen also in civilian life following catastrophes, such as automobile and train wrecks, mine cave-ins, and other accidents. Emotional shocks can produce similar effects. As an example Adler (1) has reported a study of survivors of the Coconut Grove holocaust in Boston. Here the suddenness of the calamity, along with the panic and the fact that large numbers were trapped in the blazing café, served to place many in sudden danger of death. Many of those who became so disturbed emotionally as to develop neurotic symptoms had escaped unscathed physically. The symptoms of most of the survivors subsided in a relatively short time, but many were left with residual neuroses. The most common memories of the group studied were fear of imminent death and of being choked and trampled.

It is in wartime that the acute neurotic reactions of various kinds and degree are seen most profusely, not only at the front, but in rear areas and in civilian life. The transformation of the individual from his peacetime life into one of war, with all its dangers, hardship, and stresses, tends to make unusual demands on the ego.

During the last war (according to statistics compiled by W. C. Menninger) (21) 382,000, or 34 per cent, of all the medical disability cases were neuropsychiatric. These occurred in a well-screened group. Obvious neurotics and misfits had been rejected. Of the 15,000,000 men examined, 1,846,000, or 12 per cent, were rejected for neuropsychiatric disorders. These were 38 per cent of the total number rejected for all causes. Of the remainder, 250,000 were later discharged administratively. Furthermore, 3–7 per cent of all trainees consulted the mental hygiene clinics; of this number, only 7 per cent had to be hospitalized. Unknown but large numbers consulted division psychiatrists and flight surgeons. These needed no further care or hospitalization.

## Etiology

It cannot be too strongly emphasized that the etiology of acute reactive conditions is not a matter of the individual's neurosis, latent or otherwise, but of his "fit" (Alexander) or adaptation to the particular environment. Every "normal" has vulnerabilities and may break under stress upon his specifically vulnerable spot. Conversely, a severe "neurotic" may adjust very well if his neurosis happens to fit the particular stressful situation. Thus individuals with frank chronic neuroses, such as compulsives, mild paranoids, schizoid personalities, neurotic characters, can and did adjust to combat and other situations where the external stress did not excite their specific vulnerability. Indeed, certain situations were such that a person with a certain kind of neurosis could adjust much better than a normal mature individual. For example (28):

Two professional men came into the service together. The one held to very high standards and was very adult in all his relationships. He was warmly interested in people, very much in love with his wife and children and devoted to his work. When obstacles arose to the accomplishment of what he deemed right, he invariably sought to overcome them. He was a strong, loyal man of high type and unusually mature.

The other man, although able, was of much easier virtue. Also a family man, his eye nevertheless sometimes roved. His interest in his work was noticeably overbalanced by his enjoyment of relaxation, and he never fought through obstacles or for the maintenance of standards if he could possibly avoid the trouble. In the service, as things turned out, both men went overseas and were subjected to considerable stress. The former persisted in his faithfulness to his family, strove to do the job with the utmost effectiveness and consideration and refused to compromise on his standards. As a result, he missed his family painfully but could not forget them with other women, and he had many battles to fight on his job. At the end of a year, although he maintained full control and performed efficiently, the underlying tension had so mounted that he developed disturbances of both heart and stomach and had to be evacuated.

The second man, however, took the easier way. He freely sought refuge from the frustrations of his job and personal life in wine, women and song—in his duty did no more than was expected of him, while after hours he totally forgot his troubles in the pursuit of whatever pleasures were available wherever he happened to be. A relatively lazy, irresponsible child as compared with the former upstanding, responsible, productive, independent man, he nevertheless, through his ability to escape into play, avoided enough frustration and gained enough pleasure and surcease to continue to function on this level. His ability to regress protected him, while the former man, maintaining his high level and unable to regress, broke down.

As indicated by J. Appel (3), it is probably true that every individual, if subjected to enough stress, will break down. Also many men will endure successive combat campaigns and then break down for other reasons. If the stress is sufficiently intense and prolonged, even the strongest will succumb. Some break sooner than others. Although there are basic similarities in what men feel and can stand, there are individual differences in kind and in degree of sensitivity. Everyone has vulnerabilities and breaking points.

It must be remembered that a man who breaks under a specific stress would not always do so, had he not been sensitized and his controls weakened by other experiences. This point may be clarified by the following examples (28):

A young officer complained of anxiety, irritability, and insomnia after $3\frac{1}{2}$ years of extensive combat duty aboard ship. His symptoms had developed suddenly at the termination of his leave as he was preparing to return to his ship.

Actually combat did not unduly upset him. In a way it held the same thrill as hunting. True, his emotional tension mounted continually aboard ship but not because of fear. Further exploration revealed that one of the sources of his increasing stress was being told how and when to get his hair cut. This was significant of all the restrictions aboard ship which he found eventually to be unbearable—changing his clothes for meals, standing inspection in whites after a night of enemy action, and similar infringements of his personal liberty.

He could discuss his combat experiences freely and with little discomfort, but even the memory of these minor impairments of his freedom enraged him. His resentment increased until, just before returning to his ship, he literally trembled with rage. He did not understand this and did not realize the intensity of his feelings. He was terrified only by these mysterious symptoms.

To understand this man we must go into his personal history. He was raised in the Canadian Rockies, where he enjoyed freedom beyond the realm of that known in urban or even most rural areas. At 13 his parents died and he went to live with a rigid restricting aunt, where he found conditions intolerable. Instead of giving in to her restrictions, he went off to live in a small town where he was well acquainted. He set himself up in a small cabin, worked in his spare time and went through high school. Self-reliant, and loving the freedom of the mountains, his was the personality of the independent frontiersman. It became clear why he could face danger and violence coolly but could not stand four years of supervised hair cuts. His sensitivity was restriction. He would not have broken under fear alone. In civil life he had similar but milder symptoms. Generally good natured, he had a violent temper when his freedom was impaired. Like typical combat fatigue, he suffered with insomnia and nightmares, but his dreams were not of battle. Instead, they were repeatedly of being "held down" or "fenced in."

Another man had his symptoms precipitated when his ship hit a mine. Half the crew was killed, and he was hurled 30 feet through the air. His anxiety persisted for three months, along with stomach distress and repeated nightmares, in which the scene was almost exactly the same, but the screaming of wounded shipmates noticeably worse.

He came from a poor financial background in which the necessary frugal living was a source of distress to him. In high school he was able to earn enough to have the things he wanted. He felt more comfortable and secure and resigned himself to hard work in order to get what he wanted. He thought his father could have been a better provider.

As the patient talked, it was evident that strong hostile feelings toward his father and brother were checked and controlled by a very loving and gentle attitude. This latter came from identification with his mother, who was a kindly and religious woman. He never had a fist fight, nor was he cruel to animals. He could not stand violence or bloodshed of any kind.

Here we see a young man with considerable repressed hostility which had long been inhibited because of love of his parents and careful upbringing. He could not indulge it even in reading or fantasy. In his own mind hostility could not be acted out externally but only turned against himself. Aroused by combat he could not become aggressive. His violently aroused emotion went not into hostility for others but into fear for himself.

In spite of the many complications and variations, the etiology of the acute reaction seems to boil down to a variety of internal and external factors, both physical and psychological (danger, exposure, disease, separation, anxiety, morale, etc.), which exert stresses on the individual and cause (1) general weakening and sensitization, (2) reactions resulting from specific emotional vulnerabilities, and (3) weakening and impairment of the powers of control over the symptoms.

Once a person is threatened by increasing pain, frustration, anxiety, and weakening forces of control, he reacts by physiologic and psychologic mobilization for fight or flight. This manifests itself in the various symptoms and behavior patterns common to war neuroses.

### TYPES OF STRESS AND REACTION

World War II afforded psychiatry an excellent opportunity to study the effects of stress and strain on the average person. Screened individuals from all walks of life were thrown into the common experience of military life and combat. The individual reaction to this experience depended, in a large part, upon the person's makeup and the particular kind of stresses to which he was subjected.

Combat was found to be only one of the stresses common in breakdowns. It can be a completely dissimilar experience under different conditions. A man who has been on a ship doing routine patrol, out many months without touching port, may find occasional action to be a relief from tension and boredom. On the other hand, combat can also loom horribly, and in time everyone, no matter how strong, will crack.

War affects men differently. It stirs up repressed tendencies which previously exerted some influence on a man's emotional life but by no means necessarily caused neurotic reactions. These tendencies become intensified by the stresses of war, and adequate control is lost or weakened. Irritability becomes belligerency; mild anxiety dreams become nightmares; accustomed tension becomes unbearable anxiety with startle reaction; the latent predisposition or vulnerability becomes a full-blown neurosis.

It is a matter, as we have said, of adaptation. Many very neurotic persons adjusted themselves adequately to the stress of war because their neuroses fitted the situation. A relatively normal person may succumb to neurotic illness if he finds himself unable to adapt to a particular situation. Instances of men performing heroically under tolerant officers and later breaking down under rigid discipline in the rear area are numerous.

Stresses other than those resulting from (1) combat can be roughly grouped as those arising from (2) the service itself, such as discipline, isolation, inferior assignments, and lack of recognition; (3) relations to family, such as worries about finances, marital faithfulness, illness, etc.; and (4) other relationships as to career, friends, etc.

In general, men whose emotional problems arise from aggression, guilt, and anxiety are more susceptible to breakdowns precipitated by combat or other forms of violence. One who severely inhibits his hostility is likely to have more fear and anxiety than those who accept freer expression of hostility. On the other hand, some individuals with too free hostility became murderously hostile and developed acute anxiety when their forces of control weakened.

The Achilles' heel of guilt was often seen by military psychiatrists, and frequently it was noted that the amount of guilt feelings was all out of proportion to the reality involved. Closer study often revealed that this self-blame (manifested by guilt) was because of wishes rather than deeds. For example, the death of a buddy in combat sometimes was followed by more than the usual amount of depression. The feeling tone often became one of extreme guilt, self-condemnation, and blame. Investigation frequently revealed that the accidental death of the buddy had gratified unconscious death wishes toward him.

Thus external stress acting upon the internal makeup and current emotional state of the individual can precipitate a neurotic reaction. The final appearance of the symptoms is further dependent upon the man's forces of control and his ability to cope with the reaction.

This can be summarized in the following outline which is by no means complete:

I. The intensity of the reaction is determined by:
   A. External factors
      1. Various stresses and combinations of stresses, such as loss of a buddy, decimation of a unit, severe damage to a ship
      2. The suddenness, violence, and duration of the situation
      3. Inability to express excitement by activity
   B. Internal factors (including current emotional state)
      1. Primitive instinctual impulses, such as excessive dependence or hostility
      2. Rigid superego, causing excessive guilt and fear of hostility

3. Weakness of the ego, with consequent lack of independence, self-reliance, and self-confidence

II. The strength of the forces of control and the individual's ability to cope with the reactions are determined by:

    A. His internal makeup, such as his adaptability, strength of ego, and tolerance for anxiety and hostility

    B. External factors, such as physical hardship, boredom, training, and indefiniteness; personal factors, such as understanding the reason for fighting, quality of leadership, relations with his outfit

III. Secondary reactions

Once symptoms begin to develop, the individual reactions are diverse—from minimizing the situation and hiding to complete surrender and even exaggeration

## SYMPTOMS

As with other disease processes, there may be an incubation period for emotional disorders. But, unlike certain of the acute infections, there is no specific time interval between exposure to stress and the development of symptoms. It depends upon the person's makeup and current physical and emotional state, upon the kind, amount, and duration of the stresses, and upon the outlook for the future.

The symptoms of the acute neurotic reactions are of two kinds. There are those which seem to be basic to the condition and which occur in combination in practically every case. In addition, any individual may have any other symptoms known to psychiatry. Most writers (6, 17, 22, 25) agree that the basic constellation of symptoms is as follows: (1) anxiety, (2) irritability and belligerency, (3) easy fatigability, (4) startle reaction, (5) insomnia and repetitive nightmares, and (6) difficulty in concentrating. In addition to this constellation, any individual is likely to show vegetative disturbances, depression, paranoid trends, compulsiveness, schizoid reactions, and any other symptoms which he is accustomed to developing under stress of any sort.

The typical picture seen in the last war is a fighting man recently returned from combat or the front areas. His features are distorted with fear and wan with fatigue. His normal co-ordination is troubled with gross tremors, and excessive perspiration dampens his body. Even in the quiet of the rear area, his biologic mobilization for fight or flight remains. He overreacts to ordinary noises; a low-flying commercial plane sends him into a frenzied dive for shelter. The sudden ringing of a telephone may send him leaping out of his seat, followed by hysterical crying and extreme rage at himself for such an emotional display. He is alternately passive and clinging and equally aggressive and combative on slight irritation. War movies and usual civilian noises send him into a panic, so that he becomes seclusive and prefers to remain in the ward rather than take part in the rehabilitation program. Night becomes a time of terror, when every shadow threatens danger. Even the escape into sleep is hampered by insomnia, or, when sleep does come, it ends with nightmares of his horrible experiences. His waking hours are further plagued by tension, indecision, difficulty in concentrating, headaches, gastrointestinal disturbances, dizzy spells, and other psychosomatic disturbances.

### Dynamics of Symptom Formation

Under stress every person reacts, as does every animal organism, with physiologic and psychologic mobilization for fight or flight. This may be felt subjectively as anger and/or fear. The fight impulses are manifested outwardly by irritability and belligerency. When they are repressed, they probably always generate anxiety and flight reactions, with all kinds of subsequent psychologic and somatic symptoms. These may include anxiety, paranoid trends, nightmares, cardiac palpitation, gastrointestinal disturbances, and numerous other physiologic disorders. When the flight impulses are expressed outwardly, they may become manifest in actual blind fleeing from the trauma or more unconscious and face-saving flight, such as malingering. When repressed, they may motivate misbehavior, produce physiologic symptoms designed for escape, or they may find expression in physiologic and psychologic regression to childish and infantile reactions. This may be expressed in eating disorders, enuresis, speech disturbances, motor inco-ordination, evasion of responsibility, and increase in passive-dependent-receptive demands.

Thus drives to fight and to flight, aggressive and regressive, may combine to produce any variety of impulses and tensions to reactivate childhood patterns and cause neurotic symptoms. Every neurosis, and possibly every neurotic symptom, is motivated in part by a combination of fight and flight impulses in various proportions. Long ago Freud stated that some day our psychologic understanding would rest on a physiologic basis. The understanding of hostile aggression and regression and their interplay is aided by the recognition of the physiology and biology of the fight-flight reaction (5, 31).

The basic constellation of symptoms appears to be a manifestation of the biologic fight-flight reaction, which is a mechanism common to all people and seen in one form or another throughout the animal kingdom (27). The differences are explained by the various individual ways of handling these reactions. These ways are the result of each individual's particular, highly personal endowment, training, and experience.

The study of war neuroses has contributed to a clearer understanding of the acute neurotic reactions and of the nature of neurosis in general. From it we can conclude that, if the emotional development of the individual is relatively complete, then his adaptability is high, his regressive tendencies are low, and his vulnerability is minimal. Susceptibility to neurosis thus appears to be a disturbance in the emotional development which causes specific vulnerabilities to stress and impairment of adaptability.

For a dynamic interpretation of his symptoms and as a basis for successful treatment, it is necesary to have an understanding of the man's personality and his emotional vulnerabilities, combined with the form and degree of regression, along with his characteristic methods of defense.

### General Formulation

An individual's adjustment is the result of his personality makeup interacting with his environment.

1. His makeup depends upon his heredity and congenital endowment interacting with the training, experience, and emotional influences to which he is subjected, particularly during the earliest years of childhood.

2. Every individual has certain special strengths and weaknesses in his emotional makeup.

3. These depend in large part upon how fully he matures emotionally.

4. His adjustment in any given situation depends upon how well his particular makeup fits the particular situation. If the situation fits, then an infantile or neurotic personality may adjust to it better than a mature one.

5. Breakdown can be caused by internal stresses (conflicts) or

by external ones. This chapter is concerned only with the latter, that is, the acute *reactive* neuroses.

6. When the person's makeup does not fit a given situation, the stresses of the environment generate tensions. The stresses may be general, such as overexertion and consequent fatigue; but in most cases breakdown can be understood only in terms of specific stresses acting in certain ways upon the personality makeup. Every individual has specific emotional vulnerabilities, and in most cases symptoms develop when particular stresses bear upon these.

7. Under this pressure the organism reacts to the threat with the basic biologic emergency mobilization for fight or flight. Usually, neither direct fight nor flight is possible, nor is either one a solution of the intolerable situation. Tendencies to fight and to flee must then be repressed, and they then interact to cause symptoms. The tendency to fight generally brings about powerful conscience reactions, with guilt and anxiety.

8. Psychologic regression is one form of flight. The combination of repressed impulses to fight and to flee, along with the conscience reaction and regression, give the typical picture of combat or operational fatigue—anxiety, irritability, startle reaction, catastrophic nightmares, fatigability, and a variety of other psychologic and somatic symptoms.

9. The individual struggles consciously to control his reaction (ego control).

10. The strength of the control depends upon various general factors, such as fatigue, and upon various specific factors, both internal and external.

11. As the force of the reaction exceeds the ego's capacities for control, anxiety mounts, and the symptoms are intensified.

12. Whatever the original stresses and causes of the symptoms, once they are developed, the individual can react to them in different ways. He can continue to fight against them, or he can try to exploit them for certain purposes, such as sympathy, escape, or compensation. This is called "secondary gain."

## SEQUELAE

Probably the most important complication of the acute neurotic reaction is "secondary gain": a fancied or real reward for perpetuating the illness. Theoretically, one would expect a group of symptoms precipitated by a specific stress to subside, once the stress had ceased to exist. But in every illness there is a tendency to exploit it for ulterior purposes to justify dependence on others, tyrannizing over them, and so on. Commonly this is to secure compensation. This wish is not usually a primary cause of the illness but a secondary utilization of it. It can be a very powerful motivation, however, and a long-lasting one, as is only too well known to the Veterans Administration and insurance companies, as well as to others. The secondary gain can prolong a psychologic regression from which the individual may never recover. This must be sharply distinguished from neurotic symptoms which persist for the primary reason that a man's balance of emotional forces has been upset and equilibrium never regained—for example, where so much hostility or guilt has been aroused that they are not again adequately repressed.

## Diagnosis

Usually there is no difficulty in the diagnosis of the acute neurotic reaction. One can see the stress and the individual's reaction to it. Sometimes, however, it may not be simply an acute reaction but a reactivation of a latent psychosis brought on by the stress. Usually, careful observation and the working-out of the major dynamics will reveal the true condition.

It is necessary to work out, so far as possible, the full dynamics—the patient's personality structure and major psychodynamics as they were prior to the stress and the effects of the stress upon these. It is then often found that the obvious and apparent stress was by no means the one that caused the break, but rather something quite unexpected. For example, classical war neuroses were sometimes precipitated in returning combat veterans without previous symptomatology, when they discovered evidence of infidelity, heard of the wife's pregnancy, family and financial difficulties, death of a relative or friend, and other disturbing situations.

It is well to watch for a concurrence of organic disease and psychological difficulties. Frequently, a wound was accepted with equanimity because it served as an escape from the immediate stress of combat. Soldiers were known to hope and pray secretly for a wound which would serve to initiate evacuation without loss of face. Malaria and other diseases also acted similarly and no doubt helped materially to decrease the number of psychiatric casualties by giving a rest from stress before the controls of the individual were weakened.

The syndrome "blast concussion" (20) underwent a period of popularity in the Pacific, like "shell shock" in World War I, before it was recognized to be largely psychogenic in origin. Fighting men, subjected to a near-by blast, suffered a short period of unconsciousness and, upon reviving, found their controls to be almost completely lost. The symptoms varied from regression to infantile helplessness (flight) to maniacal outbursts of completely undirected rage (fight). After a few days the patient would suddenly "awake" with a complete amnesia for all his dissociated behavior. Investigation with sodium amytal or hypnosis usually revealed the amnesia to be psychogenic and the process an acute neurotic reaction (traumatic neurosis) having the same dynamics as discussed above.

An invaluable instrument for diagnosis is dream interpretation. The dream is "the royal road to the unconscious" (9) and usually leads directly to the central theme of the acute neurotic reaction. Accurate dream interpretation, however, requires a knowledge of dynamics and special training.

## DREAMS

In acute neurotic reactions the dreams are typically repetitive catastrophic nightmares, which represent the traumatic scene. In war, with so many traumatic experiences, the repetitive scene is usually the one that precipitated the breakdown. The nightmares show the fixation to the trauma and the individual's attempt to digest it. *These dreams, which may persist indefinitely, are analyzable in exactly the same fashion as any other dreams.*

A common feature is violence usually directed against the individual but also very often or regularly against others. This violence, upon analysis, is always found to spring from the man himself. It is usually the expression in his dreams of his attempted defense by fight or flight. Often it represents mobilized hostility. It usually shows a conscience reaction aroused by the trauma. For example, a 21-month-old child was painfully injured on the leg by a falling object. That night he apparently had nightmares whenever he fell asleep. His serene features would become distorted with fear, and his arms and legs would flex. Wakened by the pain from the movement of the injured limb, he would immediately slap his father, who was trying to comfort him. One could suspect that the child was reliving the trauma repetitively in an attempt to digest it. However, his aggressive behavior on awakening is suggestive of a mobilized fight reaction as a consequence of the trauma.

Persistence of traumatic neuroses and of the nightmares signifies a failure of psychological digestion—a failure of adaptation. The reason for this failure to overcome trauma can usually be found from the dream itself in the following way: Although the nightmare typically represents the traumatic scene with great accuracy, yet some detail is usually altered. Why the individual alters this detail nearly always gives the clue to his emotional vulnerabilities and to what keeps the neurotic reaction going.

For example (28), an anxious Marine, exhausted, underweight, and jaundiced by many attacks of malaria, had become too tense to carry on. He had extensive combat service and gave a good account of himself in hand-to-hand fighting. In telling his life-story he revealed nothing which cast much light on the severity of his condition. He had a repetitive nightmare. He was in a fox-hole, and the enemy were coming at him. He reached for his rifle, but it was gone. He reached for his revolver; it was gone. He reached for his knife, but it, too, was missing. He was in a panic because he had nothing to fight with.

The dream repeated a battle scene exactly, except for the detail that the patient in reality never was caught without a weapon. The central theme of the dream is being attacked and not having weapons with which to fight. When asked to talk about this detail which differed from the reality, he revealed further facts about himself. In school he was a fine athlete. He had an athletic scholarship to a large university and an offer from a big-league baseball club. His heart was set on an athletic career, and now all his hopes were dashed by malaria. Twenty-five pounds underweight, periodically racked by chills and fever, he saw his career shattered. Without his athletic prowess he felt defenseless, and now he was reminded of the dream. He started with sudden emotion. With a burst of insight, he saw that in the dream, while asleep and off-guard, he had repeated the anxiety which tormented him *now*. As he slept and felt anxiety, rather than facing its true source, in his shattered health, career, and security, he attached it to past danger, which was no longer real.

Another Marine (28) with typical combat fatigue symptoms dreamed repeatedly of making a landing where a large number of his companions were killed, including two buddies. The dream ended with the patient himself being caught in machine-gun fire. Except for this ending, the dream repeated in minute detail the invasion scene, which, in reality, left the patient unscathed. By dreaming of being caught in machine-gun fire, this man made the scene even more terrible than the reality. A dream of killing and being killed is certainly likely to represent hostile feelings toward those who are killed, and guilt can be so great that one feels that he deserves to be killed in turn. The patient admitted that, in reality, he did wish to be killed himself, and the reason for this was that he felt so terrible about his dead buddies.

Further investigation revealed that the patient had never been at ease in his relations with people as a result of early maternal overprotection and impaired masculine freedom and security. Because of feelings of insecurity about his background, he felt uneasy and not accepted by the above-average people with whom he desired to associate. The same pattern carried over into military service, where he did not achieve the promotions he desired. He felt inferior to his buddies. This heightened his resentment, and he developed an intense underlying hostility toward his friends which he kept concealed even from himself because of his need for recognition by them. When the buddies were killed, this satisfied his unconscious hostility toward them. However, the unconscious guilt over this was overwhelming and precipitated his breakdown.

The endings of dreams are of special importance. The dream is an expression of the dreamer's feelings. Because the feelings are conflictful, the scenes are usually distorted. The ending of the dream tells something of the outcome of the patient's conflicting feelings and the kind of solution he seeks for his emotional problems.

## PROGNOSIS

The prognosis in the acute reactive neuroses is dependent on the following factors: (1) the previous emotional makeup, (2) degree of disruption of the balance of emotional forces, (3) extent of the regression, (4) promptness and adequacy of treatment, (5) secondary gain, and (6) present life-situation and future prospects.

The personality structure of the individual, with his aggressions, guilt, dependency, narcissistic needs, and other instinctual demands, and *how he handles them* in relating to reality contain the essence of the neurotic predisposition. The closer the individual was to emotional maturity prior to his illness, the better is his prognosis with rapid and accurate treatment. Individuals with low adaptability, marked regressive tendencies, and many vulnerabilities have, on the other hand, a relatively poor prognosis. The man with marked passive-dependent needs who finds gratification in his illness has little stimulus to get well. Even he often gets a therapeutic push from the hurt masculine pride which rebels at the dependency.

Frequently, people who have been able to emancipate themselves from dependency on the parents and to establish a mature independent existence will regress to childhood dependence under stress. The extent of this regression is prognostically important. It depends on the force of the trauma, the stability of his maturity, and, again, the gratification found in the regression. Long years of childhood leave a taste for carefree dependence in all of us. If a person, new to the pleasures of independence, is traumatically forced into a regression, he may never again find the confidence to leave the security of his reawakened childhood patterns.

The rapidity with which accurate treatment is instituted is also important prognostically. Men often failed to seek help because of the hurt pride involved in having a psychiatric disability and carried on in spite of severe subjective suffering. Finally, as the process progressed and they became less and less effective, they were turned in by their superiors. Many of these were found to be quite refractory to any psychotherapy. Also, the slowness of evacuation or the large number of casualties because of military exigencies often allowed weeks to go by before skilled psychiatric help was available. By that time the complications of secondary gain had set in, and this handicapped any short-term therapy. The shortage of skilled psychiatrists in the last war was another major factor in preventing rapid, accurate treatment of the acute neurotic reactions. These factors, plus many others, served to allow and to encourage regressions in these reactions. The delay in treatment allowed both conscious and unconscious recognition of the secondary gain involved and precluded any real desire on the part of the man to get well, lest he be returned to the precipitating trauma.

## PROPHYLAXIS

An excellent study by Appel and Beebe (3) involving an epidemiologic approach to prevention of the acute neurotic reactions was incorporated into the Army procedure prior to termination of the war in Europe. The senior author made a first-hand study of psychiatric casualties in Europe and concluded that practically all men in rifle battalions who are not otherwise disabled ultimately become psychiatric casualties. The average point at which the break came was from 200 to 240 aggregate combat days. The study indicated that a man reached his effective peak in 90 days and suffered a gradual fall of efficiency from then on.

It was believed that proper incentive was an important prophylactic measure, and specific measures were recommended to encourage proper motivation. It was suggested that a specific limit be set to the number of combat days, that more appropriate awards for achievement be given, that the method of evacuation screening be improved so that men still able to perform in combat would not be lost through evacuation and that the replacement system be improved so that only men trained for combat be sent in as replacements. Further suggestions included morale and emotional training, with added emphasis on independent thinking under combat situations. The importance of adequate leadership was also emphasized, especially along lines of proper maturity and attitudes, of the leaders.

The authors state that psychiatric casualties represented the result of particularly heavy enemy opposition, incompetent unit commanders, deficiencies in supply, improper training, and untoward morale influences. Similar conclusions were reached by other psychiatrists who were concerned with these problems (14). Long-range prophylaxis can aim to develop a nation of individuals with high adaptability, low regressive tendencies, and a minimum of emotional vulnerabilities. This can be achieved through the proper rearing of children emotionally so that they reach full emotional maturity.

## TREATMENT

The basis of treatment of these conditions is the same as for any neurotic condition. This can be expressed in three words—

*understand the person.* This means that one must understand the patient's emotional makeup, the stresses acting upon it, and his reactions to these stresses. With these understood, a therapeutic plan can be outlined.

The treatment of the acute neurotic reaction depends on the stage in which it is first observed and the nature and intensity of the reaction. The procedure of Grinker and Spiegel (13) was first to remove the patient from the immediate battle area. Then sodium amytal was administered, under which the patient relived with intense emotion the traumatic events. This time, however, it was only in fantasy, as he was actually in a safe place and, most important of all, he had the support and understanding of the physician. Interpretation was used where it was indicated. These authors used narcosynthesis as an adjunct, their treatment being based on psychodynamic understanding.

In the subacute stage, treatment depends chiefly upon judicious insight therapy. Interpretation, however, must be accurate. This means understanding, so far as possible, the patient's emotional makeup, his vulnerable points, and the effects of trauma on these. *The core of the emotional dynamics must be hit, since the main therapeutic objective is to help the man to understand his problem and to help himself.*

Dramatic effects can often be achieved in one to three interviews. The insight gained continues to operate for many months to come. A man's progress may even continue beyond his pre-illness adjustment. If the central theme is clearly delineated, then this insight may be enough to start him on his way out.

The therapeutic effect is largely due to the fact that a mysterious affliction is suddenly turned into an understandable problem. The terror of an unknown illness with the stigma "mental," "NP," or "psycho" turns into an understandable emotional problem that can be dealt with. The patient sees a solution if he will shift his emotional attitudes. He uses this insight for weeks and months thereafter. This can be supported by infrequent short interviews in the ensuing months. This "working-through" period is important. The insight gained must be worked over, in order to be consolidated, to insure the gains in the shift toward maturity in attitudes and satisfactory adjustment to life.

It would seem that the longer the neurotic reaction persists, the closer it comes to expressing current typical neurotic prob-

lems. The treatment then approximates the usual psychotherapeutic handling.

A great variety of accessory methods of treatment has been
tried. Reference has been made to the use of dummies for the
abreaction of rage (17). Prolonged sleep, electric shock, group
psychotherapy, repeated sodium amytal interviews, insulin sub-
shock, supportive therapy with rest, quiet, and diversion have all
been used (for detailed discussion see Grinker and Spiegel, 10).
Many of these are of great help in individual cases. Fundamentally, however, it is a neurotic reaction which is being treated, and
the same basic type of accurate understanding and psychological
treatment is required as for any other neurotic condition.

## BIBLIOGRAPHY

1. ADLER, ALEXANDRA. "Neuropsychiatric Complications in Victims of
   Boston's Coconut Grove Disaster," *J.A.M.A.*, 123:1098, 1943.
2. ALEXANDER, F.; FRENCH, T. M.; *et al. Psychoanalytic Therapy* (New
   York: Ronald Press Co., 1946).
3. APPEL, JOHN, and BEEBE, G. W. "Preventive Psychiatry: An Epidemiologic Approach," *J.A.M.A.*, 131:1469, 1946.
4. APPEL, K., and STRECKER, E. *Psychiatry in Modern Warfare* (New
   York: Macmillan Co., 1945).
5. CANNON, W. B. *Bodily Changes in Pain, Hunger, Fear, and Rage*
   (New York: Appleton-Century, 1929).
6. DUNN, W. H. "War Neuroses," *Psychol. Bull.*, 38:497, 1941.
7. FRENCH, T. M. "Insight and Distortion in Dreams," *Internat. J. Psycho-Analysis*, 20:287, 1939.
8. FREUD, S. *Beyond the Pleasure Principle* (London: Hogarth Press,
   1922).
9. FREUD, S. *A General Introduction to Psychoanalysis* (Garden City,
   N.Y.: Garden City Publishing Co., 1943).
10. FREUD, S. *Group Psychology and Analysis of the Ego* (London:
    Hogarth Press, 1922).
11. FREUD, S.; FERENCZI, S.; ABRAHAM, K.; and JONES, E. *Psychoanalysis
    and the War Neuroses* (Vienna: Vienna International Psychoanalytic
    Press, 1921).
12. GRINKER, R. R., and SPIEGEL, J. P. *Men under Stress* (Philadelphia:
    Blakiston Co., 1945).
13. GRINKER, R. R., and SPIEGEL, J. P. *War Neuroses in North Africa*
    (New York: Josiah Macy, Jr., Foundation, 1943).
14. HANSON, F. R. (ed.). *Combat Psychiatry* (Bulletin of the U.S. Army
    Medical Department, November, 1949).
15. HASTINGS, D. W.; WRIGHT, D. G.; and GLUECK, B. C. *Psychiatric
    Experiences of the Eighth Air Force* (New York: Josiah Macy, Jr.,
    Foundation, 1944).

16. HEATH, R. G., and POWDERMAKER, F. "The Use of Ergotamine Tartrate as a Remedy for 'Battle Reaction,'" *J.A.M.A.*, 125:111, 1944.

17. JASKIN, M. "Psychodynamic Aspects of the War Neuroses," *Psychiatry*, 4:97, 1941.

18. JONES, E. "War Shock and Freud's Theory of the Neurosis," *Proc. Roy. Soc. Med.*, 1918.

19. KARDINER, A. "The Neuroses of War," *War Medicine*, Vol. 1 (March, 1941).

20. LYONS, J. W. "The Blast Concussion Syndrome," *Pacific Fleet M. News*, December, 1944.

21. MENNINGER, W. C. "Facts and Statistics of Significance for Psychiatry," *Bull Menninger Clin.*, 12:1, 1948.

22. MILLER, E., *et al. The Neuroses in War* (London and New York: Macmillan Co., 1940).

23. MURRAY, J. M. "Psychiatric Aspects of Aviation Medicine," *Psychiatry*, 7:1, 1944.

24. RADO, S. "Pathodynamics and Treatment of Traumatic War Neuroses," *Psychosom. Med.*, 4:362, 1942.

25. RAINES, G. N., and KOLB, L. C. "Combat Fatigue and War Neurosis," *U.S. Nav. M. Bull.*, 41:923 and 1299, 1943.

26. SARGENT, W., and SLATER, E. "Acute War Neuroses," *Lancet*, 2:1, 1940.

27. SAUL, L. J. *Bases of Human Behavior* (Philadelphia: J. B. Lippincott Co., 1951).

28. SAUL, L. J. *Emotional Maturity* (Philadelphia: J. B. Lippincott Co., 1947).

29. SAUL, L. J. "Psychological Factors in Combat Fatigue, with Special Reference to Hostility and the Nightmares," *Psychosom. Med.*, 7:257, 1945.

30. SCHWARTZ, L. A. "Group Psychotherapy in the War Neuroses," *Am. J. Psychiat.*, 101:498, 1945.

31. SELYE, H. "The General Adaptation Syndrome," in *Textbook of Endocrinology* (Montreal, Canada: Acta Endocrinologica, Inc., 1949).

32. SIMMEL, E. "War Neuroses," *Calcutta M.J.*, 43:269, 1946.

# VII

## EMOTIONAL DISORDERS OF CHILDHOOD

### Margaret W. Gerard, Ph.D., M.D.

AN ADEQUATE description and analysis of childhood problems and their treatment would require at least a volume. In this chapter an attempt will be made only to point out the more important general principles in respect to the kind, the cause, and the treatment of childhood problems. It is hoped that the information presented here will be sufficient to stimulate readers to follow through the sources of our knowledge of emotional disorders of children in the literature now available on this subject (see references at the end of the chapter).

### HISTORICAL NOTES

Just as psychoanalysis developed a dynamic approach to the study of psychic disorders in adults, so it stimulated a similar change in the study of disorders in children. Previously, childhood problems were thought to be caused by constitutional deviations, about which little more than diagnosis could be accomplished. The discovery of Breuer and Freud (21) that, in the adult hysterical neurosis, the symptoms stemmed from reactions to previous experiences stimulated a re-evaluation of the causes of childhood neuroses and behavior disorders, since they, too, are related to environment and experiences.

In the same way, Freud's recognition that the adult personality represented a stage in a developmental continuum inevitably focused the attention of investigators upon the various stages of childhood in the search for the anlage of personality characteristics or difficulties. As Freud had related adult problems to various sexual experiences in childhood, the early psychoanalysts of children tended to interpret child problems only in terms of the sexual causes found in allied adult neurosis. Much valuable information concerning childhood sexuality was thus unearthed, which gave evidence that children did pass through various stages in which pleasurable experience had erotic elements and was focused in oral, anal, and genital areas. The importance of the genital problems of the oedipal period was emphasized in the investigation of childhood neuroses (59), just as Freud's early investigations of adult neuroses were focused on the causative role of sexual difficulties of the oedipal period.

Anna Freud offered the stimulus to investigators in Vienna to analyze the symptoms of children by means of a modified technique, which she used and taught (37). Concomitantly, Melanie Klein (67) in Berlin developed a method for the treatment of childhood disorders based upon analytic theory but quite different from that of Anna Freud. Klein's method involved hypothetical interpretation of the child's play activity as symbolic expression of inner conflicts, whereas A. Freud's method approximated more closely the more empirical method of adult analysis, in which one interpreted the meaning of an act or a fantasy only after it had been made clear through further information. This information, gained in adult analysis through "free association," was collected in child analysis through play, conversation, fantasy, etc., since the child cannot and will not associate freely in the same way as an adult. Because of the difference in the two methods, the Vienna school has produced more information concerning psychic development, which one can check in observing children and from which one can understand the causes of symptoms and of deviate activities of children of various ages.[1]

From the stimulus of the work of both schools, the child-guidance movement in this country flourished and has adapted the methods of investigation and treatment to the clinic setting. The child-guidance clinics, in turn, helped to influence education, pediatrics, and parental upbringing of children, so that, although child psychoanalysis was initiated in Europe, American child psychiatry and child care are at the present time thoroughly infiltrated with psychoanalytic knowledge.

Although most of our knowledge has been gleaned from the study in a treatment situation of children of various ages and

1. Melanie Klein has produced theories of development which deviate markedly in major points from those which are generally accepted and which are based upon collected evidence (56). Klein's theories hypothecate the occurrence of certain psychic phenomena in the early months of a child's life. There are no methods as yet to confirm or disprove these hypotheses, but one may hope the future will bring forth evidence to determine whether or not they are valid. In the meantime, the present chapter will omit discussion of her theories and thus avoid confusion.

with various problems by psychoanalytically trained therapists, in recent years various studies involving observation of infants and older children in their everyday activities have added much information to previous knowledge and have modified concepts which had been formulated by the recapitulation from memories of the early years of older children and of adults (3, 38, 39, 47, 61, 84, 89). These studies have been particularly valuable in elaborating our accurate knowledge of the environmental and constitutional influences which are responsible for the child's choice of methods of adjustment (ego mechanisms) to the variety of life-problems which he must solve at various stages in his development. The kind and quality of these early problems and the early methods of their solution form the groundwork for the beginning of childhood psychic difficulties and determine in part the constellation of adult character and its aberrations. In other words, studies of the child have aided in explaining the child and also in explaining the adult: the reverse of the original situation in which the child was described and explained by information gained through the childhood traces found in the adult. Both methods have yielded valuable results and check each other for accuracy in timing developmental events and in evaluating the importance in character formation of the quality and quantity of any one experience or of any one constitutional factor.

## ETIOLOGY

When we speak of psychic disorders in childhood, be they classified as behavior problems, neuroses, or autonomic symptoms, we are concerned in general with the disorders in adaptation to the environment in which the child finds himself. For this reason, some behavior may be considered abnormal in one environment and not in another. Anthropological studies have exposed these differences as they occur from one culture to another. Similar differences occur within a culture from one social group to another and are superficially evident in differences in manners, sexual behavior, and so forth. In even greater degree, differences occur from one age to another. What may be a serious symptom in an adult may represent normal behavior for a two-year-old and only questionable behavior for a five-year-old, as, for example, nocturnal bed wetting, temper outbursts when thwarted, fantastic lying, genital exposure. It is obvious that consideration of a disorder must always be undertaken in view of the expected or "normal" behavior of a child at the age of occurrence and with recognition that environmental demands and expectation change with the age of any child. The environment to which the child must conform not only varies from child to child but from age to age.

In chapter iv there is a discussion of the role played in personality development by the conflict between instinctual drives and environmental demands, between instinctual drives and superego standards, and between opposing instincts. When methods of solving conflicts are reached which satisfy instinctual needs, environmental expectations, and superego demands, successful and healthy adjustment follows. Symptoms, on the contrary, represent methods of solving conflicts which are unsatisfactory, because the methods do not sufficiently satisfy either the instinctual needs or the rules of social behavior or both. Any disorder, then, may be considered as evidence that the process of "structuralization" of the personality has deviated from the "norm" or from the expectancy for the particular age, to such an extent that the purpose of adaptation is only partially realized, and thus the functioning of the individual is handicapped.

These deviations are due to a variety of causes, which may operate at any or all stages of development. In chapter iv, it is pointed out that development occurs as "the interaction between the maturational processes and environmental influences." In the discussion of the development and treatment of any abnormal condition, one must consider the role which each element plays in its creation. Both the conditions of maturation and the environmental situations are changing from time to time. Yet there are certain relative constants which form the framework around which these changes occur.

One of these constants is the constitutional inheritance of the child. In 1932, Freud (42, p. 296) stated: "... we are not as yet able to distinguish between what is rigidly fixed by biological laws and what is subject to change or shifting under the influence of accidental experience." And our methods of measurement are still not sufficiently refined to differentiate accurately between a constitutional element in the production of a symptom and the modification of an inherited factor by environmental influences. However, certain basic capacities and defects are generally believed to be inherent in the individual's endowment and to influence the direction of development. Intellectual capacity—at least taken in extremes of superiority and defect—body-build, and talents of special artistic or creative superiority are generally accepted as inherited and determined by genetic patterns.

Probably there is also a constitutional variation in an individual's capacity for ego development. The development of a "strong" or well-functioning ego and superego may be partly inherent in an innate capacity. In the same way, variations in the strength of instinctual drives between one person and another may possibly be due to constitutional differences. The strength of sexual strivings as well as of aggressive tendencies, then, will play an important role in the way in which an individual can or chooses to adjust the expression of these drives to the pressure of social demands.

On the other hand, since so many other factors enter into these formulations and since it is impossible to evaluate the constitutional elements involved, practical analysis of symptom formation in this chapter will assume that variations in innate ego capacity and strength of instinct may be possible, if not probable, but are too problematic to discuss dynamically.

Of less constancy than the constitution of an individual are the personalities of the child's mother, father, and other people in his environment. Since the mother is usually the most constant individual in the child's life, particularly during the most formative years, her personality, her behavior, and her attitudes toward the child and in his presence are usually the important influences in the infant's choice of modes of impulse (instinct) satisfaction. In the absence of the mother, the person (or persons) who "mothers" or cares for the child's needs takes over this role. Other members of the family or home group come second in their influence upon his development. Thus, the family plays the role of interpreting to the developing child the rules which society expects him to obey, and teaches him the ways in which he can direct his energy to conform and still gain satisfaction for his needs. As each mother's personality is different from others', as each family's standards and habits are different, so does each child experience social pressure in different ways.

Besides the constitutional and family environmental factors which represent continuing influences on personality development, other accidental and less predictable influences also play important roles. Traumatic experiences, considered at first by

Breuer and Freud as the essential causes of the neuroses, no longer hold such prime position in the theories of causation, though they are still recognized as significant influences in the development and fixation of the pattern for certain neurotic constellations. Dynamically, an event becomes traumatic to the child when the ego is incapable of mastering the suffering and anxiety which the experience produces or of resolving the emotional conflicts created by it. This situation occurs either if the ego is weak and the event overpowering or if there is not sufficient help from parental persons in resolving the conflict. Therefore, the younger the child and the weaker his capacity for mastery, the more possible it will be to traumatize him and the more protection he needs to support his inadequacy.

Another factor which may determine the injury to the personality which a traumatic event may cause is the capacity of the event to revive a conflict which was inadequately solved at an earlier age. Hartmann (61, p. 15) has stated that the intensity of the castration fear in the oedipal phase is in direct proportion to the intensity of the oral deprivation felt at weaning.

As the child becomes older, the ego develops more adequate methods of mastering the anxiety produced by conflicts and of overcoming suffering. Hence events which could have been destructive to him when younger are no longer disturbing and may even aid in the production of adaptive techniques rather than symptoms. For example, separation of several days from a loved mother will usually cause anxiety and regressive symptoms in a one- or two-year-old child but will offer to a child of six or older an opportunity to discover that he can master many situations from habits which had previously seemed to depend upon the mother's presence. Instead of fear and regression, he gains the courage to experiment with new and even better techniques.

These more or less accidental experiences which may operate as traumas to personality development are manifold. They may occur as the result of physical illness or bodily injury; of parental losses by death or separation; of sibling births or deaths; of economic deprivation; of sexual experiences; of strong instinct temptations before the child has developed the strength to master them; of school misplacement or rejection; and so on. The way in which a child reacts to any trauma is determined by the total constellation of constitutional trend, his status of physical maturation, his integrative capacity, his previous experiences, and the type of trauma.

A final factor in the development of any symptom which must not be ignored is the influence of other symptoms and their causes which have occurred in earlier stages of development and remain as facets of the personality constellation. New symptom habits which form to meet new problems are superimposed upon old habits, the pattern of which remains interwoven with the new. Thus new symptoms partake of old symptoms, just as new skills are aided or handicapped by old skills or ineptitudes.

In childhood disorders, as in those of adults, in no instance will one cause be found for one neurotic symptom; but acting together in the production of neurotic illness are constitutional and environmental factors, degree of maturation, and previous symptoms and traumata.

### Problems of the "Oral" Period (Early Infancy)

As was discussed in chapter iv, in each phase of development the individual must solve conflicts specific for that phase, such as weaning and temporary separation from the mother in the oral phase; excretory and motor control in the anal phase; rivalry and genital fears in the oedipal phase; and so on. Only when the solutions are not adequate for self-expression and not satisfactory to meet the environmental demands do problems develop which cause the internal stress of neuroses or the external conflict of behavior difficulties. Emotional difficulties, therefore, may be differentiated according to age, as more or less inherent in the problem solving of each of the ages.

Investigations in recent years have enriched our knowledge of the importance of the early months of life in normal and abnormal personality development. Studies in the direct observation of babies under various conditions have accumulated data correlating the reaction of the infant to the type of care, or lack of it, he receives. Theoretical conclusions from the findings have added greatly to our previous understanding which had been gleaned from recapitulation in the psychoanalysis of adults.

O. Rank (82) emphasized the influence of the traumatic experience of birth upon the developing infant. Recently, speculations concerning the effect of prenatal experiences upon the postnatal personality carry the concept of environmental influence even further back and offer interesting modifications to our theories (57). Some confirmation that prenatal effects may occur was offered in a study by Sontag (85), in which correlations were found between excessive hyperactivity of the newborn (crying, sleeplessness, regurgitation, etc.) and maternal emotional stress during pregnancy, as well as between infant serenity and a normal contented pregnancy. Since it has been shown that reactions at each age are dependent in part upon the status of personality development which has grown out of reactions to previous experiences, these studies suggest that the infant probably enters the world with constitutional trends already modified by the impingement of the environment upon him while he was still in utero. In any case, there is much evidence that occurrences in the early postnatal months are very important in forming the basic patterns of reaction within which all later changes take form. It is within the security of the mother-child "symbiosis" (11) that the child's primary narcissism flourishes. Later differentiation of the concept of self from that of the mother and her breast separates love for the mother and breast from love of the self, and object love is initiated. When this "symbiotic" security is lacking, various pathological conditions develop.

Spitz (86) has shown that infants deprived of mothering in the early months of life develop a type of behavior which he calls "anaclitic depression." The child is irritable to stimuli of all kinds and develops no appropriate responses to different stimuli, becomes emaciated and marasmic. If the condition is not changed within the months of the oral phase, Spitz believes the condition is irreversible and treatment impossible. Such conclusions need to be tested by further studies directed toward adequate therapy of the child who has been so deprived, which consists of educative and ego-building techniques within the framework of affectionate personal relationship, as described by B. Rank with very disturbed children (79). However, Spitz's observations (87, 88) have clearly shown how necessary is the relationship to a mother-person for the early development of the ego. It is clear that the motherless infant, he reports, lacks any signs of adaptive mechanisms and seems to have lost even the capacity for certain reflex adaptation, such as sucking, grabbing, and pushing away.

Severe disorders in later years have been traced back, in several studies, to a pathological condition of these early months. Levy (73) and Bender (9) and more recently Bowlby (20) have described children in the latency age and in adolescence with various conduct disorders in which symptoms of extreme narcissism with affective "emptiness," defects in standards, and ego inadequacy were prominent. These children were reared in institutions with only routine care and were completely deprived of mothering.

B. Rank (80) adds a similar cause for disorganized behavior in younger children who, because of severe emotional deprivation, show indications of arrest in development such that diffuse excitability follows any sensory stimulus. For these children, object relationship is primitive and associated with the production of body sensation, as skin rubbing, rocking, sucking, etc. She has been able to relieve these conditions by a therapeutic program in which the child is given a relationship to the therapist similar to that in very early development and then led forward through the various stages as they should normally have been traveled.

Besides these severe character disorders resulting from maternal deprivation, recent researches indicate that other severe disorders—psychoses and schizophrenias in particular—and many vegetative disorders (5) can usually be traced back to markedly pathological parental attitudes, exhibited in excessive neglect, cruelty, and gross inconsistency. However, perhaps in lesser degree, the farther back our information is carried in the study of the neuroses and the behavior problems, the more we find that both psychopathological conditions and adequate personality characteristics have their roots in the experiences of the first year of life and are closely related to the types of maternal behavior to which the child is exposed or to the lack, in varying degrees, of any mothering.

This is quite understandable when we consider the factors involved in ego and superego development taken in conjunction with the fact of the organism's tendency toward repetition, which is described as the "repetition compulsion," "inertia principle," or "habit formation." If the infant in the early months has no consistent pleasant stimulus from a mother who is tender and caressing and if he is not protected adequately by her from the pain of hunger, cold, skin irritations, etc., one can easily relate to the deprivation the development of symptoms of narcissistic withdrawal, poor interpersonal relationship, and inadequate social adaptive habits described by Spitz and Bender. In the absence of a mother, the child must master his feelings of discomfort alone and satisfy his needs through autistic rather than objective activity. Once initiated, these methods become fixed through repetition into habits and ego trends, so that each new difficulty is met by turning back to one's self and thus avoiding at each step the learning of new methods of adjustment through the help of a trusted person.

A cruel and inconsistent mother offers a kind of necessity for self-sufficiency in an infant. To overcome the pain and anxiety resulting from these experiences at the mother's hand, it is possible that the child must avoid the discomfort by denying reality and avoiding object contact, at the same time creating in fantasy a world closer to "his heart's content," which forms the fabric out of which schizophrenic delusions may later be formed. Or he may localize suffering in a part of his body, the organ cathexis in psychosomatic disorders; or he may ward off awareness of pain by gross defensive motor activity, as in various hostile aggressive behavior disorders. The baby is too helpless yet to develop, on his own, adequate social habits of countering cruelty or of caring for himself independently.

In recognition of the importance of a secure, reliable, and pleasant mother-child relationship for the development of a healthy personality, concepts of child rearing have veered from the spartan ritualistic routines of the early twentieth century to immediate indulgence of the child's longing for food, for holding, for rocking, for sleeping, etc. (3, 84, 91). The term "demand feeding" is an expression of this trend. If the mother is "motherly," showing tenderness and loving gentleness, such attempts to save suffering and to foster dependence in the early months of life have proved successful for the development of emotionally secure and outgoing babies, most of whom settle soon into self-imposed routines of feeding and sleeping. If demands are then made upon them slowly to postpone bodily pleasure and gradually to modify behavior according to social needs, a continuous healthy development ensues. Difficulties occur if the demand indulgence continues too long and adaptive habits are not encouraged. Enjoyment of physical pleasure then becomes the most important goal for the child, the relationship to the mother the means toward that goal; and the pleasure of object love for the mother and from her does not grow stronger. It is pleasure from such love for the mother rather than simple sensory pleasure which encourages him to postpone physical pleasure or give it up and to master his antisocial impulses, thus avoiding the mother's displeasure and increasing her affectionate behavior. Only within this framework of love, as she differentiates for him unacceptable and acceptable behavior, does he have a guide and the incentive for ego and superego development.

Unchallenged instinct gratification continuing into and beyond the training or "anal" period deprives the child of incentives for the formation of standards (superego) and of methods for behaving according to those standards (ego). It is an important cause for later symptoms in impulsive children whose lack of ego defense mechanisms exposes them to constant anxiety produced by environmental conflicts as well as by inner instinctual conflicts which they have not the skills to resolve. The condition is similar to that of a younger child to whom a too difficult task is given; the infant is unable to meet the task because of physical immaturity; the older impulsive child cannot meet the task fitted for his chronological years because of emotional immaturity.

Another discrepancy growing out of the tendency to rely upon indulging the infant as a prevention of later difficulties lies in the role played by the mother's actual love or hostility toward her child. If she loves him, her handling is likely to be tender, painless, and unfrightening; if she rejects him or is neurotically anxious about him, no amount of indulgence can prevent the handling of her child from being painful and threatening. She hurts him or frightens him by unconscious mishandling, due to various actions—the tightness of her muscles, the awkwardness of her movements, the querulousness of her voice. To aid mothers to a better relationship to their newborn infants, closer early contact with them is encouraged more and more in obstetrical hospitals, by the "rooming-in" projects, in which prenatal and postnatal education in baby care is offered (63). Such projects help in avoiding mishandling because of maternal anxieties due to strangeness or lack of knowledge and in nourishing biological maternal love in these mothers who do not have neurotic difficulties which produce defective "motherliness." Neurotic mothers, however, who reject their children either consciously or unconsciously cannot learn adequate techniques of loving care and may even reject their children more intensely if they are expected to care for the baby during the hospital period, when they long for relief from responsibility. For the babies of such mothers, neither "rooming in" nor "self-regulating feeding" will make infancy serene; only therapy for the mother to overcome her rejecting feelings for her child will answer his needs.

Since so many emotional difficulties have their beginning in disorders of the first months of life, it is important to recognize initial symptoms, that one may know when to undertake corrective measures early before the symptoms become too fixed, and also to recognize and to understand early causative factors in later disorders, even though, at first, they may seem quite unrelated. It is important also to be able to differentiate between behavior which is normal for the maturational level and that which warns of dysfunction.

Crying in the infant is the biological response to discomfort, the purpose of which is undoubtedly to cause changes which will relieve the discomfort. It presupposes a mother-child symbiosis such that she may respond to the cry. Crying is an early action in nonspecific relationship to secure someone in the environment to relieve the suffering and satisfy the infant, and only later is it directed toward a specific person, the mother. Crying, thus, is quite normal when it is a warning and stops when appropriate relief is offered, such as feeding, warmth, or other bodily need. It is also normal, and to be expected later, when the child not only cries to gain relief of discomfort but to indicate his longing for the repetition of pleasure. This occurs often when the child has enjoyed the warmth of being held, the pleasure of caressing and rocking, both for skin and muscle sensation, and later after specific object relationship to the mother has developed. The fear of loss of pleasure and comfort then develops in separation periods, and the baby cries to bring back the loved person.

It is only when crying occurs in the absence of discomfort or in the presence of the mother or when it is excessive that one may consider the crying as a problem which has symptomatic meaning. Soon after birth, it may be indicative of trauma, both psychic and physical, resulting from difficulties during birth or possibly during the intra-uterine period, leading to what one might term "anxious expectation." In most instances, with adequate care for the infant's bodily needs, this postpartum instability passes within the first or second week. When excessive crying continues, it indicates difficulties which should not be ignored. If physical pathology is ruled out, the "emotional climate" of the mother's attitude and behavior is usually found to be at fault and may result from a variety of neurotic attitudes: frank rejection of the child with roughness in handling; impatience and forced feeding; ignoring and neglecting its needs; excessive adherence to, or marked neglect of, routine. It is common knowledge that a very young infant may cry and appear irritable and uncomfortable in its mother's arms or in her presence but will quiet down almost immediately when picked up, caressed, and spoken to gently by an experienced motherly woman, even though she be strange. This is an indication that the mother's handling is causing discomfort to the child, that the cry is in response to this discomfort, and that the infant is striving for relief from the suffering rather than for the comfort of the mother's presence which occurs later. Kris (68, p. 33) names this early relationship "anaclitic" in differentiation from true "object" relationship, which develops slowly during the first months of life.

This early period is that of "primary narcissism," in which the world seems to be accepted by the child as an extended part of himself. It is understandable, then, that discomfort and pain, if not relieved, may produce intolerable anxiety, since he has not yet learned that he alone is not responsible for his safety and that pain may be relieved by another person. Unrelieved discomfort then may start a habit of expectant anxiety, in the presence of pain or suffering of any kind. Symptoms which develop to allay this anxiety are varied. Excessive crying has been mentioned. Autistic pleasures, such as thumbsucking, head rolling, rocking, rubbing, and so forth, are very common, as if the child tries to distract attention from pain by an excess of pleasure. The danger to normal development when excessive indulgence in autistic pleasure occurs is found in the realm of object relationship and of social adaptation. Such infants grow into children and adults who turn back to themselves at the slightest frustration and difficulty; burden themselves with the task of handling life's problems alone; distrust others; are constantly anxious, with many symptoms and with restricted pleasures and restricted realms of activities.

To prevent the development of such a state, one can recognize the value of the excessive indulgence of the young infant, mentioned above, which has been in vogue for the last few years, coining the term "demand" schedule or "self-regulating" schedule to mean feeding, sleeping, caressing at the first sign of wish from the infant. A cry, then, is an "alert" to the mother to busy herself in satisfying her baby's wishes or needs. This present-day change in infant care is in direct contrast to the previous rigid schedules of almost ritualistic routine, in which the child was expected to "cry it out" and continue to fight off his discomforts until the moment arrived for his feeding or play period or other pleasure.

This change in procedure is sound certainly for the first three or four months of life. Like so many partial truths, however, it has become accepted by many physicians and parents as an essential preventive measure for later ills. To relieve early anxiety and thus to prevent severe trauma to a sensitive organism, avoidance of discomfort is essential, and the serene and healthy development of most "demand" babies substantiates the value of it. On the other hand, it is certainly not a "prevent-all," as one can recognize by the fifth or sixth or later month when the baby, now differentiating itself from his mother, is influenced by many subtle situations in this relationship. The "climate" or atmosphere produced by the mother's attitudes, in her affection, her rejection, her anxieties, her distractibilities, or even her absences becomes as essential in producing or relieving anxiety as body discomfort or its relief had been previously.

Since eating is one of the essential activities in infancy, there is need for warning that discomfort in this sphere is the most common cause of crying. However, other symptoms of feeding difficulties begin to arise early and are forewarnings of more difficult problems to come if relief is not forthcoming. The most common early symptoms are food refusal and vomiting. In both instances, if the child is physically well, the symptoms represent defense mechanisms against feeding discomfort (36). Such avoidance of an instinctual pleasure surely indicates suffering of intensity. Roughness of a mother, forced feeding beyond satiety, or too fast feeding may cause conflict between the wish for pleasure in eating and the wish to avoid suffering, in which the latter often wins out. Only by alleviating the environmental cause of the conflict—the mishandling of the child—can the symptom be resolved.

If the symptom has become fixed through automatic repetition and the mishandling occurs at the hand of the mother who cares for the child, the dawning object relationship to her becomes associated with the symptom. In such cases the first object love is ambivalent. The negative side shows up in hostility provoked by discomfort at feeding and by the consequent narcissistic suffering involved in self-denial of the satisfaction of eating. The reactive and defensive nature of this hostility becomes evident when one observes and treats such an infant. If treated in the first few months of life by substituting for the mother (or nurse) at feeding times a nursing person who is relaxed and gentle, sensitive to the baby's indications of sufficiency, one who holds him caressingly and speaks or sings gently, the symptom seems to disappear like melting ice.

As an example, a baby boy of six months entered the children's ward of a hospital with the tentative diagnosis of pylorospasm for the consideration of surgery. Since the diagnosis could not be confirmed with x-rays, the pediatrician suggested further observation on the ward in a warm emotional climate. The baby did not vomit after admission, ate and slept well, and gained weight until normal for age. He has continued well since return home under the mother's care, who, during the child's hospitalization, was given some psychotherapeutic insight into the child's conflicts and into her own attitudes and behavior which produced them and has received continued supportive and advisory aid from a social worker. The symptoms in this case were arrested during their developmental stage before fixation into a habitual defense occurred and before true object love or hostility toward the mother was well established and before the anxious attitude toward the mother who forced the food was generalized into an anxious attitude toward all people. One may hope that the early correction of this pathology may prevent further feeding difficulties.

In some instances, vomiting may occur initially as a physiological reaction to a disturbed organic condition, such as pyloric stenosis or other obstructive conditions, allergic sensitiveness to certain foods, and the like. If the organic condition is allowed to continue for months, so that vomiting is the usual sequence to food intake, an infant protects himself from the experienced discomfort by refusal to eat at all or to eat more than a minimal amount. Even if the organic condition is relieved later, an anxious expectation may be maintained and feeding continue to be invested with anxiety. This pattern of reaction to feeding and its associated experiences as to a danger is similar to the pattern produced by the rejecting mother already described. In both instances, if the baby is still within the first year of age, prevention of later neurosis with food symptoms or various symptoms derived from the "intaking" process is possible. In the one instance, correction of the organic condition must be accompanied by sensitive care in feeding, such that the child is allowed to eat at his own speed, with his own measure of quantity, and with accompanying pleasurable experience, such as tender words and caresses. In the second, similar feeding care by a motherly person may relax the baby sufficiently that the neurotic pattern is given up in favor of acceptance of food, a pattern more fitting to the "corrected" experience. Rarely does this approach fail in the early months. However, if symptoms persist in spite of physical therapy and convincingly adequate environmental change, the neurosis probably has already become integrated into the developing personality. In this case continued alertness must be used to avoid further trauma and to maintain pleasant feeding conditions. Psychotherapy may later be necessary to resolve the conflicts producing the neurotic attitude.

Thumbsucking, previously so offensive to many mothers, has become respectable in recent years. Levy's (70, 71) study of the relation between thumbsucking in infants and the length of the interval between feedings led him to conclude that sucking in itself represented a pleasure entity for which the infant strove. If insufficient satisfaction was obtained in the feeding periods, the child sucked at other times, fingers, lips, tongue, etc. The fact that babies on four-hour schedules sucked their thumbs or fingers almost universally and that those fed more frequently or whenever restless did not seek accessory sucking, he explained as due to a sucking need. This confirms Freud's description of the mouth as an erotic zone.

One does not question that stimulation of the lip and mouth mucous membrane is associated with pleasure. For the infant, it is undoubtedly the area where most pleasure is obtained, although recent studies indicate the importance of skin, muscle, and joint sensations as essential in the production of satiety reactions of the infant. Certainly, the infant may suck his thumb if he experiences insufficient pleasure in sucking at feeding. However, he sucks his thumb also for substitute pleasure when other pleasures are lacking or for solace when anxious if alone and separated from a loved person, or when actually in pain. The author has seen an eight-month-old infant, previously not a thumbsucker, suck his thumb so violently that it was cut by his teeth when he was suffering intense pain from an acute appendicitis. Following the operation, he returned to his nonthumbsucking status and did not resume the habit. Extra-feeding sucking, thus, may not always be a benign autoerotic indulgence but may be a warning that all is not well and that the child is attempting to allay the distress of undesirable experiences. The admonition so common nowadays, to let the child suck his thumb as much as he seems to wish, is certainly wise in helping a mother to overcome her own fears that sucking is evil, but if the baby is no longer a small infant and still using thumbsucking as the only pleasure in waking life, one would be as remiss to omit searching for dissatisfactions in his life which encourage the habit as to ignore vomiting or other obvious symptoms. The solution is not to let the habit continue late into latency any more than to prevent it forcefully, but to correct the cause.

Sleep disturbance often observed in early infancy is rarely or perhaps never an isolated symptom. As in later years and in adulthood, it is an indication of anxiety. The anxiousness may be from physical pain, and then sleeplessness is usually accompanied by crying; or the child may be sleepless or an excessively light sleeper because he is on his guard against an environment which has been made frightening by a neglectful, cruel, or rejecting parent. Later, sleep disturbances may be more severe or be accompanied with terrifying dreams because the dangers have been internalized. But, in general, they have their beginnings in anxious insecurity of these early months. Hence it is important to attempt to unearth the causes for the restlessness early and to relieve them before the symptom becomes habitual in order that internalization of the danger may be prevented.

### PROBLEMS OF THE "ANAL" OR TRAINING PERIOD (LATE INFANCY)

The influence of experiences in infancy upon the development of the "normal" personality and upon the kind and character of later disorders has been discussed. The child's reaction to bowel training will in part depend upon his reactions to people, especially the mother or nurse, which have become habitual in infancy. Symptoms developing in the anal period will partake of elements of symptoms which developed out of oral problems.

As the months bring maturation of the neuromuscular system, such that the anal and urethral sphincters can be voluntarily controlled, the anal phase is ushered in. At the same time, purposive activity of the skeletal muscles becomes gradually more co-ordinated into grasping, pushing, crawling, and walking. Therefore, not only is the child asked to control his excretory activities at the mother's behest, but self-expression in all aggressive[2] activity is encouraged or prohibited, as the child is taught

2. "Aggressive" is used here to mean "physically active" rather than hostile destructive aggression as is the frequent connotation in psychoanalytic literature in which aggression is used as a direct translation from the German (62).

not to touch dangerous objects or to break precious ones and to walk and crawl in circumscribed areas for his own protection.

The emotional conflicts which develop in the anal period are inherent in the prohibition and direction of the child's excretory and muscular activity which the parent as the surrogate of society imposes.

If the object relation to the mother is a pleasurable loving one, the child easily solves the conflict between his instinctual wish for free self-expression and his dependent wish for his mother's love, by modifying his activity according to the mother's demand. He defecates on the toilet and, later, urinates there instead of on the spot where the urge arises. Also, gradually he controls his grasping, walking, and other actions to accord with the permission of the mother. This is the first sign of ego development, and it represents a part of the ego described by Hartmann as "nonconflictual" (60). It is concerned with the development of adaptive skills rather than with defense against instinctual drives. The heightened pleasure which the child feels in response to his loved mother's approval of his action makes the choice of substitute outlets fairly easy. His wish to avoid her disapproval intensifies the wish to conform.

However, if the relationship to the mother has not been satisfactory either because of neglect, which intensified the need for narcissistic autistic pleasures, or because of suffering at the mother's hand, which transformed normal self-preservative aggressiveness into hostile destructive aggression toward the mother, added problems may begin to show in this training period. Negativism and stubbornness against suggestion and direction are common. The so-called "temper tantrum" becomes a reaction at each point of minor or major frustration, and the need to maintain one's will seems to be the child's concept of maintaining his integrity. He may remain incontinent and stubbornly refuse to be trained. This incontinence may be preceded by constipation, by which the child refuses to part with the product of his body until forced by physiologic bowel reflex. Playing with the stool and smearing is a common sequela in these children, who not only express hostility and rage against the unloving or severe parent by refusal to conform but actually attack with the "dirty" feces. The excreta thus become invested with value as a personal creation which affords power to ward off danger and also become an instrument of attack against the love object who has become ambivalently hated.

Less common, but sometimes beginning in this early training period, is the attempt at solution of the feared dangers by an excessive conforming obedience, in contradistinction to the aggressive temper and stubbornness. This occurs usually when the positive arm of the ambivalence toward the parent outweighs the negative hostility. The wish to maintain the love fosters conformity, but, to overcome the ever resurging hostile element of the ambivalence, the nascent ego strengthens the process of conformity so that the child may ritualize toilet activities, aggressive play, dressing, and all the other routines of life. Then, like a full-blown adult compulsion neurotic, he becomes anxious and upset if the ritual is disturbed.

In this training period one observes a dawning conscience or superego. The child with a loving dependent relation to his mother begins to differentiate "right" and "wrong" according to the mother's designation of acceptance or disapproval of his behavior. He usually can conform in the parents' presence and occasionally when alone. It has been suggested that the parent and his standards have not been truly integrated into the child's personality at this tender age, but ease of hallucinatory experiences due to his lack, as yet, of adequately differentiating reality from fantasy, brings the mother's image to him to aid in controlling his action. In those children showing exaggerated compulsive conformity, the superego seems to have a true, if precocious, existence, and in many instances the child behaves as if these standards of behavior were a separate part of himself, the parent introjected but not yet integrated. A fairly typical example of this condition was exhibited by John, a boy of twenty-six months about whom the author was consulted. He was an only child of successful parents, both of whom were perfectionistic, fairly rigid, serious persons, who believed that, with consistent discipline, one could train a child early and well. In general, John was a very obedient, friendly, serious, and undernourished child, who had been somewhat of a feeding problem from the time of the introduction of semisolid food, when he began to be fussy about the new foods and spit them out when they were forced into his mouth. He was trained for bowel control by seven months and for day wetting by ten months; he was overly clean, insisting upon hand washing with even small amounts of soiling, and had begun to be anxious at bedtime if his toys were not in a particular arrangement which he had contrived. I visited him in his own home, and, at first, he did not know anyone was there when from the hall I observed him in the family living-room where small breakable objects were placed on a low coffee table. He started to reach with his right hand for a glass dish—drew back, reached again—drew back, reached again several times until, finally, with a quick grab he picked up the dish and crashed it to the floor. He looked startled, began to cry, then with his left hand he slapped his right hand very hard, saying "Bad Johnny! Bad Johnny!"

This self-punishment indicated a precocious conscience which denied misbehavior, but a weak ego which could not control impulsive behavior. The solution then was a compromise which demanded punishment for the unacceptable act. Most children in these years can avoid disobedience when in the presence of the disciplinarian but show no sign of compunction when alone. It is as if the presence of the loved, training adult acted as both the ego and the superego. This indicates that the child as yet had not accepted as his own the standards and behavior demanded by the parents; or, in psychodynamic terms, there was a minimal internalization of the parental commands to form the superego or conscience. When the training has been too severe and too rigid for the child's maturational level, as occurred in Johnny's case, the fear of punishment and of loss of love produces control of impulsive behavior by inhibiting and punishing it before skills can be developed to express the wishes in substitute or sublimated activities. Punitive control at this stage initiates ritualistic regulation of sufficient strength for nascent compulsive symptoms, such as excessive cleanliness, orderliness, and routinization of play and toy arrangements. If the routinization is disturbed, anxiety symptoms—crying, muscle tenseness, and other symptoms—appear and indicate the fearful need for self-control which the parent has created in the infant.

Sleeping difficulties (18, 31) are not very common at this age, but they appear quite frequently in markedly conforming children. These children exhibit fear of going to bed and of being left alone and frequent wakeful crying during the night. Sometimes true night terrors occur, with dreams of injury, particularly from animals—bears and lions or tigers which eat or squeeze them. In sleep, the child is away from the protection of parental admonition, and impulses are uncontrolled by reality reminders. The superego, even though precocious, is too weak to function entirely alone, and fear that misbehavior can break through in sleep creates wakefulness or clinging to the parents in order to guard against sleep temptations. Punishment dangers then appear in the hallucinatory dream creation when sleep is yielded to.

The integration of symptoms carried over from maladjustment in the oral-dependent phase into training-period symptoms may determine the method of the resistance against training or the form of expression of hostility against the parent, or even the direction of rituals that the precocious superego takes for controlling impulses. The mouth and eating then become the areas of hostility, with malicious biting of the mother or substitute figures and objects, even biting, chewing, and swallowing toys, blankets, clothes, and all manner of objects. Feces may be eaten at this time, an indication that the continued and exaggerated investment in oral pleasure has become fused with the narcissistic meaning of the feces, the child's first "creative" production. In eating his stool, the child integrates several pleasures: eating, defying the mother whose disgust he stubbornly resists, keeping by ingestion his creative product for himself, avoiding the sense of loss which all children feel at first in the training period when they must comply with bowel control, but which deprived and severely controlled children feel severely.

A symptom one sees occasionally is interesting because it integrates eating, associated nursing movements, destructiveness, and self-punishment, that is, the twisting of hair clumps (associated with nursing), pulling the hair out (destructive and painful), chewing and swallowing it (eating). If this symptom becomes habitual, it continues into latency and may be the most noticeable symptom of a severe autistic compulsive neurosis.

### PROBLEMS OF THE "OEDIPAL" OR SEXUAL PERIOD

The oedipal period (beginning around three and lasting roughly until six years of age) is characterized by a turning of the developing sexual impulses toward the parent of the opposite sex and by an increase in sexual curiosity. Behavior difficulties which begin at this time grow out of the child's incapacity to deal with the conflicts, both environmental and instinctual, which are created by the increase in sexual impulses. The capacity to develop acceptable methods for handling the conflicts of this period is directly related to the emotional security with which the child enters this stage. If the experiences of the dependent (oral) and training (anal) periods have been wholesome and healthy and a minimum of symptoms has developed, the child meets the new conflicts with ease and with adaptive reactions. If he has been deprived, rejected, neglected, rigidly trained, or the like, his insecurity increases the problems of adaptation. Feelings of castration fear, penis envy, inferiority, and rivalry are complicated by exaggerated rage, stubbornness, dependent longing, and greed (4, 61).

Disturbing environmental experiences occurring at this time may further complicate adequate solution of oedipal conflicts, and thus aid the causation of symptoms. The birth of a sibling which may produce dependent rivalry for the mother adds to the total rivalrous feelings created by the triangular oedipal jealousy (see chap. iv) and intensifies rivalry to neurotic proportions. If the father is unusually punitive, cruel, or, in reverse, seductive toward the child, fears and exaggerated sex feelings are intensified and problems to solve are increased. Inconsistency in training and too rigid training cause trouble for the child also, for he needs help from the parent in restricting direct expression of his instincts and in guiding their expression into acceptable methods of action. That is, he needs his parents to offer superego standards and ego training. Many other experiences, familial or extra-familial, to which the child may be exposed can add to the production of neurotic symptoms. Among those most commonly found are seductive experiences, such as introduction to fellatio or sodomy; adult genital exposures; genital tampering; primal scene exposure; cruelty from other children or adults; exposure to accidents and death; and the loss by death or long absence of a loved one, such as mother, father, sibling, nurse.

The genital sensations turn the child's interest toward the pleasure he experiences in this area. Masturbation begins often as a result of exploration and may then be repeated, from time to time, by any normal child for the autistic pleasure itself, or as a momentary solace, when lonesome, bored, or in pain. Masturbation may become excessive and take on all the characteristics of a compulsive neurotic habit. In this case, it serves the purpose of allaying anxiety which may stem from a variety of causes. Frequently the rejected or neglected child who has solved his fear of insecurity and discomfort by various infantile autistic pleasures, such as thumbsucking and fecal smearing, will turn to masturbation as a more satisfactory solace. The average mother finds it often more difficult to sanction masturbation than other autistic indulgences, but the rejecting mother is likely to be extremely incensed with the child for the act. This increased rejection intensifies his need for masturbation to relieve his fear, and as a result he stubbornly continues to indulge himself.

In other instances, compulsive masturbation may result from a fear of injury; persistent handling of the genitals is a reassurance of their intactness. This fear may result from threats of injury, which parents and nurses so frequently offer if the child is seen to handle himself, or from some traumatic experiences, such as fellatio or rough play with the child's genitals by another child or adult; or from the poor reasoning of a little boy who first sees a girl and thinks her injured; or from an expectation of retaliation from the father whom he wishes to displace in his mother's exclusive love.

A little girl also may masturbate compulsively for reassurance, but with less evidence to comfort her. She, too, becomes more interested in her genitals with increasing hormonal production. Exploration of the area discloses that she has less than her brother or little boy playmate. Repetitious compulsive handling of her genitals seeks for the missing penis. Since it is never found, excessive masturbation may continue because the pleasure offers some relief from the anxiety which arises from the feelings of inferiority and envy. As has been described previously, under healthy conditions for normal feminine development, these feelings are fleeting and are resolved in the little girl by an identification with her mother, who accepts the advantages of feminine love and maternity. Penis envy and inferiority feelings, however, may become intense and obvious symptoms in the little girl who is already disturbed in her relationship to her mother (4, 61). Insecurity which was initiated in the oral-dependent phase and continued into the training period expresses itself in the oedipal stage through an added despair of personal inadequacy. Oral envy or deprivation thus reinforces penis envy or feeling of genital incompleteness. The person she has turned to for love, that is, herself, when she was unloved or rejected by her mother, thus is believed to be an injured or imperfect person, unworthy of love. Despair develops again when her dawning sexual feelings long for love from her father. She who was unloved by her mother now finds herself unlovable, and in her childish reasoning must be completely incapable of competing for her father's love.

These feelings of unworthiness and these fears of injury may get out of bounds and lead to the exaggeration of other activities, normal for the age in mild form but presenting disturbing symptoms when intensified, as "peeping," exhibiting of genitals, "tomboy" behavior of girls, or "sissy" behavior of boys, and excessive rivalry and jealousy. These symptoms are usually part of an attempt to deny the knowledge of genital anatomy and to get reassurance that all is not as inadequate or as dangerous as experience has seemed to indicate. The peeper keeps looking and looking compulsively, after he has seen enough to know the facts, because of the persistent wish to find evidence to assure him that he is not injured or inferior. Similarly the child persistently exposes his genitals as if to say, "See, I am all right, adequate, and uninjured." But his belief to the contrary discredits reassurance, so that the act is continued again and again.

Denial of genital facts is carried even further in fantasy when the little girl insists that she has a penis, acts like a "tomboy," and refuses to accept her feminine status. The roots of later serious masculine identification are seen in her excessive aggressiveness, her competitive hostility toward boys, and even in attempts to urinate like a boy. As one little four-year-old girl confided to her therapist, "I am sure I have a 'peenie,' for I can make my 'wee wee' go straight into the toilet like Johnny does—if I stand close and pull my skin tight in front." The little boy denies his feelings of inadequacy by fantasying himself with enormous genitals to match his father's, bragging of strength and bigness, and, like the girl, expressing his fantasied exaggerated masculinity in excessive aggressiveness and competitive hostility, a forewarning of aggressive, destructive behavior problems in years to come. His denial, when fear of injury is excessive, may take the opposite form, and he fantasies himself a girl with no penis to be injured. Concomitantly, he gives up masculine aggressiveness; becomes passive, shy, and feminine, a "sissy" who is afraid of all boyish activities and prefers a feminine role. As a boy of five and one-half shyly said to his mother, as he tucked his penis between his legs, "See, mom, I look just like Mary!" When questioned further he answered, "I do it when I am afraid at night, or when Dad scolds me, or any old time."

Anxiety symptoms may begin to be excessive at this period, with repetitious nightmares and fear of the dark, of new situations, and of strange persons. Phobias with special objects to fear may arise to displace the more generalized anxiety. Anxiety is always in evidence when conflicts are not yet solved. It is, therefore, present always in one form or another during childhood, a period of continuous need for new solutions of new problems. Anxiety may become excessive in the oedipal period when circumstances historical and present make an acceptable solution impossible. The anxiety produces protection against danger of injury or punishment by creating a wariness which aids in the avoidance of dangers. This wariness may be so intense that the child becomes more and more withdrawn and autistic, with regression to thumbsucking, fecal play, and such. More common, however, is the allaying of free-floating fearfulness by the production of symptoms, which, if they offer some comfort by partial solution of the conflict or conflicts, become habitual. In latency one finds these symptoms organized and integrated into the personality as habits of living, so that the conflicts are allayed in part by repression and in part by other defense mechanisms involved in the symptom formation. Further healthy development, however, is handicapped by the fact that much energy must be expended in maintaining the symptom, energy which should be available for the development of adaptive skills, and by the fact that the symptom itself interferes with normal behavior.

These neurotic symptoms which begin to show embryonic organization in the oedipal period become obvious handicaps in the latency period. Phobias and compulsive rituals are early symptoms. Pathological motor activities, such as stammering and tics, may begin. Some autonomic symptoms commonly arise early, such as asthma, enuresis, constipation, colitis, and a variety of feeding difficulties, such as food sensitivity and aversion, neurotic vomiting, and anorexia, as well as bulimia with obesity. Indications of some unacceptable behavior symptoms are often found at this time, such as sadistic cruelty and masochistic submission, uncontrollable stealing and lying, insatiable demanding with concomitant selfishness.

### Problems of the "Latency" Period

The term "latency," originally used to delineate those years between the sexual period of the oedipal phase and the sexual maturation of adolescence, assumed that sex impulses remained latent during this time. Freud (44) described the period as one in which the recession of instinctual drives is accompanied by the consolidation of the superego; and Anna Freud (33, 35) elaborated this description by emphasizing the role of ego development in which the ego gradually assumes superiority, directing the behavior of the child according to the exigencies of reality, while the sex drives remain latent. The study of neurotic manifestations in these years, between about six and twelve, indicates that there is not truly a recession of sex impulses at this time (23), but an increasing tendency toward their repression, with renunciation of erotic activity. This change results from the gradual strengthening of the ego, which directs sexual energy into substitute and sublimated channels according to the behest of the superego, which becomes increasingly organized, and of the environment, which makes increasing demands for conformity to social rules.

Latency, then, may be considered for practical purposes as that period in which the child develops standards of behavior, which he accepts as his own (superego) and in which he gradually develops skills, mental and physical, to serve the purpose of adaptation (ego). This process passes through various experimental attempts, so that symptoms may occur transiently and then give place to more adequate behavior. Only when a symptom remains fixed in spite of its adaptive inadequacy do we consider the condition pathological in childhood. It is an indication that the ego can find no solution more satisfactory and that the repetition compulsion has crystallized the symptom into a habitual reactive pattern, more or less permanent.

Just as neuroses in adults have their origin in unsolved—or one might say "mis-solved"—conflicts in childhood, so do the neurotic and behavior problems of latency stem from prelatency conflicts. One will find the same neurotic constellations in childhood as in adulthood. Analyzing the dynamic structure of the childhood conditions, one finds the same causative conflicts, the same defense mechanisms involved, the same standards enforced as are known to occur in comparable adult neuroses. Various differences, however, are disclosed when one compares, in detail, similar neuroses of different age periods. These differences are directly related to the stage of maturation of the individual, which, grossly, is related to his chronological age. Hence, in the adult, the neurosis is much more firmly integrated into the character of the patient; and the younger the child, the less fixed has it become as a mode of reaction. In the young child both ego and superego are still influenced by the behavior of the parents and others in the environment, so that a change of environment may modify the strength or kind of superego-ego actions. The older the child, the firmer is the character pattern, the less influence has the environment in changing it, and the closer is the total neurotic constellation to that of the adult. This variation is significant both in the prognosis and the responsiveness to therapy and in the modification of treatment techniques to fit the needs of the particular age, as well as the needs of the particular neurosis.

Just as the neurosis is less fixed in childhood, its dynamic pattern is less complicated by secondary defense mechanisms which may have developed to resolve secondary problems created by the neurosis itself. For that reason, the analysis of childhood symptoms can offer clarification as well as confirmation of the dynamic mechanisms involved in the production of the similar adult neuroses.

In childhood one finds in one form or another, or at one time or another, all the adaptive and defense mechanisms which are revealed in adults. These appear weaker and more vulnerable, however, in the nascent forms of childhood, and, as the neurosis progresses, one or another mechanism may be displaced or complicated by more efficient mechanisms, or at least more adequate to the solution of the problems. This change occurs as needs vary according to problem changes during maturation and as the integrative capacity of the ego is strengthened through education as well as through growing ability to adapt both mentally and physically. Symptoms may therefore be transient or may be replaced or enhanced by other symptoms; mechanisms may change; and superego standards vary so that latency displays a slow kaleidoscopic change, but always with inherent trends traceable to early infancy which form the framework within which the variations are built.

The earliest mechanisms observed are denial and inhibition, which show in the prelatency period in lying and in control of impulsive activity, particularly in the presence of adults. A small child may raid a prohibited candy box when no one is around but never touch it during a parent's presence, or innocently insist he had not touched it later when evidence of a candy-smeared mouth reveals the act.

Repression which progresses from denial and inhibition may

be observed first in the oedipal period, as destructive impulses and sexual impulses are found to be unacceptable to the child, since they are incompatible with each other and are unacceptable to those whose love he wishes to maintain. In latency, repression becomes increasingly firm and forms the basis from which other mechanisms form and then produce neurotic solutions of the repressed instincts, feelings, and superego standards.

Projection also begins early, at first as conscious lying, i.e., "Johnny broke the chair, not I," and later as true projection seen so commonly in latency, when the child, already guilty from the pressure of his standards of behavior, never lets himself feel responsible for fights, sex play, or other misbehavior and really believes "Johnny started it!" or "Johnny made me do it!" Re-action formation—a frequent defense against hostility and un-requited love—is typical of the late oedipal and early latency periods, either as a normal phase of development or in exagger-ation as a symptom. The child then "adores" the rival siblings or "hates" the parents of the opposite sex. Substitution of activity or of objects occurs early at the behest of others, but only well into latency does it become a technique integrated into the personality and voluntarily accepted. It represents the effect of a fairly consistent and firm superego and an ego strong enough to enforce renunciation of intense wishes.

Sublimation occurs as an even later refinement of substitution and may indicate sturdy adjustment or a too restricted adaptation with many concomitant symptoms. Displacement, also, arises in the oedipal period, and at first it is seen in simple form, as when the little boy becomes fearful of losing a leg or a finger instead of a penis or indulges in nose boring instead of anal or genital play. One child of four, a nose-borer whenever he was anxious, said once, when fantasying smearing feces all over the world, "I have no bowel hole, none at all; I don't make 'B.M.' at all; if I had a hole, I'd push it back up." In latency, displacement becomes in-creasingly an important method of solving conflicts growing out of unacceptable body wishes, and forms an important part of all the autonomic symptoms of this period as well as of adulthood.

The use of a part for the whole, as seen in fetishism, is quite common in childhood both as a phase in normal development and also in problems of compulsive rituals. A little girl of seven, to ward off dangers of "murdering burglars" at night, took to bed with her a pine-needle pillow of her mother's; she said, "the small and firm feel of it makes me feel safe and cozy." Introjection—perhaps one of the earliest methods of solving the discomfort arising out of separation from the mother—becomes an important way in latency of solving and accepting the demands of the parents. It is responsible also for depressions seen frequently in late latency or preadolescence.

Causative factors in the emotional problems of latency are multiple. The same attitudes of parents which produced problems in infancy, if unchanged, continue to interfere with normal or adequate development: lack of love, neglect, rejection, cruelty, perfectionistic demand for good behavior, inconsistency, and the like. Added problems grow out of personal inadequacies of physical and mental ability, traumatic experiences, and, particularly important in latency, differences in moral and behavior demands between those of the parents and those of the larger environment into which the child enters at five or six. Finally, one should emphasize again the handicaps of earlier neurotic difficulties with which the child enters latency and which form the foundation on which he builds new habits to meet new experiences.

In this short chapter, it would be impossible to describe and discuss in detail all the problems and their kaleidoscopic configurations which occur in latency. An attempt will be made only to designate the more common difficulties, their general causes, and the more important dynamic factors involved in their organizations. As is well known, disorders do not occur in isolation, nor do they result from one cause. Any one child may present a variety of problems, any one of which may seem in the ascendancy at one time, another at another time, but all of which are interrelated and interdependent. For practical purposes, the psychic disturbances of childhood are classified here according to the realms of interference rather than according to classical symptom categories or even dynamic constellations. Groupings chosen are (1) infantile phenomena or marked developmental immaturity, (2) motor disorders, (3) conduct problems, (4) common neuroses, (5) vegetative disorders, and (6) psychoses.

Infantile phenomena include various mouth activities of thumb or finger or object sucking or biting, anal or urine incontinence, and excessive masturbation. Causes of these activities have been discussed earlier. If they continue into latency when the attitude of persons, such as parents, teachers, and friends, in the child's environment tends to disapprove and criticize, it usually indicates a marked insecurity in respect to love and protective needs and to self-esteem. He clings to old autistic pleasures for solace and stubbornly refuses to give them up for more mature satisfactions because he is afraid of loss or suffering. Sometimes incontinence continues not only from unwillingness to give up the pleasure of excretion at his own will but because there has not been sufficient incentive to control himself. Mothers who allow "self-regulation" of the excretions as they wisely allowed self-regulation of feeding earlier and offer no special approval as incentive for cleanliness may be responsible for prolonged incontinence, which, in turn, fixes pleasure-seeking at the anus and urethra. Such fixation then causes withholding of interest in the pleasure of substitute activities acceptable in latency, as play, learning, exploring. In reverse, incontinence may result from negativism, a defense against pressure from a too rigid, too demanding parent, in an attempt at survival and for self-esteem or narcissistic wishes. The conflict is simple instinct versus environment, with instinct conquering when environment offers no comparable gratification or when other gratifications are too dangerous because they are punished. Nocturnal enuresis, however, if not simple incontinence and not accompanied by diurnal wetting, is a conversion symptom and represents a substitute for masturbation. It may occur as a regressive phenomenon after training for cleanliness has been accomplished (7, 52, 53, 66).

Various infantile activities, such as thumbsucking, incontinence, or excessive masturbation, occur as regression phenomena in a child who may have achieved development up to his age expectation of five, six, seven, or older, when traumatic experiences are severe enough to break down his feeling of personal adequacy or his expectation of parental love and protection. Such trauma may be sudden loss of a loved parent through death or disaster, the birth of a sibling who monopolizes the mother's care and love, serious physical illness or operation, with separation from a mother by hospitalization. These regressions often cause sufficient disintegration of the still weak and insecure ego to retard development and to give access only to neurotic solutions, which build cramping symptoms rather than healthy adaptive techniques.

Motor disorders may occur as generalized: excessive purposeless activity, inhibition of movements, awkwardness, and repetitive organized, purposeless movements like rhythmic movements, tics, and stammering.

Hyperactivity often occurs as one phase of other serious difficulties in conduct or in neurosis. It is usually accompanied by lack of concentrated thought and always indicates an anxiety state in which the underlying fear is near the surface and is not resolved by organized symptom formation or goal-directed activity. One common cause of this excessive motion is inconsistency in training accompanied by cruelty and often neglect. The child is constantly afraid of his own instincts, the expression of which may bring punishment. He is afraid of suffering from deprivation or just from irrational, unexplained rage in a parent. He can learn no defense against this suffering either from precept or from experience, and he moves constantly, as if to move is to get away from suffering, partly to drain off unacceptable instinctual energy, and partly to avoid pain. Neurotic hyperactivity must be differentiated from that found in organic disorders, in which other signs of organic involvement will be found (10), and also from the hyperactivity often seen in epileptics (55), in which both the convulsive occurrences and electroencephalogram tracings will aid in the differential diagnosis.

Inhibitions of movements and awkwardness often result from fear of various instinct expressions in which the parental restrictions are consistent and firm, and inactivity is rewarded by various signs of acceptance. Such inhibitions may cause slowness in walking, in the use of hands in skills, and is usually accompanied by psychic withdrawal into fantasy when impulses may be surreptitiously indulged in autoerotic satisfactions. In extreme cases, such inhibitions may interfere seriously with social adjustment and reality adaptation.

Rhythmic movements of various kinds may result from movement restrictions in infancy (74). Such restriction interferes with more versatile movement and directs motor impulses into the one or more possible movements, such as rocking and head rolling. In latency the child may continue the habit for solace or to express, through displacement, new but unacceptable wishes like masturbation, so that erotic satisfactions become so combined with infantile muscle pleasures that the one movement expresses through condensation two primitive needs. Many so-called "bad habits" fall into this category, such as nail biting, ear pulling, hair twisting, nose boring, teeth grinding.

Tics are inappropriate movements similar to the rhythms mentioned above but are different, in that they are usually defined as fleeting spasms of small muscles representing a physiological unit movement, such as eye blinking, grimacing, tongue clicking, head jerking. Since psychotic mannerisms are often confused with tics, various dynamic explanations have been suggested (30, pp. 161–65). Those cases carefully analyzed in which the precipitating experience was known disclosed the tic as a part of an inhibited grosser defensive movement which occurs at a point of excessive trauma in children with fairly severe superegos, who are inhibited in large-muscle activity by restrictive but warm parents. The partial movement, then, later takes over the meaning of a defense in other anxious situations to which it is not appropriate (54). An example is that of the little boy with eye blinking initiated as a defense against seeing, first, an uncle with an empty eye socket and, second, a little girl's genitals with a slit instead of a penis. The blinking at first represented an attempt at denial of the unacceptable fearful knowledge, and later occurred whenever he was frightened. Stammering is probably a form of tic. It has been variously described as a displaced anal constipation (25, 26, 29), a partial inhibited obscenity of verbal hostile aggression. But, whatever the conflict may be against which stammering defends, the form of partial spasmic motion is ticlike.

Conduct problems cover a variety of difficulties which interfere with the child's social living both at home and in the larger world of school and neighborhood. Withdrawn behavior, in which the child avoids as much as possible relationship with persons, both adults and children, and acts more or less as an automaton, is a problem which one sees occasionally. When severe, it may be the precursor of a psychotic state, or, when only an occasional occurrence, it may indicate a tendency toward a fantasy solution of problems when a reality solution is too difficult. It has its roots in the autistic pleasures of infancy, intensified by deprivation of pleasure in the relationship to the mother. When analyzed, such children show a strong narcissistic tendency, with poor affective relation to others. They conform outwardly to demands made upon them but live in a rich fantasy life involved with both destructive activity and pleasurable indulgence. Such children are often described in such terms as "I can't seem to get close to him" or "nothing I do or say seems to affect him, but he's a good enough child." The superego in such children seems to be only a reflection of those in his environment at the time. His standards for reality behavior change from good, to bad, to indifferent as a chameleon changes his color. He is imitative but not creative except in his fantasies. Because so much energy is absorbed in autistic fantasies, skills develop slowly, and school achievement is far below ability. As causative, neglect is found to be the most pertinent factor. Levy called it "affect hunger" (73); Rabinovitch (78) described such cases as resulting from maternal deprivation; and one can believe that many of the deprived children described by B. Rank as "atypical" (79) continue to develop the autistic inaccessibility of these withdrawn children. In some cases, if the child is not allowed to withdraw into fantasy but some strong stimulus from the outside forces him to respond for protection, explosive destructiveness or sexual indulgence may break into action with all the energy previously used in fantasy creation. Such a child then changes from passivity to a severe impulsive behavior problem. When the defense is broken, the capacity for mastery is impaired. It is probable that some of the adult criminals described by Alexander belong to this category (6). When this occurs, anxiety reasserts itself, and the child becomes fearful of the consequences of his untamed impulses.

A withdrawn boy of ten, when attacked by a gang of boys who teased him by whipping him with ropes, calling him "sissy," "goody, goody," suddenly became violently aggressive, kicking, punching, and screaming. At home, later, and until taken into a protective institution for treatment after several months, he hit at everyone who came near him, had screaming nightmares, and evidenced excessive sweating and palpitation at sounds or movements. Previously fairly moderate in eating, he began to eat excessively and wolfishly, and soiled and wet himself occasionally. This extreme regression occurred in a child when his only defense was broken, because he could depend in no way for help and comfort upon parents who had always neglected him and given only necessary routine care, without love.

Aggressive conduct disorders range from those mild ones of disobedience and stubbornness to more serious delinquencies. The dynamic factors in the milder disorders are similar to those in the delinquencies, with similar, if more exaggerated, symptoms. It is pertinent, therefore, to outline some of the more common delinquent symptoms, with the psychodynamics involved, and say only for the less extreme symptoms that they may occur as reactions to a provocative environment; but if they remain untreated or if conditions continue to provoke the child, these milder symptoms may be only the precursors to the development of delinquent character and delinquent behavior.

Delinquencies may occur as a result of the pleasure-seeking of children incapable of controlling a wish to steal, to burn, to destroy, and in some instances to kill. The impairment of ego control may or may not be accompanied by a rigid or corruptible superego. In the case of the rigid superego, the delinquency is likely to be followed by self-punishment, either in depressive phenomena or in self-destructive activities, such as observed in the child who always stumbled, hit his head, or was otherwise hurt when he beat his little sister. More often, however, the child's standards are corruptible, and consequent behavior is likely to be directed toward avoidance of punishment and continued delinquency. Lack of superego patterns altogether is most unusual.

Delinquencies from neurotic reasons are fairly frequent (6, 46, 64). Stealing may be compulsive, a defense against the feeling of deep oral deprivation, when the object stolen is only a symbol for the love wished from the mother. It may occur also as an attempt to obtain objects to substitute in a symbol for the longed-for penis in the case of the little girl, or the more potent father's penis in the case of the little boy. One boy who stole fountain pens for this purpose had accumulated 113 before he was apprehended. The delinquent act had become the means of allaying temporarily the anxiety created by the oedipal conflict.

Destructive cruelty, such as beating a playmate or a dog, may similarly express destructive wishes toward a sibling, a father, or a mother. The satisfaction of the act then fuses the cruelty with love wishes which may also be directed toward the same pattern, and a sadist is born.

Sexual delinquency is rarely serious in the latency period, except as it may indicate a method of solving conflicts and allaying anxiety which, if maintained, may cause serious consequences in adolescence or adulthood. Peeping may be the normal result of unanswered questions, or it may be a compulsive and repetitive method of attempting to overcome a castration fear. The same may be true for exhibitionism and other perverted activity. The dynamics are similar to those of the adult perverts' exhibitionism and peeping, sodomy, and fellatio. In the child, however, the erotic drive is less intense, and, through wholesome education or through adequate treatment, the symptoms are less malignant than of those of the adult in whom the perversions have become a fixed pattern.

Under common neuroses are included the various neurotic constellations which are described under adult neuroses: phobias, compulsions, hysterical phenomena, learning inhibitions, etc. The description of symptoms and dynamic analysis need not be repeated in this chapter. It should be mentioned, however, that in the latency period symptoms may occur transiently as temporary methods of problem solving, but may be discarded in favor of more adequate methods when and if they become available. An example of a transient neurotic symptom is the compulsive avoidance of cracks in a sidewalk entered into by many children at a time when conflicts involving hostility versus tender feelings for a mother are being solved. This crack-jumping is accompanied by a revealing poem, "If you step on a crack, you will break your mother's back." Such experimental solutions, however, may remain permanent and a childhood compulsion neurosis develop, quite similar to that in the adult.

Disturbances of the vegetative functions (5) are also found in childhood. Allergic disorders occur and exhibit various manifestations at different times, disclosing the same mechanisms of causation as have been found in adults. Change in symptoms with change in maturation levels is particularly interesting and probably due to changes in the problems the child must solve. The change from eczema to asthma is an example. Although the majority of the vegetative symptoms investigated have been found to have their onset most commonly at adolescence or later, still instances are unearthed quite frequently in any large pediatric practice or clinic. One sees ulcerative colitis, diabetes, asthma, skin disorders, alopecia areata, rheumatoid arthritis, hyperthyroidism, and duodenal ulcer.

The psychoses, like the organic disorders with emotional etiology, are less common in childhood than among adolescents and adults. However, cases with classical symptoms disclosing severe pathological ego defects, disorientation to reality and delusional life have been described and analyzed. They show mechanisms similar to those of adults (8, 28, 50, 51), and have been described as occurring in children with basically disturbed relationship to the mother (76). Whether or not these conditions represent lack of development beyond primary narcissism or regressive phenomena is not yet clear. However, accuracy in diagnosis and analysis of the total development of the child may aid in better understanding of the conditions described by various authors and lead to a more accurate differential diagnosis between psychoses and organic brain symptoms, a subject still confused in the literature.

## TREATMENT

Psychoanalytic treatment of children, like that of adults, is based on the uncovering of the unconscious psychic conflicts which, in the ego's attempt at solution, are responsible for the development of the symptoms. The more mature ego is capable of finding more adequate methods of adaptation. Anxiety initiated in infancy is easily resolved after it is disclosed and recognized as inherent in the infant's incapability of avoiding suffering but as no longer appropriate to the abilities and facilities for adaptation accessible to the mature human being. The child's ego is still in the making, and the younger the child, the less fixed the patterns and the less secure the standards to guide him. It is this difference in ego capacity which is responsible for an important difference between the technique of child analysis and that for adults. The analyst must not only aid the patient in resolving the unconscious conflicts which cause difficulty, but he must educate the child in methods of adaptation for use of the free energy in skills and social life. The child's superego, unlike that of the adult's, has not arrived at true independence and still relies upon adult guidance and precept. He cannot find more acceptable standards of behavior methods of adaptation without help. The analyst may be called upon to set standards and goals.

Anna Freud (37) discusses the importance of the analyst in education of the child's ego during the analytic process and describes various educational aids. By her honesty, her consistency, her understanding of the child's wishes, and by offering him acceptable ways of satisfaction she temporarily functions as a parent, a wise parent in lieu of the unwise real ones. Therefore, as the pathological patterns are broken down and the impulses freed from repression, re-education into healthy expressions and standards takes place. The educational process is improved by manipulation of school, home, and recreational facilities, to create new impressions and new outlets for the child and to revise the demands made upon him by the outside world. Often the parents are encouraged to seek treatment for themselves, so that they no longer have the original neurotic attitudes toward the child and may create more easily a new home environment. At times, "collaborative therapy" of two analysts, one for parent, one for child, is recommended (65, 95).

Another significant difference between the child and the adult which influences the technique of treatment is the difference in mode and capacity of communication. Free association in the sense of adult analysis is impossible to the child except in late latency, when verbal facility is advanced. When the child recognizes suffering as coming from internal rather than external circumstances, his therapeutic wish may be sufficiently great to aid him in co-operation with the analyst. Most children and particularly those with emotional problems distrust adults as a result of past experience and therefore refuse the confidences inherent in verbally free associative activity. Not only the fear of adults but also the child's fear of his own impulses which have been "tamed" so recently and with such difficulty offer another resistance to free speaking which might easily uncover those wishes he fears. For most children, however, the analyst unravels the elements of the neurotic constellation as they are revealed in the child's play or verbal and pictorial fantasies, in his attitudes toward the analyst, the parents, other adults, children, animals, and the like.

Different also is the role of the analyst in the psychoanalytic process. Although Melanie Klein (67) contends that the relationship to the child analyst is that of a transference neurosis similar to the transference of the adult, the experience of most analysts has shown that it is only in part a transference neurosis and is also in part a new realistic relationship, as described by Anna Freud (37). This difference is due to the fact that, in general, children in treatment are still living with and reacting to their own parents and have not yet such fixed patterns of reaction that they transfer them to each new person. The younger the child, the less fixed the pattern and therefore the weaker the transference neurosis.

It has been shown that this new relationship must be one in which the analyst is found to be sympathetic, friendly, and useful, different from the destructive characteristics of the parents.

To be confidential, the child must have a minimum of hostile feelings toward the analyst. A positive, dependent relationship is the most auspicious for cure (37). To create this positive feeling in the child, it is not only essential that the analyst behave differently from the parents, but he must also like the child, since the child is dependent upon the feelings of adults in his environment for security and comfort and he is more sensitive than most adults to the actual feelings of other people. He senses intuitively and quickly ambivalence, rigidity, rejection on the part of the analyst. An introductory period for the development of this positive relationship is usually necessary in each child analysis. Anna Freud suggests that this period vary from one to several months, depending on the specific child's fear of persons. In this period the analyst makes himself as useful and necessary to the child as possible, as a good companion in play, as an aid in making equipment, models, dolls' clothes, or the like, and as a teacher of skills when the child so wishes. Once liking and confidence have been achieved, the little patient can confide more easily his fears and his attitudes and so work through feelings and conflicts which have developed through his relationship to his parents under whose influence he is still suffering. In the framework of this good relationship he avoids a major part of the transference neurosis and acts out his feelings toward the original objects upon whom he is still dependent.

Sickness insight on the part of the child, if it may be obtained, is an advantage in the progress of treatment. A very young child is incapable of such insight, for his intellectual capacity is not yet developed sufficiently to differentiate adequate and inadequate social techniques, or relative suffering. The older the child, however, the greater capacity he has to understand that his suffering stems from within and from unsuccessful behavior habits. His insight then creates a longing for change and a willingness to suffer the discomfort of further communication for the purpose of future happiness. To help the child to this sickness insight, a good relationship to the analyst is essential; for, before he is willing to face his weakness, he must know that, unlike the parents, the therapist will sympathize with rather than criticize his difficulties.

Sickness insight aids the child in understanding the relationship of the symptom to the conflict at its root, and in facing the original anxiety which grew out of it. As with the adult, to understand is the first step in the resolution of an infantile conflict and is the basis for viewing it as no longer pertinent to the present stage of development. Thus before the child's energy can be freed for use in adequate adaptation, interpretation is as essential as for freeing the adult. Direct interpretation may be possible in some instances if the evidence is clear, when, either because of his age or previous analytic aid, the child's ego has become sturdy enough to face the anxiety which he could not face at the time of the onset of the symptoms, and when his wish to get well is great enough to give him courage to view previously unaccept-able facts abou himself. This situation rarely occurs, and, until nearly the end of treatment, most children shy away from a direct interpretation until it has become palatable by indirect methods. The indirect methods used are many and varied and depend to some extent upon the skill and bent of the analyst, partly upon the interest of the patient. Sometimes a story may be used in which the situation of the patient is portrayed in the characters of the tale. In other instances a correlation is made between the child's fantasies and his own life, and yet again a comparison between others' experiences and those of the patient, or a generalization that all children "feel that way sometimes" may introduce an interpretation. But, eventually, as in adult analyses, the interpretations will include explanation of origins and causes leading the child back to the forgotten traumas of earlier years and to the recognition of the present unreality of the anxiety.

The frequency of treatment periods and the duration of treat-ment tend to vary much more in recent years than when child analysis was first developed. The five periods a week has been modified, depending on the optimum frequency and also on the actual difficulties of time taken in transportation, taken out of school or out of other healthy activities. To maintain an optimum condition for a good relationship and analytic progress, the child must not give up so much that he feels deeply deprived. He must not sacrifice too much of companionship or suffer too much of ennui and discomfort, to make him dislike going to the treatment. Therefore, the optimum frequency is sometimes sacrificed for optimum co-operation. If not too infrequent, however, thorough analysis may be entered into even if the child is not seen daily. The author has found that at least twice a week is the minimum for progress. In general, one finds that the young child progresses better, the greater the frequency. The frequency necessary for the older child varies according to the kind of difficulty and to the capacity of the child to maintain a continuous analytic relationship during intervals.

The details of analytic techniques will vary from age to age, as has been indicated. The younger the child, the more play will be used for communication and the less complicated will be the interpretations; the older the child, the more likely that the analysis will be conducted verbally in conversation, fantasies, dream retailing, and the like, even though play or constructive activity may occur concomitantly, and the more direct and inclusive the interpretations. Other modifications also are necessary in the treatment of the child and will depend upon the variations in the constellation of the character. Only a few may be mentioned here. Aichhorn (2) has described in detail the modification he developed for the treatment of delinquents who possessed corrupt superegos and weak or criminal egos. He found the creation of a loving, dependent, needful relationship even more necessary in these cases, and thus made himself not only a desirable person but an absolutely necessary person to such a child. For other forms of defective ego problems, as with many acting-out impulsive children, modifications also are used, in which the analyst, for a long time, acts in place of the ego for the child, protects him by kindly restriction and direction from acting out directly either destructive or erotic impulses. Also in the treatment of psychotic children the analyst may play a very active role, attempting to make reality sufficiently interesting to lure the child from his narcissistic and unrealistic autism.

## Diagnosis

Although, for practical purposes, classification of the child's problems is made according to the area of disturbance, such symptom diagnosis is not all that is necessary for the planning of treatment. Of even greater importance is an evaluation of the dynamic causes of the symptoms, including the basic conflicts involved; the ego mechanisms used in attempted solution; the historical experiences which produced the conflicts; the development of the symptoms and concomitant personality characteristics; and, finally, the effectiveness of the ego and superego functions relative to the normal expectation for the age of the child.

From these data one can evaluate the capacity of the child to relate himself to the therapist, his capacity for insight, the severity of the illness, and the strength of resistance to treatment he may offer.

For such a dynamic diagnosis, a careful developmental history from the parents is valuable. Many projective tests, based on psychoanalytic principles, such as the Rorschach, Szondi, and Thematic Apperception tests, may be useful, for they give detailed information concerning kinds of fears, conflicts, and automatic solutions. Finally, and probably of greatest value, is the preliminary period with the child, when the analyst may explore the child's social attitudes, his fears, and his methods of self-protection as they occur in the new situation.

## PREVENTION

A word on prevention should not be omitted. The more we know of the emotional experiences during development which initiate psychic disorders and of those which maintain the pathology, once it is started, the wiser we can be in promoting healthy development and avoiding personality distortion. Obviously, healthy, loving parents are essential in our society, in which the child is reared in the family unit. Therefore, anything which promotes adult mental health is a cornerstone in the building of child mental health, be it adult education, adequate facilities for work and play, economic security, or psychotherapy.

Equally important is knowledge of the child's needs, which the loving parent, the teacher, and the physician can use to avoid the traumata of sudden pleasure deprivation, painful separation, demand of performance beyond his capacity, physical pain without protective sympathy, and the like. The more wisely the child is fed, is trained, is guided and taught, the greater his facilities for learning social skills to expend his energy; the fewer catastrophic experiences he is exposed to; and the more likely he is to grow into a sturdy, happy, creative person. It is obvious, however, that one cannot offer any child ideal conditions, and, in spite of good preventive measures, problems may develop. If they do, prevention then of future difficulties is possible if early diagnosis is made and treatment is provided, before the patterns are so fixed that the crippling is only partially reversible.

## BIBLIOGRAPHY

1. ABRAHAM, K. "Contributions to the Theory of the Anal Character," in *Selected Papers* (London: Hogarth Press, 1927), chap. xxiii.
2. AICHHORN, A. *Wayward Youth* (New York: Viking Press, 1945).
3. ALDRICH, C. A., and ALDRICH, M. *Babies Are Human Beings* (New York: Macmillan Co., 1939).
4. ALEXANDER, F. "Concerning the Genesis of the Castration Complex," *Psychoanalyt. Rev.*, 22:49, 1935.
5. ALEXANDER, F. *Psychosomatic Medicine* (New York: W. W. Norton & Co., Inc., 1950).
6. ALEXANDER, F., and HEALY, W. *Roots of Crime* (New York: Alfred A. Knopf, 1935).
7. ANGEL, A. "From the Analysis of a Bed Wetter," *Psychoanalyt. Quart.*, 4:120, 1935.
8. BENDER, L. "Childhood Schizophrenia: A Clinical Study of One Hundred Schizophrenic Children," *Am. J. Orthopsychiat.*, 17:40, 1947.
9. BENDER, L. "Infants Reared in Institutions; Permanently Handicapped," *Bull. Child Welfare League of America*, Vol. 24, No. 7 (September, 1945).
10. BENDER, L. "Organic Brain Conditions Producing Behavior Disturbances: A Clinical Survey of Encephalitis, Burn Encephalopathy, and the Traumatic States," in *Modern Trends in Child Psychiatry* (New York: International Universities Press, 1945).
11. BENEDEK, THERESE. "The Psychosomatic Implications of the Primary Unit: Mother-Child," *Am. J. Orthopsychiat.*, 19:642, 1949.
12. BERES, D., and OBERS, S. "The Effects of Extreme Deprivation in Infancy on Psychic Structure in Adolescence: A Study in Ego Development," in *The Psychoanalytic Study of the Child*, 5 (New York: International Universities Press, 1950), 212–35.
13. BERGMAN, P., and ESCALONA, S. "Unusual Sensitivities in Very Young Children," in *The Psychoanalytic Study of the Child*, 3/4 (New York: International Universities Press, 1949), 333–52.
14. BERNFELD, S. "Psychoanalytic Psychology of the Young Child," *Psychoanalyt. Quart.*, 4:3, 1935.
15. BLANCHARD, P. "Psychoanalytic Contributions to the Problems of Reading Disabilities," in *The Psychoanalytic Study of the Child*, 2 (1946) (New York: International Universities Press, 1947), 163–87.
16. BORNSTEIN, B. "The Analysis of a Phobic Child; Some Problems of Theory and Technique in Child Analysis," in *The Psychoanalytic Study of the Child*, 3/4 (New York: International Universities Press, 1949), 181–226.
17. BORNSTEIN, B. "Clinical Notes on Child Analysis," in *The Psychoanalytic Study of the Child*, 1 (New York: International Universities Press, 1945), 151–66.
18. BORNSTEIN, B. "Phobia in a Two-and-a-half Year Old Child," *Psychoanalyt. Quart.*, 4:93, 1935.
19. BORNSTEIN, S. "A Child Analysis," *Psychoanalyt. Quart.*, 4:190, 1935.
20. BOWLBY, J. *Maternal Care and Mental Health: A Report Prepared*

*on Behalf of the World Health Organization as a Contribution to the United Nations Programme for the Welfare of Homeless Children* (Geneva: World Health Organization, 1951).

21. BREUER, J., and FREUD, S. *Studies in Hysteria* (New York: Nervous and Mental Disease Publishing Co., 1936).

22. BURLINGHAM, D. "Child Analysis and the Mother," *Psychoanalyt. Quart.*, 4:69, 1935.

23. BUXBAUM, E. "A Contribution to the Psychoanalytic Knowledge of the Latency Period," *Am. J. Orthopsychiat.*, 21:182, 1951.

24. BUXBAUM, E. "Exhibitionistic Onanism in a Ten-Year-Old Boy," *Psychoanalyt. Quart.*, 4:161, 1935.

25. CORIAT, I. H. *Stammering: A Psychoanalytic Interpretation* (New York: Nervous and Mental Disease Publishing Co., 1928).

26. CORIAT, I. H. "A Type of Anal-erotic Resistance," *Internat. J. Psycho-Analysis*, 7:392, 1926.

27. DESPERT, J. L. "Play Analysis in Research and Therapy," in *Modern Trends in Child Psychiatry* (New York: International Universities Press, 1945), pp. 219–55.

28. DESPERT, J. L. "Psychotherapy in Child Schizophrenia," *Am. J. Psychiat.*, 104:36, 1947.

29. FENICHEL, O. *Outline of Clinical Psychoanalysis* (New York: Psychonalytic Quarterly Press and W. W. Norton & Co., 1934).

30. FERENCZI, S. *Further Contributions to the Theory and Technique of Psycho-analysis* (New York: Boni & Liveright, 1927).

31. FRAIBERG, S. "On the Sleep Disturbances of Early Childhood," in *The Psychoanalytic Study of the Child*, 5 (New York: International Universities Press, 1950), 285–309.

32. FREUD, A. "Aggression in Relation to Emotional Development; Normal and Pathological," in *The Psychoanalytic Study of the Child*, 3/4 (New York: International Universities Press, 1949), 37–42.

33. FREUD, A. *The Ego and the Mechanisms of Defence* (London: Hogarth Press, 1948).

34. FREUD, A. "Indications for Child Analysis," in *The Psychoanalytic Study of the Child*, 1 (New York: International Universities Press, 1945), 127–49.

35. FREUD, A. "The Latency Period," in *Introduction to Psychoanalysis for Teachers* (London: George Allen & Unwin, Ltd., 1931).

36. FREUD, A. "The Psychoanalytic Study of Infantile Feeding Disturbances," in *The Psychoanalytic Study of the Child*, 2 (1946) (New York: International Universities Press, 1947), 119–32.

37. FREUD, A. *The Psycho-analytical Treatment of Children: Technical Lectures and Essays* (London: Imago Publishing Co., 1946).

38. FREUD, A., and BURLINGHAM, D. *Infants without Families: The Case for and against Residential Nurseries* (New York: International Universities Press, 1944).

39. FREUD, A., and BURLINGHAM, D. *War and Children* (New York: Medical War Books, 1943).

40. FREUD, S. "Analysis of a Phobia in a Five-Year-Old Boy," in *Collected Papers*, Vol. 3 (London: Hogarth Press, 1946).

41. FREUD, S. *Beyond the Pleasure Principle* (London: Hogarth Press, 1948).
42. FREUD, S. "Female Sexuality," *Internat. J. Psycho-Analysis*, 13:281, 1932.
43. FREUD, S. "On Narcissism: An Introduction," in *Collected Papers*, Vol. 4 (London: Hogarth Press, 1949).
44. FREUD, S. "The Passing of the Oedipus-Complex," in *Collected Papers*, Vol. 2 (London: Hogarth Press, 1924).
45. FREUD, S. *Three Contributions to the Theory of Sex* (4th ed., New York: Nervous and Mental Disease Publishing Co., 1930).
46. FRIEDLANDER, K. *The Psycho-analytical Approach to Juvenile Delinquency: Theory, Case-Studies, Treatment* (New York: International Universities Press, 1947).
47. FRIES, M. "Interrelationship of Physical, Mental, and Emotional Life of a Child from Birth to Four Years of Age," *Am. J. Dis. Child.*, 49:1546, 1935.
48. FRIES, M. "Play Technique in the Analysis of Young Children, *Psychoanalyt. Rev.*, 24:233, 1937.
49. FRIES, M. "Psychosomatic Relationships between Mother and Infant," *Psychosom. Med.*, 6:159, 1944.
50. GELEERD, E. "A Contribution to the Problem of Psychoses in Childhood," in *The Psychoanalytic Study of the Child*, 2 (1946) (New York: International Universities Press, 1947), 271–91.
51. GELEERD, E. "The Psychoanalysis of a Psychotic Child," in *The Psychoanalytic Study of the Child*, 3/4 (New York: International Universities Press, 1949), 311–32.
52. GERARD, M. W. "Child Analysis as a Technique in the Investigation of Mental Mechanisms," *Am. J. Psychiat.*, 94:653, 1937.
53. GERARD, M. W. "Enuresis: A Study in Etiology," *Am. J. Orthopsychiat.*, 9:48, 1939.
54. GERARD, M. W. "The Psychogenic Tic in Ego Development," in *The Psychoanalytic Study of the Child*, 2 (1946) (New York: International Universities Press, 1947), 133–62.
55. GIBBS, E. L.; GIBBS, F. A.; and FUSTER, B. "Psychomotor Epilepsy," *Arch. Neurol. & Psychiat.*, 60:331, 1948.
56. GLOVER, E. "Examination of the Klein System of Child Psychology," in *The Psychoanalytic Study of the Child*, Vol. 1 (New York: International Universities Press, 1945).
57. GREENACRE, P. "The Biologic Economy of Birth," in *The Psychoanalytic Study of the Child*, 1 (New York: International Universities Press, 1945), 31–51.
58. GREENACRE, P. "The Predisposition to Anxiety," *Psychoanalyt. Quart.*, 10:66, 610, 1941.
59. HALL, J. W. "The Analysis of a Case of Night Terror," in *The Psychoanalytic Study of the Child*, 2 (1946) (New York: International Universities Press, 1947), 189–227.
60. HARTMANN, H. "Ich-Psychologie und Anpassungsproblem," *Internat. Ztschr. f. Psychoanal. u. Imago*, 24:62, 1939.

61. HARTMANN, H. "Psychoanalysis and Developmental Psychology," in *The Psychoanalytic Study of the Child*, 5 (New York: International Universities Press, 1950), 7–17.

62. HARTMANN, H.; KRIS, E.; and LOEWENSTEIN, R. M. "Notes on the Theory of Aggression," in *The Psychoanalytic Study of the Child*, 3/4 (New York: International Universities Press, 1949), 9–36.

63. JACKSON, E. B. "Pediatric and Psychiatric Aspects of the Yale Rooming-in Project," *Connecticut M. J.*, 14:616, 1950.

64. JOHNSON, A. "Sanctions for Superego Lacunae of Adolescents," in *Searchlights on Delinquency* (New York: International Universities Press, 1949), pp. 225–45.

65. JOHNSON, A. M., and FISHBACK, D. "Analysis of a Disturbed Adolescent Girl and Collaborative Treatment of the Mother," *Am. J. Orthopsychiat.*, 14:195, 1944.

66. KATAN, A. "Experiences with Enuretics," in *The Psychoanalytic Study of the Child*, 2 (1946) (New York: International Universities Press, 1947), 241–55.

67. KLEIN, M. *The Psycho-analysis of Children* (London: Hogarth Press, 1932).

68. KRIS, E. "Notes on the Development and on Some Current Problems of Psychoanalytic Child Psychology," in *The Psychoanalytic Study of the Child*, 5 (New York: International Universities Press, 1950), 24–46.

69. LEITCH, M., and ESCALONA, S. "The Reaction of Infants to Stress: A Report of Clinical Observations," in *The Psychoanalytic Study of the Child*, 3/4 (New York: International Universities Press, 1949), 121–40.

70. LEVY, D. M. "Experiments on the Sucking Reflex and Social Behavior of Dogs," *Am. J. Orthopsychiat.*, 4:203, 1934.

71. LEVY, D. M. "Fingersucking and Accessory Movements in Early Infancy," *Am. J. Psychiat.*, 7:881, 1928.

72. LEVY, D. M. "Maternal Overprotection," in *Modern Trends in Child Psychiatry* (New York: International Universities Press, 1945), pp. 27–34.

73. LEVY, D. M. "Primary Affect Hunger," *Am. J. Psychiat.*, 94:643, 1937.

74. LEVY, D. M. "On the Problem of Movement Restraint: Tics, Stereotyped Movements, Hyperactivity," *Am. J. Orthopsychiat.*, 45:644, 1944.

75. MENNINGER, W. "Characterologic and Symptomatic Expressions Related to the Anal Phase of Psychosexual Development," *Psychoanalyt. Quart.*, 12:161, 1943.

76. PIOUS, W. L. "The Pathogenic Process in Schizophrenia," *Bull. Menninger Clin.*, 13:152, 1949.

77. PÖRTL, A. "Profound Disturbances in the Nutritional and Excretory Habits of a Four and One Half Year Old Boy: Their Analytic Treatment in a School Setting," *Psychoanalyt. Quart.*, 4:25, 1935.

78. RABINOVITCH, R. D. "Round Table: The Psychopathic Delinquent Child," *Am. J. Orthopsychiat.*, 20:232, 1950.

79. RANK, B. "Adaptation of the Psychoanalytic Technique for the Treat-

ment of Young Children with Atypical Development," *Am. J. Ortho-psychiat.*, 19:130, 1949.

80. RANK, B. "Aggression," in *The Psychoanalytic Study of the Child*, 3/4 (New York: International Universities Press, 1949), 43–48.

81. RANK, B., and MacNAUGHTON, D. "A Clinical Contribution to Early Ego Development," in *The Psychoanalytic Study of the Child*, 5 (New York: International Universities Press, 1950), 53–65.

82. RANK, O. *The Trauma of Birth* (New York: Harcourt, Brace & Co., 1929).

83. RIBBLE, M. "Anxiety in Infants and Its Disorganizing Effects," *Modern Trends in Child Psychiatry* (New York: International Universities Press, 1945), pp. 11–25.

84. RIBBLE, M. *The Rights of Infants* (New York: Columbia University Press, 1943).

85. SONTAG, L. "Differences in Modifiability of Fetal Behavior and Physiology," *Psychosom. Med.*, 6:151, 1944.

86. SPITZ, R. "Anaclitic Depression: An Inquiry into the Genesis of Psychiatric Conditions in Early Childhood. II," in *The Psychoanalytic Study of the Child*, 2 (1946) (New York: International Universities Press, 1947), 313–42.

87. SPITZ, R. "Hospitalism: A Follow-Up Report on Investigation Described in Vol. I, 1945," in *The Psychoanalytic Study of the Child*, 2 (1946) (New York: International Universities Press, 1947), 113–17.

88. SPITZ, R. "Hospitalism: An Inquiry into the Genesis of Psychiatric Conditions in Early Childhood," in *The Psychoanalytic Study of the Child*, 1 (New York: International Universities Press, 1945), 53–74.

89. SPITZ, R. "Relevancy of Direct Infant Observation," in *The Psychoanalytic Study of the Child*, 5 (New York: International Universities Press, 1950), 66–73.

90. SPITZ, R., and WOLF, M. "Autoerotism: Some Empirical Findings and Hypotheses on Three of Its Manifestations in the First Year of Life," in *The Psychoanalytic Study of the Child*, 3/4 (New York: International Universities Press, 1949), 85–120.

91. SPOCK, B. *The Common Sense Book of Baby and Child Care* (New York: Duell, Sloan & Pearce, 1946).

92. STERBA, E. "Analysis of Psychogenic Constipation in a Two-Year-Old Child," in *The Psychoanalytic Study of the Child*, 3/4 (New York: International Universities Press, 1949), 227–52.

93. STERBA, E. "Excerpt from the Analysis of a Dog Phobia," *Psychoanalyt. Quart.*, 4:135, 1935.

94. SYLVESTER, E. "Analysis of Psychogenic Anorexia and Vomiting in a Four-Year-Old Child," in *The Psychoanalytic Study of the Child*, 1 (New York: International Universities Press, 1945), 167–87.

95. SZUREK, S.; JOHNSON, A. M.; and FALSTEIN, E. "Collaborative Psychiatric Therapy of Parent-Child Problems," *Am. J. Orthopsychiat.*, 12:511, 1942.

# VIII

## CONTRIBUTIONS OF PSYCHOANALYSIS TO THE STUDY OF ORGANIC CEREBRAL DISORDERS

### Henry W. Brosin, M.D.

#### Review of Studies Other than Psychoanalytic

BECAUSE of the high cost, emotional and financial, of personality disorders, increased concern has been expressed about the failure of the behavioral sciences to make more significant progress in their prediction and control. The full story of this failure must be left to the future, but a brief survey may present some of the more obvious barriers to progress. The crucial lack of quantitative and more flexible, yet useful, methods is probably the most important handicap. This seems to be especially true in those human organisms whose central nervous system and total personality organization are under the stress of cerebral organic deficit. Psychiatrists and neurologists in the past did not as a rule devote themselves intensively to the psychological study and treatment of organic cerebral disorders after the diagnosis was made, because treatment was often difficult and unrewarding. The malarial treatment of paresis and the successes of Goldstein, Poppelreuter, and others in treating the head injuries of World War I called attention to the fact that many of these supposedly hopeless cases were amenable to expert treatment by trained personnel.

Some progress has been made recently in methods of treatment through the utilization of complex hospital settings with specialized equipment and newer methods of group and individual therapy. However, the long, arduous training regimes required for treating head-injury cases are too consuming of time and energy to permit most physicians to make this a major lifework, with the consequence that these duties have been relegated to new classes of well-trained lay therapists who do most of the exacting work (58, 135). Unfortunately, this shift in responsibility as well as in method of treatment to lay therapists results too often in separating the patient from his physician to such a degree that the latter loses intimate working knowledge of his patient. This lack of working together results in impoverished experimental investigation of patients with organic deficit, even though they are among the most challenging and baffling "experiments of nature." In spite of much good treatment in the latter years of World War II, relatively few new insights were gained. This fact is almost as amazing as the circumstance that, in spite of thousands of studies by hundreds of competent workers, there is only confusion and contradiction about both facts and theories. Goldstein, who published his first paper on aphasia in 1906, ascribes this lack of unanimity to the extreme importance of a personal bias (subjective attitude) in the methods of examining the patient, reporting observations, and making interpretation (58, p. x).

Many protocols are valueless because the facts recorded are not comparable; the focus of interest varies from gross anatomic localization to cleverly controlled experimentation and sophisticated interpretation from many points of view. Unfortunately, the organic psychoses and the disturbances of the language function which are often their outstanding symptoms are not easily explicable by one hypothesis but must be studied as total-personality involvements. This requires knowledge of the important properties of the organic deficit, of the kind of person the patient is and of the defenses which have been called out to protect the patient against his deficit, and, finally, of the genetic-dynamic developmental history which makes this interplay more intelligible, including the pertinent physical, intellectual, and social factors in both past and present. The fragmentation of opinions is so intimidating that, in spite of extensive activity before 1910, only five publications have dared to make a comprehensive survey of the field of aphasia during the last forty years (58, p. vii).

This brief introduction will help explain why psychoanalysts, most of whom are private practitioners preferring ambulatory cases with a more favorable prognosis, have not been more active in this field. The glorious beginnings of nineteenth-century neurology failed their promise when confronted by the anatomic, physiologic, and psychologic complexities exhibited by these cases. The simple reflex circuit diagrams and their

associated concepts were inadequate to support the myriad contradictory facts which intensive clinical examination produces.
Although many early analysts were trained in neurology, they
were, in the early days of analysis, in no better position economically to study these cases than were their colleagues in psychology or neurology. In addition, they were handicapped by the
fact that they had few hospital appointments to facilitate this
work and that the prognosis was so poor that it was not practical
for them to spend their time in this way, especially since other
fields of treatment were much more attractive for both theoretical and practical reasons.

The theoretical and practical gaps which kept experimentalists
and clinicians, especially analysts, apart no longer seem to be
such formidable barriers. The more comprehensive attitudes
currently growing at an accelerated rate in both groups present
more than a mere hope that productive collaboration is possible.
Tangible experimental work projects already under way before
1943 in the field of objective studies of psychoanalytic concepts
number well over one hundred, while a survey of the literature
on experiments with the psychoanalytic process itself and on
mechanisms such as aggression and substitution reveals over
eighty studies (150, 151). While Sears concludes that experimental psychology has not yet made a major contribution to
these problems, he asserts that some progress has been made in
understanding the dynamics of personality. He doubts the ap-
propriateness of any attempt of experimental psychology to test
psychoanalytic theory, since "available techniques are clumsy,"
and advises experimentalists to get as much help as they can from
psychoanalysis in order to build up a system based upon behavioral, instead of experimental, data (150). The more recent
work of Levy (108) on affect hunger and the studies of Spitz
(157, 158, 159, 160, 161), and Bowlby (22) on the depressions
in babies brought on by separation from the mother and by maternal deprivation, and similar studies by J. P. Scott (148), of the
Jackson Laboratories, on puppies are examples of the more integrated type of experimentation. The collection of essays, *Organization and Pathology of Thought*, edited by David Rapaport
(133), is an excellent introduction to the problems before us.

Even though many problems of psychoanalysis are not yet
amenable to rigorous experimental verification, there are many

signs that the entire field of research in personality is becoming more adapted to problems at the human level. Leading psychologists, although not concerned with psychoanalysis, are broadening their experimental horizons and methods so that they can deal with data which will be significant to the clinician. These advances are not fully reviewed here,[1] but several representative workers will be mentioned, in order to furnish the student with a few guideposts for his own exploration.

It has been said that psychoanalysis and "learning theory" have contributed most to the advances in personality study (101). Each year sees a new series of books and papers substantiating this view, though at this time a truly unified theory cannot be offered. A critical survey of learning theories by E. R. Hilgard (81) points out their similarities and differences and the experimental work which gave rise to them. Such work gives hope to those clinicians who need sound psychological theories dealing with data on perception, memory, motivation, learning, etc., even though at this time "there are no laws of learning which can be taught with confidence" (81, p. 326). Hilgard points out that, while psychology is a young science, much work has been done since Ebbinghaus gave it a good start in 1885. Hilgard cites the following reasons for the lag:

The concepts appropriate to this field are not ready, since motivated control of learning and more careful delineation of different types of learning are not given the necessary prominence. There has been too much inappropriate quantification. Most psychologists and psychiatrists welcome sound quantification, but they deplore the execution of crude experiments which do violence to the real problem in order to achieve quick quantitative results. Psychologists and psychiatrists alike need new methods to deal with significant subject matter rather than trivial content which yields superficial quanta. The preoccupation with comparative methods needs to be put in proper perspective. Animal experiments are valuable if they shed light on human behavior; but since humans are able to use language more complexly than animals, they probably learn differently. Therefore, as much work as possible should be done on humans, with careful attention to those animal experiments which will be useful for comparison. The importance of animals for surgical work and for genetic studies on heredity is self-evident, but in many other areas too great a price has been paid for insignificant results [81].

This judgment is supported by an intensive analysis of the statistical studies of Rorschach Test results by a statistician, who

1. See chap. xiv.

points out the inadequacy of older methods for dealing with projective techniques (31). Direct physiological experimental approaches are highly desirable, and, when new electronic devices permit, they will furnish vital information about the complex processes involved in thinking. Possibly more skilful work on lower animals would permit crude beginnings even now. In all justice, though, we have no reason to believe that neurophysiological data would alter the problems of memory and learning in ordinary life-settings. The way most people live together probably will not be greatly illuminated by electronic descriptions of behavior, even though they may explain the origin of some diseases.

One typical citation from such leaders of neurophysiology as Sherrington (154), Adrian (7), and Lashley and Wade (105, 106) regarding the inadequacy of neurology may suffice to help the understanding of problems of thinking:

> At the present time nothing whatever is known concerning the nature of the alterations in the nervous system which constitute memory traces. Knowledge of cerebral physiology is in fact so limited that it does not even lend a greater plausibility to one than to another of the many speculations concerning the organic basis of memory with which the literature is burdened. Association with direction of flow of nervous excitation or with a ratio of excitation is neither more nor less fantastic as a physiological theory than is association between hypothetical conditioned-reflex arcs. The only relevant facts are those of psychology ... [106, p. 86].

Lashley does not share Sherrington's pessimism about understanding the relations between mind and brain; he believes that the principle of organization and an operational point of view make a connection possible. Factors supporting Lashley's view are the physiological discoveries concerning the intricacy of cortical organization and the experimental demonstration of recurrent or reverberatory circuits by Lorente de Nó (113, 114, 115), a demonstration which greatly enlarges the previously limited picture of central nervous system organization as a primitive set of reflex connections. Electrophysiologic studies of the cortex support this more flexible view and open up further possibilities for understanding psychological activity as independent of particular nerve cells. Lashley's experiments require central nervous system organization in which there is reduplication of functional elements, that is, an equivalence of parts which permits "functional effects which are independent of the particular structural elements transmitting the pattern." Such a model permits study of problems in perception, even though they have not led to a common description of organization.

A second point of convergence of physiology and psychology is motivation. The work of Beach (14, 15) suggests that "destruction of parts of the cerebral cortex reduces the intensity of the sexual drives, somewhat in proportion to the extent of damage. Males with more than half of the cortex removed may show no reaction to a receptive female. Large doses of testosterone, however, will restore them temporarily to normal interest and activity." Similarly, revival of the maternal drive has been achieved by hormone injections by Wiesner (177). In rats "these primitive drives, chemical, environmental, and central nervous factors are somewhat interchangeable. The ultimate mechanism is the nervous organization of which the excitability may be increased by (1) the hormone, (2) appropriate stimulation or (3) some factor which correlates with the amount of nervous tissue intact" (14).

A third common interest is in the organization of intellectual functions. Heretofore, interest had largely centered on *what* has been done, rather than *how* it was done or *how* the functions are related. It has been common practice heretofore to group together a series of patients' performances to given tasks, such as serial addition, block manipulation, picture reproduction, or interpretation of test material. The groupings are called by such names as "recent" and "remote" memory, "perception," "emotion," "imagination," "reasoning," and "abstraction." It is possible that these artificially created classes do not represent similar functions (processes), and this would help to explain why it has not been possible to understand or classify in these terms the mental defects from organic brain injury. Numerous criticisms exist of the fact that one cannot understand loss of memory for names of common objects (amnesia, aphasia), inability to form individual words (verbal aphasia), inability to comprehend spatial or temporal or other relations when presented in words, and related symptoms in terms of these classical academic categories. A new psychology of language and a new neurophysiology are required to make these complex facts intelligible.

Another example of possible co-operation is the use of factor analysis, as developed by Spearman and Thurstone (172). It is not unlikely that detailed analytic data on such common activities as eating, working, dreaming, and menstruation not only would reveal a dynamic picture of a kind which is well known to psychoanalysis but would, in addition, provide the factor analyst with data which might throw some additional light on the problems of thinking in aphasics and normals. However, before major insights can be expected from this type of analysis on large groups, the groundwork will probably have to be laid by persistent re-examination of the single case. No less an experimentalist than J. B. Watson, the behaviorist, said that he preferred to do one thousand tests on one rat rather than one test on one thousand rats, thus expressing the preference of most analysts; but for scientific purposes it will be essential to pursue several methods of inquiry.

Lashley is confident that an understanding of thinking is possible in terms of organization of both mental and physiological elements. "Perhaps the most important contribution of psychologists to this problem has been the realization that the characteristics of the mental can be stated meaningfully only as a structure or organization of elements which are themselves as purely conceptual as is the energy of physics. Such a notion was foreshadowed by the growth of behaviorism, but it remained for the logical positivists to develop a critique of scientific thinking which gives it rigorous formulation" (105).

Further evidence that the resolution of some problems of thinking lies in the search for correspondence of organization between mental and neurological functions is perhaps given by the statement of an electrophysiologist, Gibbs: "The behavior of brain waves seems more psychological than physiological" (55).

## FREUD AS NEUROLOGIST

It is a historical curiosity that, according to Brun (24), Freud, the father of psychoanalysis, should also have been "the most significant predecessor of von Monakow" in neurology. In thirty publications, Freud demonstrated his creative talent in making significant contributions to the study of the development of the posterior roots of the spinal cord, the genetic development of unipolar from bipolar cells, the fibrillar structure of the axis cylinder, and the motility of the protoplasm in the nucleus. Thus he gave an improved picture of central nervous system function and structure, foreshadowed the neuron theory, and invented a microscopic method for tissue preparation and a new microscopic stain (gold chloride for axis cylinders)—not to mention his cocaine research and clinical investigations on the cerebral diplegias in children, bleeding in scurvy, syringomyelia, acute multiple neuritis, early hemianopsia, etc. (24, 59, 92). For this chapter, however, his most important monograph is *Zur Auffassung der Aphasien* (46). Here Freud, after his work with Meynert in cerebral anatomy, takes sharp issue with the then commonly accepted localization theories of Wernicke-Lichtheim and writes in favor of a more functional view of the central nervous system, which inclines toward Hughlings Jackson's conceptions. In much that he wrote before 1893, Freud anticipated the findings and interpretations of neurologists who followed him. His concepts of ego function, while crude, are not unlike those of leading neurophysiologists today (7), and they may be more useful for some time to come. He began at the ground floor and developed a discipline and rigorous attitude which served him well when he dared explore alone the dread world of the unconscious. In spite of his pioneer work on aphasia, neither he nor his pupils returned to it seriously. Later historians may chart the ebb and flow of fashions in this as in other sciences. Perhaps the dearth of interest up to now will presently be replaced by new activity with better techniques and more suitable cases.

The vocabulary in this chapter will illustrate current difficulties in exposition: Ferenczi's libido theory and his description of ego function will not satisfy those with newer definitions, nor will "regression," "sexual fixation," "castration" or "oedipal" phenomena please those who speak in broader terms, but I shall try to transcribe accurately the intentions of a few of the older writers, in their own vocabularies.

## GENERAL PARESIS OF THE INSANE

For years before Noguchi and Moore demonstrated the spirochete in the brain of paretics in 1913, shrewd clinical psychiatrists, through observing the mental status, had guessed that some of the symptomatology was due to organic deficit and related compensatory mechanisms. Unfortunately, psychological test methods were not sufficiently developed to demonstrate organic deficits neatly, and this caused most clinicians to lose interest in the problem. They also neglected the study of the content of the delusions and hallucinations because they felt that there was no sense in trying to understand these fragments of an organically disordered brain, even though highly respected psychiatrists like Bleuler and Jung had demonstrated the meaningfulness of schizophrenic delusions in 1906.

In 1925, Hollós and Ferenczi (85) advanced earlier considerations markedly by examining more closely whether such disordered functions as the dementias, memory loss, grandiosity, and use of numbers in paretics were arbitrary or whether there were psychological determinants. They cite numerous examples to support the latter hypothesis, meanwhile building up, both explicitly and implicitly, a picture of the ego as an organ of the central nervous system. That the preferential use of numbers and the content of the delusions are related to life-experiences is relatively easy to accept, but to appreciate that the repression in a paretic is a repression of his awareness of his sickness is a step forward which helps us understand mental states in severe chronic diseases, such as advanced tuberculosis and multiple sclerosis. The description of the return of the repressed in symptomatic behavior, together with the wish-fulfilment fantasies based upon early life-experiences, makes much confusing behavior more intelligible. Hollós and Ferenczi point out specifically that such behavior is possible "only by an infantile regression of the critical faculty" (85, p. 16). The relation of this observation to others that the principal cortical changes in paresis may be in the frontal lobes (80, 141, 176) needs more psychologic and psychoanalytic experimental verification, especially in the lobotomy series.

Ferenczi then developed a further theory that injury to, or disease of, the body or an organ causes withdrawal of libido (in Fenichel's terms, "supplies" of love, affection, interest) from the ego's attachments to objects in the outer world and focuses them on the sick area. The concentration of energies upon the self may recapitulate the infantile state of narcissism before object relationships were established. That such redistribution of energies is important for healing is asserted by Ferenczi in discussing war wounds. Soldiers who had a severe flesh wound did not have such severe psychological difficulties as did those who were not organically maimed. Presumably this bound energy, says Ferenczi, is not free to move about and thereby cannot be used to cause neurosis. Furthermore, he points out that severe organic injury to a highly erogenous zone may cause a psychotic reaction, such as are seen in puerperal psychoses, and that major psychoses caused by psychological conflicts (manic-depressive disease and schizophrenia) are cured by some severe trauma or intercurrent infectious disease. That this occurs occasionally is attested by reports and verbal communications. Perhaps our current experience with shock and surgical procedures causes us to be skeptical of a single simple explanation which really does not explain, namely, that the surplus libido is bound in the diseased area. Nevertheless, Ferenczi makes the daring jump to envision paresis as a cerebral pathoneurosis, that is, the brain becomes an erogenous zone by a complex system of displacement upward, which when injured causes a neurotic reaction of the entire personality. It is carefully emphasized that the somatic signs and symptoms in all body systems due to the physical injury are of primary importance. These symptoms may be expressions of the loss of brain tissue or the restitutive efforts of the organism to such loss. In addition, however, there are those functional disorders which express the disorder of "the equilibrium in the housekeeping of the narcissistic libido" (85, p. 34).

Ferenczi thinks that, of the various phases of paretic progression (cf. Bayle's initial depression, maniacal excitement, paranoid delusions, terminal dementia), only the early "neurasthenic" symptoms are attributable to organic defect. For example, diminished potency is interpreted as withdrawal of libido from sexual objects for some other use; that it is not simply organic is shown in its later return. The frequent hypochrondriacal complaints are probably expressions of the ingoing libido. Euphoria and enhanced interest in objects are only overcompensations, masks to hide the twofold damage to the body and the ego. Melancholia becomes the rule when the ego is forced to recognize the injury, and the familiar dynamics of Abraham (2) and Freud (50) help explain the further progress of the impoverished ego. The ego can compensate (withdraw into a pathoneurotic hypochondria or expand in a reactive euphoria) so long as the loss involves only various peripheral organs, but when the destructive process attacks the "most highly estimated activities of the ego—the intellect, morality, esthetic sense—the self-observation of such a deterioration must draw after it the feeling of impoverishment of the sum total of narcissistic libido, which according to our suggestion, is connected with the supremacy of the higher psychical functions" (85, pp. 37–38).

This latter state is a crucial blow to the self-esteem, which, with other complications, leads to melancholia. Apparently much body destruction can be tolerated if the ego's activities furnish libidinal satisfaction, but if both body and psychological gratifications are lost, the pain to the ego becomes sufficiently intolerable to accept psychotic solutions such as: (*a*) mania (dissolution of ego ideal into narcissistic ego) or (*b*) delusions of grandeur (hallucinatory wish-fulfilments).

How can systematic, albeit disordered, processes such as these affect an ego disintegrating under attack by an organic disease? Ferenczi's explanations are clear enough, but the reader must recall that his paper was written before Freud published *The Ego and the Id* (49) and lacks the more specific definitions of ego and superego functions to which we are now accustomed.

The ego develops from its early stages of unrestrained or hallucinatory omnipotence, through the stage of magic gestures, later to phases when the reality principle gradually becomes dominant.[2] Through this development, the ego is enabled to separate personal wishes from those demanded by forces outside itself; to master adaptive processes, such as alertness, cleverness, prudence, wisdom, and morality, and yet at the same time to remain elastic for new adaptations. This comes about gradually through a series of interpersonal relations, of identifications with superior figures into a more or less integrated superego (ego ideal), which in time also becomes to the ego functions an object like outside reality and the id. Reality testing remains a function of the ego; with every new mastery of function there are numerous rewards, such as the attainment of an ideal, narcissistic gratification, improved prestige to the ego, and the well-being which comes with recovery from a tension state. In paresis, with decline of ego mastery, there occurs regression to the earlier states of infantile omnipotence. "General paresis seen from the psychoanalytic viewpoint, is really regressive paresis" (85, p. 41). These hypotheses confirm Freud's prediction that the analysis of the psychoses will show conflict and substitution mechanisms in the sphere of ego psychology similar to those found in psychoneuroses, namely, conflicts between the functions of the ego and one of its objects. An overly simplified formula states that in neuroses the conflict is between the ego functions and the id functions, while psychoses are major maladaptations because of similar disturbances between the ego functions and the environment. Repression in neuroses may be replaced by a manic phase in paresis, the mechanisms of

2. For a detailed summary of ego development see chap. iv.

the latter being "sequestration" of the noxious ideas, thus protecting the ego from further diminution of self-esteem. The "sequestration" may expand into compensatory delusions of grandeur, power, potency, the patient's age before illness, or a projection of his illness. There may be highly active perverse sexual activity. There may appear in paresis a kind of melancholia which is different from the psychogenic type which mourns the loss of an ideal, but becomes a grief over the successive organic loss of one level of identification after another, a dissection, as it were, of one ideal from another as in dreams and psychoses, showing how multiple identifications are integrated into the ego-superego systems and how they may retain independence (separate identity) under these circumstances.

The explanation of why one patient develops a manic or depressive or quickly progressive demented phase follows the familiar lines of presupposing constitutional and environmental factors, stressing the latter in the genetic dynamic sense. The weak links, interpersonal relationships, in ego and libido organization, the fixation points in development, and the specificity and severity of the trauma are points of departure which help us to understand the development of a pathological process. Habitually egocentric characters will develop different clinical forms of paresis from those individuals with numerous liberal relations to others; those patients with strong genital primacy will differ markedly from those who regress easily to the polymorphous perverse sexual practices of childhood. The speed of the organic paretic process may be significant, since sudden loss may occasion a more violent grief reaction, which is less likely to bring on a paretic mania or melancholia than in a slowly progressive disease. A more complex analysis may show that, if the basic "ego nucleus" of Ferenczi (superego) survives the paretic destruction to both physical and psychological functions, there will be stronger psychotic reactions (compensations). If these superego and ego functions are also involved, then there will be proportionately greater evidence of simple deterioration. The excited manic paretic or the incessantly melancholic one is not so devoid of insight as was commonly written into hospital records. From this it appears that the prognosis in these types after the various malarial or pyretotherapies is much better, with only slight defects remaining. The so-called "galloping" or "agitated" clinical types are perhaps best explained, according to Ferenczi, by assuming that the disease process begins in the "ego-nucleus," not in the "ego-periphery," and that the psychological forces which normally hold the various elements of the personality together, even against noxious attacking forces, are failing to function, thereby permitting the patient to slip into various fragmented identifications and personifications. This process also exists in acute toxic deliria for similar reasons. Could it be that in these patients the prefrontal lobes are predominantly involved? "These speculations on a stereo-chemistry of the psyche" are offered provisionally by Ferenczi, with the belief that "many psychotic manifestations of general paresis, as well as the entire course of this disease, prove themselves to be not inaccessible to psychoanalytic explanation" (85, p. 48) and that psychoanalysis can offer much to the study of organic cerebral disorders.

Most experimental psychologists and psychoanalysts will agree that the data from patients as translated into the Freudian idiom give unified understanding to otherwise fragmented clinical insights. The picture of the ego as an organ, under stresses internal and external, fighting to maintain the integrity of its functions—perceptive, receptive, integrative (organizing), and executive (motor)—even under savage onslaught, like a well-disciplined, though damaged, army in retreat, is a useful metaphor, however crude it may be for later refined study. Some of the experiments suggested, namely, those dealing with the types of ego disintegration in relation to physical damage to brain tissue as to both mass and location, have first-rate quality; the clinical dissection of the symptoms into those which are specific organic brain deficits, those due to general tissue destruction and debility, those due to psychological realignment of personality forces, and those due to numerous compensatory reactions deserve much more attention from clinicians and laboratory workers. Lobotomy and lobectomy cases are especially good controls which enable workers to study at length and in adequate numbers the correlations here suggested (73, 75).

Although Ferenczi's provocative hypotheses were widely commented upon, few analysts continued work directly on this problem. Schilder (147), concentrating on a method of studying dementia in these cases, told paretic patients short stories and then requested reproductions. The errors, omissions, and substitutions in the patients' distorted recall furnished Schilder with data which caused him to assert that the paretic mental processes were essentially those in the Freudian unconscious, with some resemblances to and some differences from schizophrenic thinking. Most important was the avoidance of reality by schizophrenics, whereas paretics made desperate efforts to maintain contact. Schilder felt that the schizophrenic also uses archaic material, while the paretic uses only actual material. Because of these convictions, Schilder denied Ferenczi's thesis of regression. Far more observation is essential to verify the larger meaning of both propositions. Perhaps the dispute is founded in a failure to define the terms adequately, for Schilder is right when he states that the paretic ego resists regression but wrong if he denies libido regression (97). If we adopt Freud's description of ego regression, as evidenced by the frank exhibition of unconscious mental mechanisms, then by Schilder's experiments we would consider ego regression present. Katan takes this position after examining some paretics both before and after malarial therapy. He does not support Schilder in the latter's assertion that regression is not present until after malaria, for he thinks that both the dynamics of the content and the mental status are evidence of regression; but he agrees that patients treated with malaria show many more symptoms, leading him to a suggestion that there must be attempts at recovery before one can see symptoms of regression. Since 1918 the use of malaria and pyretotherapy has spread so widely that we see relatively few severely regressed paretics; furthermore, they are treated so quickly that no prolonged pretreatment study is possible; it is likely that appropriate methods to study dementia will be developed in other diseases (152).

W. C. Menninger (118) has reported work on forty-three cases of juvenile paresis observed personally and has reviewed 610 cases recorded in the literature. Since 40 per cent are feeble-minded and most of the remainder confused or regressed to simple dementia, with inadequate emotional response and restless purposeless behavior, there was little opportunity to study the dynamics of regression. Grotjahn (69, 70), reporting 57 cases, describes the essential unity of personality and reintegration of the ego, even with somatic defects, under malarial treatment. Both Menninger and Grotjahn examine the dynamics of the disturbed behavior in order to make it more intelligible. Menninger finds progressive regression of both ego development and libido distribution as observed by Katan. Since in most cases the personality is not well developed, there is little evidence of acute symptom formation such as is seen in adults, but fragmented unconscious insights, depression, grandiose delusions, and other psychotic mechanisms are occasionally observed. Autoerotic phenomena are frequent. Grotjahn (70) extends the description and develops the dynamics of the symptom formation of juvenile paretics in terms similar to Ferenczi.

Hartmann and Schilder (79) were able to hypnotize mildly ten of fourteen paretics with the aid of medinal and paraldehyde but were unable to produce catalepsy, amnesia, or real sleep. They speculate upon the cortical and the ventricle damage present and hypothecate its effects upon the damaged ego structure or the failure of the sleep apparatus in lieu of a tenable neurophysiological hypothesis, which will come only with new data.

Coriat (30) summarizes his experience in terms of tissue destruction, which causes damage to the ego apparatus, the preconscious system, and the libidinal mechanisms of the id and hence makes possible delusions and hallucinations which are akin to the formations of dreams. When the repressive functions of the ego are diminished, the wish-fulfilment impulses of the id force their way into awareness. In this sense paresis, an organic disease, says Coriat, is dynamically similar to a major functional psychosis. For when the ego functions are impaired, that is, unable to maintain equilibrium with the outer and inner forces according to the reality principle, then there occur the regressive phenomena of the pleasure-principle level of infancy. It is not so easy for us now to say, as Coriat does, that an acquired dementia is an organically conditioned fixation, since we take a more complex view of these concepts and are less friendly to such mechanical models or personalized entities. Even in the vocabulary of interpersonal relations, however, these models cast some light on clinical events. Rapaport's publications (132, 134) on the psychoanalytic theory of thinking and the papers by other authors in *Organization and Pathology of Thought* (133) will be helpful to those who pursue the elusive questions just described.

## EPILEPSY

Clinical psychological examinations of epileptic patients indicate that (*a*) the organic lesion is permanent, with crippling effects upon mental and physical behavior; (*b*) the handicap to the person is dependent on his personality organization, as well as on the size, location, and nature of the lesion; (*c*) the personality disorganization may be directly caused by the lesion or only modified by it in various ways, both direct and indirect.

If the ego is conceived as the organ of the mind with perceptive, integrative, and executive functions with which the mind meets internal and external reality, it will be under stress when its habitat, the body, is injured. Not only does the ego have a defective instrument with which to do its work, but it suffers itself a loss of well-being and completeness, and therefore seeks recompense by self-love and self-protectiveness—a process which has been described as withdrawal of the libido from outside interests. The narcissistic investment of the ego is often present in any type of organic illness, and, while useful to promote healing, it is unattractive because of the resultant selfishness, dependence, querulousness, demandingness, and critical complaining. Usually the ego draws to itself more libido than is necessary for healing, thereby diminishing the amount of energy available for outside activity, productive work, and mature human relations. There is another penalty when excess libido is bound inwardly, for, as was seen in the patients with general paresis, this energy must be used in some fashion. The accumulating energy may build up tensions which precipitate or augment epileptic attacks. In so far as some of the inwardly bound energy may be destructively oriented, the already weakened ego energy is unable to turn this into socially acceptable channels and suffers even more damage.

Psychotherapy, then, may be highly useful in reducing attacks by reducing the accumulation of ego-bound (narcissistic) libido. This can be done through encouraging constructive activities which drain off this libido and permit the patient to be healthier and more efficient and to achieve higher levels of satisfaction. A long educative process may be necessary to permit the patient to persuade himself on his own initiative that he may abandon his magical defenses and autoerotic narcissistic gratifications for small but solid achievement.

Following Freud's exposition in 1928 of the affective components in the convulsive disorders in "Dostoevsky and Parricide" (48), analysts have been interested in the psychological determinants of this disease. Although Freud distinguished sharply between organic and affective epilepsy, it is clear that he regarded convulsion as a relatively nonspecific somatic reaction which permits discharge of large masses of stimuli that cannot be handled psychically. Other clinicians have commented that practically anyone under proper circumstances may be forced into some form of epileptic reaction: petit mal, staring, absent-mindedness, sleep starts, outbursts of rage, teeth-grinding, jaw clenching, numbness (13, 62, 95, 107, 155). Accumulations of hostile destructive forces which cannot find appropriate outlets will in predisposed individuals be expressed as epileptiform or convulsive states. More detailed expositions of the interpretations of individual symptoms in concrete cases can be found in the articles cited.

## Hypnosis in the Brain-injured

Earlier workers have found that most brain-injured patients were not amenable to hypnosis, nor could suitable results be obtained with those showing some susceptibility. Hartmann and Schilder (79), using medinal and paraldehyde for induction, were able to hypnotize ten of fourteen patients with paresis, many of them with severe dementia. Apparently, only O. Vogt had attempted to do this earlier, and he stopped with superficial (light) induction. Hartmann and Schilder found only light induction possible, usually without real hypnotic sleep, amnesia, or motor phenomena. Suggestions to hallucinate and inability to open eyes were successful. Hartmann and Schilder were impressed by the sensory phenomena (hallucinations) and the suggestibility in the sphere of judgment and thinking, and, after careful trials, did not believe that the hallucinations were merely paretic confabulations. The failure to induce real sleep, catalepsy, and amnesia was striking, reflecting genuine cortical damage, and, these authors thought, gave evidence of loss of control over third-ventricle structures. Psychologically, it is postulated by them that, in the hypnotically induced state, the paretic can concentrate energy and respond to some suggestions but that, in the spheres of motility and sleep, suggestions are not effective. Hartmann and Schilder suggest that the failure to produce amnesia represents a failure of the repressive processes, which indicates the failure of a damaged ego structure with its now meaningless motives for forgetting, or may be related causally to the failure to induce sleep. More data are needed to develop this suggestion into a tenable neurophysiological hypothesis.

Hartmann and Schilder (79) cite four cases of head injury which had a Korsakoff-like syndrome. All four denied the fact of head injury with elaborations about the accident and later events. This observation raises questions regarding the relation of thinking disturbances to dementia, to retrograde amnesia, possible psychogenic and physiogenic causes, and differences and similarities between Korsakoff's disease and dementia. Many complex questions are also introduced: the efforts of the ego to maintain the fiction of the integrity of the person; similarities between hysterical and "organic" amnesias; relations between memory, sleep, and dream functions; the steplike nature of recall; the psychological representation of an organic limitation (which they prefer as an explanation to a simple organic deficiency); the probability of retention of memories, even though recall is not possible under current circumstances (since it may be available under other conditions).

Hartmann (77) reaffirms his earlier work and that of others in Korsakoff's disease, stating that, while an organically induced amnesia is an entity, it has some resemblances to a functional amnesia, since learned material which is not otherwise available can be recovered under hypnosis, even under intensive examination. He points out that these relationships need further study. After review of earlier work by Bonhoeffer, Brodman, Gregor, Pick, Pötzl, Poppelreuter, Riklin, Roemer, J. H. Schultz, and others, Hartmann (78) expands previous dynamic explanations to show that patients with Korsakoff's syndrome will repeat stories in keeping with the pleasure principle and that some repressive mechanisms, physiological or psychological, are at work. In addition to the usual studies of difficulties of "attention," "retention," "recall," "recent memory," "disorientation," the confabulation is further studied as an emotionally centered device to reduce unpleasant tensions, aimed at protecting the patient from realization of the memory defects. The confabulations are conceived as the effort of an organically damaged ego system to protect itself. The similarities to fantasy and dream production support this belief. The possible importance of midbrain lesions must be kept in mind.

## Aphasia and Head Injuries

The vast literature on these subjects shows some psychoanalytic insight which is slowly finding increased application. The myriad complexities involved in studying the problems of thinking, memory, and allied processes do not make the task of communicating this insight any easier, since we lack good models for "brain-mind" and a vocabulary which can convey accurately our observations and deductions. In brief, psychoanalysts have noted that patients with head injuries also utilize repression, suppression, substitution, and symbolism in much the same way as patients with neuroses, traumatic neuroses, psychoses, and deliria do. Not all difficulties in thinking (e.g., Korsakoff's syndrome) are due to conflictful emotions, but some are.

The ego functions of perceiving, storing, categorizing, repressing, and initiating motor action are seen to be intelligible even in the absence of an organic deficit. Sharp distinctions between sensory-receptive, motor-expressive, amnesic aphasias, and combinations of these appear to be artifacts created by our limitations in understanding the basic processes of thinking. While aphasia is defined as a disorder of the language functions, it is essential to note that it involves the total organization of the person in a physical-social setting, which includes his historical development. Some patients with severe language disorders are practically normal in their practical and social behavior, while others with minimal language impairment show marked changes in character, attitudes, and ability to adapt themselves to ordinary life-situations. These differences in patients are not easily defined in terms of peripheral ego functions which are amenable to experiment, although the rise of the projective techniques and more subtle experimental settings are advancing this area considerably (9, 58, 122). An excellent example of the applications of these techniques to other organic diseases is the work of Apter and Halstead (9, 10, 11) on brucellosis and hypertension. Injury to the cerebral cortex means injury also to the ego functions, not only mechanically but psychologically, for the cerebral functions are highly valued by man, and any diminution in their efficacy causes apprehension and concern, which in turn arouse defensive measures to protect the total organism from pain and harm. An organism uncertain of its spatial-temporal-social relations (disturbance of the comprehension of the environment), as brain-damaged cases are, is much more vulnerable to suffering than the normal person, even though much of the basic core of the ego be intact—as it so often is. In fact, the essential stability of the ego, even though the brain is severely damaged, is one of the outstanding impressions one gathers from these patients; yet it is easy to see that anxiety, perplexity, confusional states, caution, constriction, uncertainty, distractibility, and emotional lability in combination can obscure this basic stability. Pointed therapeutic skills have done much to prove this view. Pötzl (129) has shown that in these patients the imagery and thinking under emotional pressures have marked similarity to dream productions and are analyzable in the usual manner.

The elucidation of the development of the post-traumatic syndrome and the evaluation of current symptoms have benefited considerably from psychoanalytic observations and reconstructions. Following Freud's descriptions of a traumatic situation (47), in which he emphasized the subject's admission of his own helplessness in the face of a much stronger force, succeeding writers, including Betlheim (18), Ferenczi (37), Stengel (164, 165), Schilder (143, 144, 146), Kardiner (95), Kelman (100), Fenichel (36), Bender (16), Bychowski (26), and Grinker and Weinberg (67), expanded the dynamic interpretations of the interplay between organic and emotional trauma. Kardiner emphasizes those ego activities which aim at controlling both incoming stimuli and the internal equilibrium so that the organism can master both external and internal needs at an optimum. The traumatic neurosis represents, then, a failure of older patterns of adaptation, together with "persistent and unrelenting efforts at restitution" (95). The patient's failure to attain internal mastery, made worse by sensory and motor disorders, causes loss of confidence in the self-system, which, in turn, generates heightened anxiety, anticipatory tensions, masochistic imagery, and fantasies in both day thoughts and night dreams. These forces are held to be responsible for the psychological symptoms created in the manner familiar in the conventional neuroses. The studies mentioned are of importance for the understanding of malingering, accident proneness, and "war neuroses." Continued refinements can be expected as more careful delineation becomes possible (66).

We can hope that, with increased skills, there will be improved methods for the study of neurotic or psychotic reactions engendered by ACTH, cortisone, toxicity, psychosurgery and shock, vagotomy and sympathectomy. Hollós and Ferenczi (85) stressed that almost everyone wants to be intelligent, competent, and responsible. As the ego or self-system is injured, it constricts itself in order to organize its defenses. These may take the form of active or passive patterns or combinations of both. The withdrawal of outgoing energy may impede the very recovery so valiantly sought, because it prevents the maintenance of bonds to other people essential to well-being and increases the suffering due to deprivation. Where there is a physical injury to use as an alibi, however, the ego integrity will be protected from self-accusing guilt. Regression to earlier patterns of dependent working relations (passivity) is then more respectable. The physical illness is utilized by the patient both consciously and unconsciously to increase his prestige with himself and others, in spite of the fact that he is making a worse adaptation than is necessary.

### Surgical Lesions of the Cortex (Psychosurgery)

At the International Neurological Congress in London in 1935, Fulton and Jacobsen (54) reported behavioral changes in two chimpanzees following bilateral removal of the anterior of the frontal lobes. The lobectomized chimpanzees had shown less irritability and overreaction to frustration, which seem to be common in psychotic human behavior. Egas Moniz, a neurologist, and Almeida Lima, a surgeon of Lisbon, during 1935-36 performed the operation on human subjects for the relief of marked anxiety states. Freeman and Watts (45) introduced the prefrontal lobotomy operation into the United States in 1936 (76). In spite of relatively little experimental work, nearly ten thousand radical lobotomies had been done by January, 1949 (8). The voluminous literature on the subject is confusing in many respects, but several reviews are helpful in obtaining a bird's-eye view of various current opinions. The most useful are probably those of Kolb (102), Lewis (111), Greenblatt (60, 61), Fulton (52, 53), Mettler (119), G.A.P. Report No. 6, V.A.T.B. 10-46 (130), and Crown (32).

In a searching review of the psychological studies on patients following prefrontal leucotomy, Crown (32) concludes that some psychological changes can be found on careful testing. Although he excludes some studies, such as the Columbia-Greystone project, because it is concerned with cerebral topectomies, he includes the excellent reviews of Fleming, Kisker, Walker, Patridge, Klebanoff, and Robinson. Fleming's (38) latest review is probably of most interest to clinicians. Crown (32) writes that the syndrome following prefrontal leucotomy is characterized by "apathy, lack of spontaneity, fatuous equanimity, absence of finer emotional response, thoughtlessness and, at times, euphoria. In the selection of cases which will respond well to the operation, the presence in the symptomatology of signs of emotional responses is considered generally to be the most important criterion." He shows that both intellectual and nonintellectual functions are altered by surgery and discusses the research design of future psychometric studies.

Although a few psychiatrists who are also psychoanalysts have published observations on lobotomized patients, it is unfortunate that there is no systematic psychoanalytic study of this group, for the sake of basic science research as well as for clinical evaluation (102). The skeptical view of many psychotherapists is expressed well by Nolan D. C. Lewis (111), who sharply criticizes the indiscriminate use of psychosurgery without adequate study and a rationale. He is supported in this position by Winfred Overholzer, superintendent of St. Elizabeth's Hospital, and Harvey Tompkins, chief of the Veterans Administration Psychiatric Division (*Newsweek*, December 12, 1949, and personal communication). Halstead, Carmichael, and Bucy (76), in 1946, upon reviewing available lobotomy reports, remark: "Unfortunately, aside from their value as vital statistics, it is impossible to assess the validity of these findings. At no point have there been other than superficial attempts made to standardize the criteria for the pre-operative and post-operative clinical status of the patients. Not a single patient has been adequately studied. For a moral and social responsibility to do this, there has been substituted a phenomenal array of case statistics. Unfortunately, the pyramiding of unknowns is scarcely a pathway to knowledge. This is no less true in those few instances where clinical opinion has been supplemented by psychometric devices" (76, pp. 217–18). Kolb (102) and Lewis (111) both stress the need for detailed information, to make study and comparison possible on such basic considerations as type of illness and duration, age, prepsychotic personality, hereditary and familial factors, constitutional type, results from previous therapies, accurate description of the exact surgical procedure with verification wherever possible, a full description of the postoperative psychotherapy and long-term follow-up of the patient's adaptations. There is increasing recognition that the surgical procedures themselves must be standardized, and it is hoped that careful open topectomies, thalamotomies, or gyrectomies will replace the cruder radical lobotomies, transorbital lobotomy, or cortical undercutting. Without such information, there can be no rational selection of therapy. In fact, it is not clear that there is "any statistical proof that operation in early cases affords a higher percentage of results than can be obtained by other methods of therapy or from so-called spontaneous recovery" (102, 111).

The mental status of the patient after psychosurgery has been described frequently (if inadequately in most cases) to reveal the loss of important ego functions, with replacement by new defenses familiar to students of frontal lobe deficit. The variabilities reported are probably functions of greatly different operations with regard to the location and amount of brain tissue involved and the personality organization of the patient, including his past history and the postoperative course. The alterations in the patterns of thinking, feeling, and acting in relation to time, energy, money, hobbies, religion, work record, domestic and sexual habits, and other interpersonal relations can be studied to good advantage by psychoanalysts who are accustomed to applying the microscope of analysis to the data of everyday life. Psychoanalysts could supply some categories of information with greater skill than others if they utilized the techniques of free association and dream analysis. As members of a team including neurologists, psychiatrists, and experimental psychologists, they could provide data which would help decide some gross questions and focus attention upon basic questions pertinent to learning, memory, levels of ego organization with respect to organic injury (76, 102), etc. In spite of the models available in other clinical areas, there is no current record of such close study of a case following psychosurgery.

From a survey of two hundred cases of prefrontals, Frank found "a poverty or entire lack of dreams, and a thinning, or disappearance of dereistic experience—they cannot daydream about their wishes, or be abstractly angry in a sustained fashion. They become, owing to this emotional asymbolia, more plain, matter-of-fact like. In many ways this has a resemblance to slight senile personality changes. Owing to the emotional desensitization, the passions and conflicts which are expressed in their psychoses gradually shift out of focus, very much as old men can look serenely upon the follies of their youth. Again, as in senile personality changes, post-leucotomy patients do not like adventure, but want to remain in a more or less stereotyped routine of activities. The learning ability for new knowledge is, as some patients complain, reduced. In the old involutional melancholic the paradox occurs that the desperate loneliness of oncoming senility is alleviated by reaching sooner the state of a happy dotage. . . . The fundamental personality pattern remains unchanged after leucotomy; it has less legend only" (42, p. 508). Four years later after "contact with more than 300 cases of lobotomy" Frank states: "I think the only clinical criterion which remains available for the indication of lobotomy, considering the many variables, is the intensity and duration of the suffering of the patient. To summarize: The emotional asymbolia caused by lobotomy drains away a psychic dimension. The forebrain, so far as gross functional representation goes, is an important instrument for the integrity of the preconscious system. Lobotomy, by the subsequent defensive hypercathexis and constriction of the ego-boundary, enables the psychic apparatus in some cases to ward off the flooding by id derivatives. Schizophrenics who after the operation have nobody to accept them cannot make an adjustment outside a hospital" (43, p. 42).

From my own observation of over fifteen cases and from personal communications received from three analysts, I can report that dreams are uncommon in most patients in the period immediately following psychosurgery but that in three to six months there is an increasing number of dreams in many patients who previously were able to dream. In two patients there were no dreams a year after the operation, although they had had some dreams before the operation. The form and content of free associations and dreams in this group will furnish valuable comparative data to evaluate the various types of psychosurgery and to help us understand better the dynamics in these patients. Upon extended acquaintance with these patients the inertia, lack of spontaneity, retardation and perseveration, decreased humor and lightheartedness, and the denial of injury become much more apparent.

Experimental psychologists and analysts would have a much better opportunity to examine the intricacies of thinking if data on recovery from the various types of psychosurgery, especially topectomies, were available. The differences in clinical outcome as correlated with the location, plane, and size of the lesion promises much more fruitful research. Grinker (63, 64), like Lewis (8), equates cortical function with abstract thinking and ego functions, whereas the hypothalamus and related structures are the principal centers for id or instinctual functions. The rhinencephalon promises to be more important in these operations than heretofore assumed. Here are ideal opportunities to study differential growth and defenses in the organism under stress. The nature of the basic endowment; acquired action-systems; the interaction between various parts of the personality when different parts of the cortex take over new motor or sensory functions; the more definite understanding of such concepts as anxiety level, regression, and feed-back regulation to main equilibrium—all will help us build a better conceptual model of a "mind in action."

## POSTENCEPHALITIS AND PARKINSONISM

An outline of a few leading articles in this field must suffice for the time being, until a more integrated exposition based on careful observations on more cases is feasible. Nevertheless, it is stimulating to read of the psychoanalytic interpretations offered for these diseases. Smith Ely Jelliffe (in 1925) was one of the first to call attention to the possibilities. After further study he published a monograph, *Psychopathology of Forced Movements and Oculogyric Crises of Lethargic Encephalitis* (90), which has received interested, if not altogether approving, opinion. The searching review by Kubie (103) and Jelliffe's (91) reply are worth mentioning for the purpose of illustrating the need for better clinical and psychological writing. Jelliffe, after pointing out that such non-Freudians as A. N. Whitehead and H. Bergson also understood the meaning of total-personality organization and repression, attempts to demonstrate the usefulness of Freudian concepts in explaining the "positive symptoms" of Hughlings Jackson, the Gestalt phenomena of Wertheimer and Goldstein, and the emergents of Morgan. These concepts, he says, help provide a background for understanding the compulsive phenomena of postencephalitic oculogyric crises. Organic disease (in the sense of irreversible structural changes) in such diseases as postencephalitis causes the total machine to function less efficiently in its adaptation to reality; but this fact may be less vital than its corollary that the machine as a whole continues to function in spite of damage to a part. A blind or lame man may continue to walk by means of the healthy total organism which may make adequate compensatory adaptations. Jelliffe credits improved insight into the complexities of these adaptations to

Von Monakow, Goldstein, Schilder, Hollós and Ferenczi, and W. A. White.

The specific problems of compulsions as fixed patterns of discharges are found in many areas, from the physicochemical to intricate mass sociological reactivity, such as religious rituals. A common factor in all compulsions, whether muscular, ideational, or sociological, is "ambitendence" or ambivalence (20). Oculogyric spasms are somewhat allied to compulsive tics, even though the crises are extreme manifestations of drives in one direction, while tics are "short cramp states with more or less ambitendent characteristics" (90). This bipolarity, the rapid yes-no quality, Freud thought to be an essential element in compulsions, whereas patients with symptoms of conversion hysteria carry out opposites in a single symptom simultaneously in space and time. Some single aspects of oculogyric crises may even function as conversion symptoms, but this does not make the disease an hysteria any more than a conversion symptom in a general paretic alters the basic nature of this disease. That eye movements, like much other synergistic body behavior, must be studied as a part of the total adapting person and not as a single body reflex is supported by detailed studies of numerous neurologists, whose work also illustrates the fallacy of incomplete generalizations from limited data. Eye movements including the oculogyric crises do not occur as isolated phenomena. It is profitable to consider them, at least in many cases, as compulsive phenomena, that is, as substitutive actions occurring in a highly anxious patient who is looking away from some dreaded object of actual or symbolic reality or is forced to stare at it. This is often but not invariably accompanied by a slowing of thought processes (bradyphenia), probably related to inhibition from repression, an anxious emotional state inducing hypervigilance (hypertonia) of the striped and unstriped musculature, and in increased vigilance of the conscious state. Examples are cited of evidence that conscious control and placebos can alter the crises and that fixed psychological situations can induce them, usually accompanied by emotions such as depression, guilt, hostility, and anxiety. Pain may or may not be present. Kubie (103) points out that it is uncertain from the material whether these manifestations are due to the pre-encephalitic personality, from the specific localized organic lesions, or from the effect of the latter upon the personality, in that the instinctual drives are forced to a distorted expression through an injured central nervous system. The relation of compulsive phenomena to tics and clarification of the criteria distinguishing two possible kinds of tics, one basically organic and the other psychogenic, are not developed. Other studies by Jelliffe on Parkinsonian body posture and its unconscious defensive meaning are of passing interest (89). The following authors develop various aspects of this problem: Stekel (168), Bürger and Mayer-Gross (25), Stengel (166, 167), Bender (17), Marshall (116), Shaskan *et al.* (153), Sands (140), and Booth (21).

Booth's use of the Rorschach (21) Test and handwriting specimens to aid his diagnosis and interpretations of the psychodynamics in Parkinsonism is a development which deserves attention in this and other disorders. In 66 cases, Booth found evidence to believe that the Parkinsonian personality, both senile and postencephalitic, is characterized by "urge toward action, expressed through motor activity and through industriousness; striving for independence, authority, and success within a rigid, usually moralistic, behavior pattern" (21, p. 13). Some factors shaping this personality structure and governing the appearance of symptoms are suggested, together with hints for psychotherapy.

Hoffer's analyzed case illustrates the rewards of intensive work with a severe cerebral deficit (84). For five years, a twenty-eight-year-old woman had had spells every four or five days compelling her to smoke thirty or more cigarettes. She was seen in analysis for ten months, thus allowing Hoffer to compare the ego constriction and defense theories of Jelliffe with the increased drives postulated by Stengel (166, 167), as well as to examine the idea that the basic drives in Parkinsonian patients are intensified by the illness in the direction of increased aggressivity and the defenses against it.

## KORSAKOFF'S SYNDROME

Since Korsakoff's disorder is a nonspecific clinical picture found as a sequela to various kinds of cerebral disease (head injury, senility, paresis, presbyophrenia, alcoholic avitaminosis, etc.), it furnishes another experimental setting in which to study the relation of gross organic cerebral tissue loss to the total function of an organism. Here, as in some of the convulsive disorders and general paresis, the central memory loss and resultant defenses can be shown to be due in part to repression and rationalization. Betlheim and Hartmann (19) read to patients a story with frank sexual descriptions which were reproduced by the patients in conventional ways, with deletion of the sexual material and with familiar elaborations in the form of dream symbols, such as "climbing the stairs" and "putting the knife into the sheath" for coitus, and cigarette and knife for penis. These confabulations show clearly that strong underlying affects are operative in determining what material is accepted, how it is reworked, and what is remembered by those having organic disorders of the cortex as well as by normal persons. With the current interest in geriatrics, these studies are of more than academic interest, for they hold some promise of help to therapists in finding more ways to increase the efficiency of the aging ego, even though the organic loss of tissue is present. Psychoanalytic studies on problems of old age were suggested by Karl Abraham (1) in 1926, but there are few such studies. Grotjahn's "Psychoanalytic Investigation of a 71-Year Old Man with Senile Dementia" (71) is an example of the dynamics of improvement with psychotherapy. Such diseases as Pick's and Alzheimer's, which are now being studied more for the metabolic than for the morphologic changes in the brain, have received relatively little attention from Americans. According to Polatin, Hoch, *et al.* (128), Alzheimer's disease was not adequately mentioned in any English-language textbook prior to 1927, and the first *intra vitam* diagnosis of Pick's disease was not published until 1934, when E. Kahn reported one case.

### The Effects of Shock Therapy
#### upon Psychological Behavior

In spite of the thousands of patients who have received various types of "shock" therapy since Sakel (in 1933), Meduna (in 1935), and Cerletti and Bini (1937-38) introduced these methods, there has not been an active psychoanalytic study of these methods. It is perhaps notable that intensive psychodynamic investigations of the prolonged narcosis treatment with barbiturates (Klaesi in 1922), carbon dioxide (Lowenhart *et al.* in 1929), nitrogen (Himwich *et al.* in 1938), oxygen (Hinsie *et al.* in 1934), refrigeration (Talbott and Tillotson in 1941), and electric narcosis treatment (Thompson *et al.*, 1944) have been uncommon (94). The lack of good physiological explanations for the behavioral changes observed in patients undergoing these stresses does not simplify the attempt to find psychological reasons for these changes. The best lead may be the work of Himwich (82, 83) and his colleagues on insulin patients suggesting that reduction of cerebral metabolism and hypoxia are the key processes involved. Unfortunately, there has been no comprehensive study linking this clinical work with the large amount of research on hypoxia on airmen and the high-altitude studies which were stimulated by the war. The reader is referred to the work of Sakel, Meduna, Georgi, Angyal, Ewald, Gellhorn, Stief (94), Weigert (175), Moriarity and Weil (121), Grinker and McLean (65), Rennie (136), Katzenelbogen (98), and others for further review of the several physiological theories offered in explanation of the efficacy of shock and psychosurgery.

Whatever the nature of the physiological stress, powerful psychological consequences are observed. Klaesi, Maier, Flinker, Humbert, and Friedman (94) were among the earliest to recognize the psychological importance of physical procedures. Many patients regard the therapy as a threat to life, and consequently they turn with dependence to the attending staff. Clow and Prout studied 100 patients who had severe physical illness. Eighteen of these also had electroconvulsive therapy (E.C.T.), and 3 had insulin shock. From these patients, Clow and Prout were able to form more definite opinions regarding the clinical observation that some patients improve with physical illness and to relate this empirically to the shock therapies:

> This study of a group of 100 patients definitely suggests that one factor determining the mental improvement often associated with intercurrent physical disorder is a stimulation of the patient's interest towards the realistic goal of recovery through a threat to his physical existence. It is as if the aggression and interest which is withdrawn from external reality and turned inward into the relatively useless fabric of mental illness can often be organized ... by the fear of death which is phylogenetically perhaps his most fundamental concern [28, p. 184].

Schilder (145) recommended early that advantage be taken of the patient's dependence upon the physician immediately after the highly threatening shock, although, along with Weigert (175), he does not believe this phase to be central to remission. The initial anxiety and complications of increased passivity and dependence have been described by Millet and Mosse (120). They also stress the melancholic patient's masochistic view that the treatment is a fitting punishment administered by a judicial doctor-father. Mosse further describes shock as a battering-down of the patient's defenses, with consequent need of psychotherapy and support and reintegration, even though the essential process of the treatment is the atonement for guilt. This process (which may explain why only some psychoses are more amenable to treatment than neuroses), he says, strengthens the ego, increases potency, and liberates libido. There is a paradox involved in the postshock confusional state with its attendant memory defects, in that some memories are definitely "forgotten" while others are liberated. This paradox is implicit in the conflicting reports under review.

Since some patients show extensive erotic behavior, Ligterink (112) suggests that this is an important factor in remission, but opinion is divided about its prevalence and its significance.

Silberman (156) describes some of the inner experiences reported by patients during shock, in terms of the fear of traumatic death and euphoric rebirth. Plaut (127) reports seven cases with initial resistance to the passive role, followed by increased dependence to such a degree that the patients feared to leave the hospital. Jelliffe (94) favored the theory that the threat of death followed by reawakening mobilizes the forces of the ego to overcome the autism and regression. Tanner (171), Moriarity and Weil (121), Schilder (145), Weigert (175), Grotjahn (72), and Kaufman (99) amplify this thesis in various ways.

Glueck (56, 57), regards the accelerated catharsis and ego reintegration as vital processes; Bychowski (27) apparently supports the latter hypothesis, although he speaks of insulin as facilitating the victory of the healthy ego over the pathological one. Weigert (175), after a historical introduction and discussion of dynamics, attempts to explain the apparently contradictory views of Jelliffe and Glueck about the effect of shock upon the ego.

Scott (149) amplifies Jelliffe's theory from his observations on 67 patients. After noting the ambivalent threat to life and integrity, he describes the "gradual concentration of psychic contents into objects in the immediate vicinity." He believes that the actual nearness to death during the depth of the insulin coma may be more important than the apparent consciousness of death, because the fear itself may be unconscious. He also compares the experience of rebirth during emergence from coma with initiation rites. Rubenovitch (94) states that fear of the treatment, short of the threat of death, was the primary agent in insulin treatment, and this opinion became more popular with the use of metrazol. Schilder (145) attempted to combine the psychologic and organic views by utilizing the formulation of the awakening after an epileptic seizure as a victory over death, an elation at rebirth, but expressly states that metrazol is much more than a psychologic agent in the ordinary sense; it is an organic agent, the physiologic action of which affects those "more labile organic structures which serve emotions and which are damaged by the process of schizophrenia." Orenstein and Schilder (123, 124) observed that shock therapies stimulated objective, but not psychodynamic, insight. Abse (3, 4, 5, 6) describes a schizophrenic patient who improved because the repressive force of the E.C.T. satisfied his need for punishment and hence enabled him to reject ego-alien impulses. This is not thoroughgoing therapy because the patient's adaptation is unstable, in response to the anxiety which results in repression and regression. Great care must be exercised to protect such a patient in his post-treatment environment, or more substantial psychotherapy should be employed.

Fordham (41) describes a patient with schizophrenia in whom he believed that the psychoanalytic therapy went counter to the E.C.T. because "the shocks produced an adaptation based on an infantile mechanism and prevented the development of the individuation process upon which the success of the analysis depended."

It is Flescher's (39, 40) thesis that the motor component of the different shocks has not been sufficiently stressed. He cites the psychological value of epileptic convulsions as outlets for aggression and also mentions the cure of traumatic war neuroses by Simmel, who provided a dummy as an outlet for their aggressions, and concludes that E.C.T. is superior to insulin in depressive cases. Flescher believes that E.C.T. works on a primary instinct, that is, on an element which is partly psychic and partly organic. The destructive instinct is freed from inhibition by the convulsions and permits a subsequent liberation of other libidinal energies for more constructive ends. In keeping with this belief, he does not think E.C.T. is valuable when the hostility is reactive, that is, "due to motives of resistance or defense against impulses of a different instinctual origin."

Cohen (29) finds that the fear produced by the prolonged

injection of metrazol which does not result in a convulsion is without therapeutic effect. A. E. Bennett's (94) demonstration that metrazol therapy can be effective when the convulsive phase is controlled with curare offers another challenge to investigators.

Attention should be called to the sedative use of insulin for the treatment of anxiety states as described by Rennie (137) and later by Martin (117). Although a different problem from those under immediate review, the experimental and therapeutic possibilities deserve further attention.

Frosch and Impastato (51) combine a number of earlier suggestions, including those of Schilder, Ferenczi and Hollós, and Nunberg to offer the theory that repeated shock therapy brings about organic processes which shatter the ego. The resulting confusional state associated with anxiety is the result of the disturbed somatopsychic homeostasis and the dissolution of the usual ego boundaries. In attempting to re-establish an equilibrium, the ego may be more or less successful, thus producing various clinical syndromes. If relatively unsuccessful, the ego may regress to archaic narcissistic levels of operation, with attendant weakened defenses, and thereby become more vulnerable to influences from both within and without. If the ego can master the anxiety and the regressive processes in the intervals between shocks, it may be able to bring its adaptations to previous or even higher levels of achievement. Because restitutive defense measures are variable, they will appear as different kinds of reactions.

Even after fifteen years' experience with many cases, it is apparent that there is a wide range of opinion about the efficacy, mode of operation, and prognosis after shock treatment. Lack of space prevents a more detailed discussion of such topics as the importance of the convulsion itself, the appearance of spontaneous convulsions after treatment, and the presence or utility of overt anxiety; but it is worth while to point out some judgments about the relevance of psychotherapy. Some writers, like Sachs (65) or Myerson (65), have interpreted the results from physical agents to mean that physical means alone can cure psychosis. Grinker and McLean (65), Levy *et al.* (110), Moriarity and Weil (121), Wilson (179), Weigert (175), Rennie (136), Kaufman (99), Karliner (96), and Eissler (33) are among those who hold that psychotherapy is a useful and even indispensable adjunct if permanent results are to be obtained. The deep misgivings of some therapists regarding the abuse of shock will be apparent from Eissler's paper:

Sullivan, when discussing recent advances in the physical treatment of psychoses, says that "these sundry procedures, to my way of thinking, produce 'beneficial' results by reducing the patient's capacity for being human. The philosophy is something to the effect that it is better to be a contented imbecile than a schizophrenic. If it were not for the fact that schizophrenics—in my sense—can and do recover and that some extraordinarily gifted and therefore socially significant people suffer schizophrenic episodes, I would not feel so bitter about the therapeutic situation in general and the decortication treatments in particular." This statement succinctly expresses what I have tried to say. Freud's advice, although given with respect to the treatment of neuroses, is, in my opinion, equally applicable as a guiding principle to valid therapy for the functional psychoses: "After all," writes Freud, "analysis does not set out to abolish the possibility of morbid reactions, but to give the patient's ego freedom to choose one way or the other" [33, p. 81].

Weigert concludes:

The result of our observation leads to a very reserved application of convulsion therapy. In favorable cases we abstain from every sort of artificial interference with the exception of psychotherapeutic help which supports the natural healing process of the psychosis. If this natural healing process is retarded we prefer the milder sleep treatment as an attempt to overcome the impasse to which the emotional conflict has led. Only if the sleep treatment fails do we feel justified in applying shock or convulsion therapy as a desperate attempt to overcome the patient's inward conflicts by catering to his need for punishment and self-destruction.

Doing this, we know, we reinforce the patient's hopeless belief in a cruel response to destructive drives. In most cases we do not break through the vicious circle of uncontrolled drives, need of punishment and expiation leading back to unmastered greed, the extremes of manic-depressive dynamics, that evade the maturing development by renunciation. Shock and convulsion therapy is opposed to the main striving of psychoanalytic therapy: to mitigate the cruelty of an archaic superego and to help the patient to endure the necessary, but not the unnecessary, hardships of reality [175, p. 209].

Grinker and McLean (65) take the more neutral position that the various shock therapies have often enough shown beneficial results and of such proportions that they deserve close study. In their thoughtful review, they report the psychodynamics of a depressed woman treated with metrazol during the course of psychotherapy, and they present a psychophysiological theory that either physical or psychological shocks of sufficient intensity may alter the inhibited pathways "between the cortex (ego) and diencephalon (biological drives)."

They are supported in their greater willingness to use shock by a group of psychiatrists who have carefully studied the current results (74). This committee found shock most useful in the patients with depression (involutional melancholia; manic-depressive psychosis, depressive type; psychoneurosis, reactive depression; and depression associated with certain organic brain disorders). Shock may be helpful in some cases of manic-depressive psychosis, manic type; a few acute cases of schizophrenia, organic psychosis with excitement. Shock seems contraindicated in psychosomatic conditions, psychoneuroses with the exception of neurotic depressions, psychopathic personalities, and the behavior problems of children. The committee finds, from accumulated experience, that there are no absolute physical contraindications to electro-shock therapy. The need for adequate safeguards in giving out-patient electric shock therapy is stressed.

From experience with insulin, metrazol, and electric shock therapy, the writer has been impressed with the relationship which exists between the patient and doctor and others of the attending staff, whether or not the patient shows overt convulsions, anxiety, guilt, or hostility. There is good reason to believe that some insulin patients owe much of their recovery to a good relationship with a nurse or other significant figure. Some nurses on insulin wards have a significantly higher number of recoveries. If successful patients are followed therapeutically after shock, one finds ample evidence that many of their problems are still with them. Whatever the physical agent employed, there usually remains the challenge to improve the adaptation of the patient after the initial confusion and memory changes decrease, and to prevent relapses which are often present even when shock is given in full dosages. Because of uneven results with the new methods of shock therapy, no firm recommendations can be made at this time.

There is lively interest, but little agreement, in the signs of intellectual impairment after shock therapy of more than a few weeks' duration since the reports by Levy, Serota, *et al.* (12, 109, 110, 125, 181). Landis (104) summarizes much of the experimental work up to 1949. He finds that ordinary psychometric instruments do not detect a loss of intelligence or show how temporary is the change in memory functions or whether there is a permanent decrease in affect. More recently Janis (86, 88) reports persistent retroactive circumscribed amnesias beyond the usual period of recovery, during which the temporary organic reactions to the treatments clear up. Analysis of his data provides support for the hypothesis that these amnesias may be related to the changes in affect, not as a primary factor reducing affective disturbances, but providing another defense akin to repression which makes other defensive symptoms unnecessary.

The review by Stainbrook (162) in 1946 summarizes earlier work. Interested students will find Ellis' essay, "Toward the Improvement of Psychoanalytic Research" (34), valuable for clarifying their studies. The dynamically oriented clinician can contribute significantly in these studies on affect and symptom alteration as well as in the detailed studies on the more localized, specific loss of thinking functions which are puzzling the experimentalist. Long-term follow-up studies by experimental psychologists and psychoanalysts are needed to reveal more accurately the changes in thinking and in ego dynamics attendant upon shock therapy. It is probable that better hypotheses for all mental activity are required in order to clarify the major issues presented by observations (132, 134).

## BIBLIOGRAPHY

1. Abraham, K. "The Applicability of Psycho-analytic Treatment to Patients at an Advanced Age," in *Selected Papers* (London: Hogarth Press, 1927), pp. 312–17.
2. Abraham, K. "Notes on the Psychogenesis of Melancholia," in *Selected Papers* (London: Hogarth Press, 1927), pp. 453–64.
3. Abse, D. W. "A Case Illustrating the Limits of the Cure Following Convulsion Therapy," *Brit. J. M. Psychol.*, 22:194, 1949.
4. Abse, D. W. "Psychology of Convulsion Therapy," *J. Ment. Sc.*, 86:95, 1940.
5. Abse, D. W. "Rationale of Convulsion Therapy," *Brit. J. M. Psychol.*, 19:262, 1940.
6. Abse, D. W. "Theory of the Rationale of Convulsion Therapy," *Brit. J. M. Psychol.*, 20:33, 1944.
7. Adrian, E. D. *The Physical Background of Perception* (Oxford: Clarendon Press, 1947).
8. "Anglo-American Symposium on Psychosurgery," *Proc. Roy. Soc. Med.*, Vol. 42, Suppl. 1949.
9. Apter, N. S.; Eisele, C. W.; et al. "Cerebral Pathology in Brucellosis: A Combined Medical, Neuropsychiatric, and Experimental Psychological Study," *Tr. Am. Neurol. A.*, 73:39, 1948.
10. Apter, N. S.; Halstead, W. C.; et al. "Cerebral Complications in Essential Hypertension," *Tr. Am. Neurol. A.*, 74:219, 1949.
11. Apter, N. S.; Halstead, W. C.; et al. "Impaired Cerebral Functions in Chronic Brucellosis," *Am. J. Psychiat.*, 105:361, 1948.

12. BARRERA, S. E.; LEWIS, N. D. C.; *et al.* "Brain Changes Associated with Electrically Induced Seizures," *Tr. Am. Neurol. A.*, 31–35, 1942.
13. BARTEMEIER, L. H. "Concerning the Psychogenesis of Convulsive Disorders," *Psychoanalyt. Quart.*, 12:330, 1943.
14. BEACH, F. A. "Effects of Cortical Lesions upon the Copulatory Behavior of Male Rats," *J. Comp. Psychol.*, 29:193, 1940.
15. BEACH, F. A. "Effects of Injury to the Cerebral Cortex upon Sexually-receptive Behavior in the Female Rat," *Psychosom. Med.*, 6:40, 1944.
16. BENDER, L. "Organic Brain Conditions Producing Behavior Disturbances: A Clinical Survey of Encephalitis, Burn Encephalopathy, and the Traumatic States," in *Modern Trends in Child Psychiatry*, ed. N. D. C. LEWIS and B. L. PACELLA (New York: International Universities Press, 1945).
17. BENDER, L. "Post-encephalitic Behavior Disorders in Childhood," in *Encephalitis: A Clinical Study*, ed. J. B. NEAL (New York: Grune & Stratton, 1942), pp. 363–84.
18. BETLHEIM, S., and HARTMANN, H. "Über Fehlreaktionen bei der Korsakoffschen Psychose," *Arch. f. Psychiat.*, 72:275, 1924.
19. BETLHEIM, S. "Zur Frage des zwangsmässigen Greifens bei organischen Hirnerkrankungen," *Monatschr. f. Psychiat. u. Neurol.*, 57:141, 1924.
20. BLEULER, E. *Textbook of Psychiatry* (London: George Allen & Unwin, Ltd., 1923).
21. BOOTH, G. "Psychodynamics in Parkinsonism," *Psychosom. Med.*, 10:1, 1948.
22. BOWLBY, J. *Maternal Care and Mental Health* (Geneva: World Health Organization, 1951).
23. BROSIN, H. W. "Emotional Aspects of Organic Disease," *Wisconsin M. J.*, 48:607, 1949.
24. BRUN, R. "Sigmund Freud's Leistungen auf dem Gebiete der organische Neurologie," *Schweiz. Arch. f. Neurol. u. Psychiat.*, 37:200, 1936.
25. BÜRGER, H., and MAYER-GROSS, W. "Über Zwangssymptome bei Encephalitis lethargica und über die Struktur der Zwangserscheinungen überhaupt," *Ztschr. f. d. ges. Neurol. u. Psychiat.*, 116:645, 1928.
26. BYCHOWSKI, G. "The Ego of the Brain Wounded," *Psychoanalyt. Rev.*, 36:333, 1949.
27. BYCHOWSKI, G. "Psychoanalyse im hypoglykämischen Zustand: Versuche zur Therapie der Psychosen," *Internat. Ztschr. f. Psychoanal.*, 23:540, 1937.
28. CLOW, H. E., and PROUT, C. T. "A Study of the Modifications of Mental Illness by Intercurrent Physical Disorders in One Hundred Patients," *Am. J. Psychiat.*, 103:179, 1946.
29. COHEN, L. H. "The Therapeutic Significance of Fear in the Metrazol Treatment of Schizophrenia," *Am. J. Psychiat.*, 95:1349, 1939.
30. CORIAT, I. H. "A Psychoanalytic Interpretation of the Mental Symptoms of Paresis," *Psychoanalyt. Rev.*, 32:253, 1945.

31. CRONBACH, L. J. "Statistical Methods Applied to Rorschach Scores: A Review," *Psychol. Bull.*, 46:393, 1949.
32. CROWN, S. "Psychological Changes Following Prefrontal Leucotomy: A Review," *J. Ment. Sc.*, 97:49, 1951.
33. EISSLER, K. R. "Schizophrenia: Structural Analysis and Metrazol Treatment," *Psychiatry*, 6:75, 1943.
34. ELLIS, ALBERT. "Toward the Improvement of Psychoanalytic Research," *Psychoanalyt. Rev.*, 36:123, 1949.
35. "Evaluation of the Results of Surgical Procedures Undertaken for the Relief of Psychoses," *Surg., Gynec. & Obst.*, 92:601, 1951.
36. FENICHEL, O. *The Psychoanalytic Theory of Neurosis* (New York: W. W. Norton & Co., 1945).
37. FERENCZI, S. "Disease or Patho-neuroses," in *Further Contributions to the Theory and Technique of Psycho-analysis* (London: Hogarth Press, 1926).
38. FLEMING, G. W. "The Neurosurgical Treatment of Mental Illness," *Recent Progress in Psychiatry*, 2:661, 1950.
39. FLESCHER, J. "The Discharging Function of Electric Shock and the Anxiety Problem," *Psychoanalyt. Rev.*, 37:277, 1950.
40. FLESCHER, J. "Further Contributions to the Psychodynamics of Convulsive Treatment," *J. Nerv. & Ment. Dis.*, 109:550, 1949.
41. FORDHAM, M. "A Comparative Study between the Effects of Analysis and Electrical Convulsion Therapy in a Case of Schizophrenia," *Brit. J. M. Psychol.*, 20:412, 1946.
42. FRANK, J. "Clinical Survey and Results of 200 Cases of Prefrontal Leucotomy," *J. Ment. Sc.*, 92:497, 1946.
43. FRANK, J. "Some Aspects of Lobotomy (Prefrontal Leucotomy) under Psychoanalytic Scrutiny," *Psychiatry*, 13:35, 1950.
44. FREEMAN, W. "Psychosurgery," *Am. J. Psychiat.*, 106:534, 1950.
45. FREEMAN, W., and WATTS, J. W. *Psychosurgery in the Treatment of Mental Disorders and Intractable Pain* (2d ed.; Springfield: C. C. Thomas, 1950).
46. FREUD, S. *Zur Auffassung der Aphasien* (Wien: F. Deuticke, 1891).
47. FREUD, S. *Beyond the Pleasure Principle* (London: Hogarth Press, 1922).
48. FREUD, S. "Dostoevsky and Parricide," in *Yearbook of Psychoanalysis* (New York: International Universities Press, 1946), pp. 231–49.
49. FREUD, S. *The Ego and the Id* (London: Hogarth Press, 1923).
50. FREUD, S. "Mourning and Melancholia," in *Collected Papers*, 4 (London: Hogarth Press, 1925), pp. 152–70.
51. FROSCH, J., and IMPASTATO, D. "The Effects of Shock Treatment on the Ego," *Psychoanalyt. Quart.*, 17:226, 1948.
52. FULTON, J. F. "Neurophysiology, 1942–1948," *New England J. Med.*, 240:883, 920, 1949.
53. FULTON, J. F.; ARING, C. D.; *et al. The Frontal Lobes* (Baltimore: Williams & Wilkins, 1948).
54. FULTON, J. F., and JACOBSEN, C. F. "Functions of the Frontal Lobes: Comparative Studies in Monkeys, Chimpanzees, and Man," *Abstr. Second Internat. Neurol. Congress* (London, 1935), p. 70.

55. GIBBS, F. A. and E. L. *Atlas of Electroencephalography* (Cambridge: Addison-Wesley, 1945).

56. GLUECK, B. "The Effect of the Hypoglycemic Theory on the Psychotic Process," *Am. J. Psychiat.*, 94:171, 1937.

57. GLUECK, B. "Psychopathologic Reactions and Electric Shock Therapy," *New York State J. Med.*, 42:1553, 1942.

58. GOLDSTEIN, K. *Language and Language Disturbances* (New York: Grune & Stratton, 1948).

59. GRAY, H. "Bibliography of Freud's Pre-analytic Period," *Psychoanalyt. Rev.*, 35:403, 1948.

60. GREENBLATT, M.; ARNOT, R.; *et al. Studies in Lobotomy* (New York: Grune & Stratton, 1950).

61. GREENBLATT, M., and MYERSON, P. G. "Psychosurgery," *New England J. Med.*, 240:1006, 1949.

62. GREENSON, R. R. "On Genuine Epilepsy," *Psychoanalyt. Quart.*, 13:139, 1944.

63. GRINKER, R. R. "A Comparison of Psychological 'Repression' and Neurological Inhibition,' " *J. Nerv. & Ment. Dis.*, 89:765, 1939.

64. GRINKER, R. R. "Hypothalamic Functions in Psychosomatic Correlations," in *Studies in Psychosomatic Medicine*, ed. F. ALEXANDER and T. M. FRENCH (New York: Ronald Press Co., 1948), pp. 46–84.

65. GRINKER, R. R., and McLEAN, H. V. "The Course of a Depression Treated by Psychotherapy and Metrazol," *Psychosom. Med.*, 2:119, 1940.

66. GRINKER, R. R., and SPIEGEL, J. P. *Men under Stress* (Philadelphia: Blakiston Co., 1945).

67. GRINKER, R. R., and WEINBERG, J. "Neuroses Following Head and Brain Injuries," in *Injuries of the Brain and Spinal Cord and Their Coverings*, ed. S. BROCK (Baltimore: Williams & Wilkins, 1949), pp. 329–41.

68. GRODDECK, G. *Die psychische Bedingtheit und psychoanalytische Behandlung organischer Krankheiten* (Berlin: S. Hirzel, 1917).

69. GROTJAHN, M. "Zur Klinik und Psychologie der juvenilin Paralyse," *Monatschr. f. Psychiat. u. Neurol.*, 92:299; 93:19, 1936.

70. GROTJAHN, M. "Psychoanalysis and Brain Disease: Observations of Juvenile Patients," *Psychoanalyt. Rev.*, 25:149, 1938.

71. GROTJAHN, M. "Psychoanalytic Investigation of a 71-Year Old Man with Senile Dementia," *Psychoanalyt. Quart.*, 9:80, 1940.

72. GROTJAHN, M. "Psychiatric Observations of Schizophrenic Patients during Metrazol Treatment," *Bull. Menninger Clin.*, 2:142, 1938.

73. GROUP FOR ADVANCEMENT OF PSYCHIATRY, *Research on Prefrontal Lobotomy* (Rept. No. 6 [June, 1948]).

74. GROUP FOR ADVANCEMENT OF PSYCHIATRY, *Revised Electro-Shock Therapy Report* (Rept. No. 15 [August, 1950]).

75. HALSTEAD, W. C. *Brain and Intelligence* (Chicago: University of Chicago Press, 1947).

76. HALSTEAD, W. C.; CARMICHAEL, H. T.; *et al.* "Prefrontal Lobotomy: A Preliminary Appraisal of the Behavioral Results," *Am. J. Psychiat.*, 103:217, 1946.

77. HARTMANN, H. "Zur Frage organische Amnesie und Hypnose: Versuche an Korsakoffkranken," *Wien. klin. Wchnschr.*, 40:1507, 1927.

78. HARTMANN, H. "Gedächtnis und Lustprinzip: Untersuchungen an Korsakoffkranken," *Ztschr. f. d. ges. Neurol. u. Psychiat.*, 126:496, 1930.

79. HARTMANN, H., and SCHILDER, P. "Hypnoseversuche an Paralytikern," *Jahrb. f. Psychiat. u. Neurol.*, 44:194, 1925.

80. HASSIN, G. B. *Histopathology of the Peripheral and Central Nervous Systems* (New York: Paul B. Hoeber, Inc., 1940).

81. HILGARD, E. R. *Theories of Learning* (New York: Appleton-Century-Crofts, 1948).

82. HIMWICH, H. E.; BOWMAN, K. M.; *et al.* "Biochemical Changes Occurring in the Cerebral Blood during the Insulin Treatment of Schizophrenia," *J. Nerv. & Ment. Dis.*, 89:273, 1939.

83. HIMWICH, H. E.; FROSTIG, J. P.; *et al.* "The Mechanism of the Symptoms of Insulin Hypoglycemia," *Am. J. Psychiat.*, 96:371, 1939.

84. HOFFER, W. "Analyse einer postencephalitischen Geistesstörung," *Internat. Ztschr. f. Psychoanal. u. Imago*, 25:264, 1940.

85. HOLLOS, S., and FERENCZI, S. *Psychoanalysis and the Psychic Disorder of General Paresis* (New York: Nervous and Mental Disease Publishing Co., 1925).

86. JANIS, I. L. "Psychologic Effects of Electric Convulsive Treatments. I. Post-treatment Amnesias," *J. Nerv. & Ment. Dis.*, 111:359, 1950.

87. JANIS, I. L. "Psychologic Effects of Electric Convulsive Treatments. II. Changes in Word Association Reactions," *J. Nerv. & Ment. Dis.*, 111:383, 1950.

88. JANIS, I. L. "Psychologic Effects of Electric Convulsive Treatments. III. Changes in Affective Disturbances," *J. Nerv. & Ment. Dis.*, 111:469, 1950.

89. JELLIFFE, S. E. "The Parkinsonian Body Posture: Some Considerations on Unconscious Hostility," *Psychoanalyt. Rev.*, 27:467, 1940.

90. JELLIFFE, S. E. *Psychopathology of Forced Movements and the Oculogyric Crises of Lethargic Encephalitis* (New York: Nervous and Mental Disease Publishing Co., 1932).

91. JELLIFFE, S. E. "The Psychopathology of the Oculogyric Crises and Its Funeral by Dr. Lawrence Kubie," *Psychoanalyt. Quart.*, 4:360, 1935.

92. JELLIFFE, S. E. "Sigmund Freud as a Neurologist: Some Notes on His Earlier Neurobiological and Clinical Neurological Studies," *J. Nerv. & Ment. Dis.*, 85:696, 1937.

93. KALINOWSKY, L. B. "Experience with Electric Convulsive Therapy in Various Types of Psychiatric Patients," *Bull. New York Acad. Med.*, 20:485, 1944.

94. KALINOWSKY, L. B., and HOCH, P. H. *Shock Treatments and Other Somatic Procedures in Psychiatry* (New York: Grune & Stratton, 1946).

95. KARDINER, A. "The Bio-analysis of the Epileptic Reaction," *Psychoanalyt. Quart.*, 1:375, 1932.

96. KARLINER, W. "Present Status of Electric Sleep Treatments," *M. Rec.*, 159:87, 1946.
97. KATAN, M. Quoted by J. H. W. VAN OPHUIJSEN in "Organic Psychoses," in *Psychoanalysis Today*, ed. S. LORAND (New York: International Universities Press, 1944), pp. 287-94.
98. KATZENELBOGEN, S. "A Critical Appraisal of the Shock Therapies II (Insulin)," *Psychiatry*, 3:211, 1940.
99. KAUFMAN, M. R. "Factors in Psychotherapy: A Psychoanalytic Evalution," *Psychiat. Quart.*, 15:117, 1941.
100. KELMAN, H. "Character and Traumatic Syndrome," *J. Nerv. & Ment. Dis.*, 102:121, 1945.
101. KLUCKHOHN, C., and MURRAY, H. A. (eds.). *Personality in Nature, Society, and Culture* (New York: A. Knopf, 1948).
102. KOLB, L. C. "Evaluation of Lobotomy and Its Potentialities for Future Research in Psychiatry and Basic Sciences," *J. Nerv. & Ment. Dis.*, 110:112, 1949.
103. KUBIE, L. S. Review of *The Psychopathology of Forced Movements and the Oculogyric Crises of Lethargic Encephalitis* by S. E. Jelliffe, *Psychoanalyt. Quart.*, 2:622, 1933.
104. LANDIS, C. "Experimental Methods in Psychopathology," *Ment. Hyg.*, 33:96, 1949.
105. LASHLEY, K. S. "Coalescence of Neurology and Psychology," *Proc. Am. Phil. Soc.*, 84:461, 1941.
106. LASHLEY, K. S., and WADE, M. "The Pavlovian Theory of Generalization," *Psychol. Rev.*, 53:72, 1946.
107. LENNOX, W. G. *Science and Seizures* (New York: Harper & Bros., 1941).
108. LEVY, D. M. "Maternal Overprotection (*Concluded*)," *Psychiatry*, 5:63, 1942; also in *Modern Trends in Child Psychiatry*, ed. N. D. C. LEWIS and B. L. PACELLA (New York: International Universities Press, 1945), pp. 27-34.
109. LEVY, N. A., and GRINKER, R. R. "Psychological Observations in Affective Psychoses Treated with Combined Convulsive Shock and Psychotherapy," *J. Nerv. & Ment. Dis.*, 97:623, 1943.
110. LEVY, N. A.; SEROTA, H. M.; *et al.* "Disturbances in Brain Function Following Convulsive Shock Therapy; Electroencephalographic and Clinical Studies," *Arch. Neurol. & Psychiat.*, 47:1009, 1942.
111. LEWIS, N. D. C. "Comments on Psychosurgery," read at the November, 1949, meeting of the Washington, D.C., Psychiatric Society (also personal communication).
112. LIGTERINK, J. A. T. "Drawbacks of Convulsion Therapy Produced by Metrazol Administration in Schizophrenia," *Psychiat. en neurol. bl.*, 41:633, 1937.
113. LORENTE DE NO, R. "Analysis of the Activity of the Chains of Internuncial Neurons," *J. Neurophysiol.*, 1:207, 1938.
114. LORENTE DE NO, R. "Studies on the Structure of the Cerebral Cortex. I. The Area Entorhinalis," *J. f. Psychol. u. Neurol.*, 45:381, 1934.
115. LORENTE DE NÓ, R. "Studies on the Structure of the Cerebral Cortex.

II. Continuation of the Studies of the Ammonic System," *J. f. Psychol. u. Neurol.*, 46:113, 1934.

116. MARSHALL, W. "The Psychopathology and Treatment of the Parkinsonian Syndrome and Other Postencephalitic Sequelae," *J. Nerv. & Ment. Dis.*, 84:27, 1936.

117. MARTIN, G. J. "Sedative Insulin Treatment of Anxiety in the Anxiety Neurosis," *J. Nerv. & Ment. Dis.*, 109:347, 1949.

118. MENNINGER, W. C. *Juvenile Paresis* (Baltimore: Williams & Wilkins, 1936).

119. METTLER, F. A. (ed.). *Selective Partial Ablation of the Frontal Cortex* (New York: Paul B. Hoeber, Inc., 1949).

120. MILLET, J. A. P., and MOSSE, E. P. "On Certain Psychological Aspects of Electroshock Therapy," *Psychosom. Med.*, 6:226, 1944.

121. MORIARITY, J. D., and WEIL, A. A. "Healing Mechanisms in the Shock Treated Neurotic Patient," *J. Nerv. & Ment. Dis.*, 101:205, 1945.

122. OBERHOLSER, E. "Zur Differentialdiagnose psychoneurotischer u. organischer Zustände nach Schädeltrauma mittelst des Rorschachschen Formdeutung Versuches," *Ztschr. f. d. ges. Neurol. u. Psychiat.*, 136:452, 1931.

123. ORENSTEIN, L. L., and SCHILDER, P. "Psychological Considerations of the Insulin Treatment in Schizophrenia," *J. Nerv. & Ment. Dis.*, 88:397, 1938.

124. ORENSTEIN, L. L., and SCHILDER, P. "Psychological Considerations of the Insulin Treatment in Schizophrenia," *J. Nerv. & Ment. Dis.*, 88:644, 1938.

125. PACELLA, B. L., and BARRERA, S. E. "Spontaneous Convulsions Following Convulsive Shock Therapy," *Am. J. Psychiat.*, 101:783, 1945.

126. PARKER, G. M. "Analytic Views of the Psychic Factor in Shock," *New York M. J.*, 108:12, 58, 1918.

127. PLAUT, A. B. J. "Some Psychological Observations on E.C.T.," *Brit. J. M. Psychol.*, 21:263, 1947–48.

128. POLATIN, P.; HOCH, P. H.; *et al.* "Presenile Psychosis: Report of Two Cases with Brain Biopsy Studies," *Am. J. Psychiat.*, 105:96, 1948.

129. PÖTZL, O. "Über einige Wechselwirkungen hysterischer und organischer zerebraler Störungmechanismen," *Jahrb. f. Psychiat.*, 37:269, 1917.

130. *Prefrontal Leucotomy: An Evaluation* (V.A.T.B. Rept. No. 10-46) (Washington 25, D.C., May 21, 1948).

131. "Anglo-American Symposium on Psychosurgery," *Proc. Roy. Soc. Med.*, Vol. 42, Suppl. 1949.

132. RAPAPORT, D. "On the Psycho-analytic Theory of Thinking," *Internat. J. Psycho-Analysis*, 31:161, 1950.

133. RAPAPORT, D. (ed.). *Organization and Pathology of Thought* (New York: Columbia University Press, 1951).

134. RAPAPORT, D. "Toward a Theory of Thinking," in *Organization and Pathology of Thought*, ed. D. RAPAPORT (New York: Columbia University Press, 1951), pp. 689–730.

135. *Rehabilitation of Chronic Neurologic Patients* (V.A. Pamphlet No. 10–29 [May, 1949]).
136. RENNIE, T. A. C. "Present Status of Shock Therapy," *Psychiatry,* 6:127, 1943.
137. RENNIE, T. A. C. "The Use of Insulin as Sedation Therapy," *Arch. Neurol. & Psychiat.,* 50:697, 1943.
138. *Research on Prefrontal Lobotomy* (G.A.P. Rept. No. 6 [June, 1948]).
139. *Revised Electro-Shock Therapy Report* (G.A.P. Rept. No. 15 [August, 1950]).
140. SANDS, I. J. "Type of Personality Susceptible to Parkinson's Disease," *J. Mt. Sinai Hosp.,* 9:792, 1942.
141. SCHAFFER, K. "Die werktätigen Prinzipien in der Histologie organischer Hirn-Geisteskrankheiten," *Arch. f. Psychiat.,* 85:16, 1928.
142. SCHILDER, P. *Introduction to a Psychoanalytic Psychiatry* (New York: Nervous and Mental Disease Publishing Co., 1928).
143. SCHILDER, P. "Language and the Constructive Energies of the Psyche," *Scientia,* March, April, 1936, pp. 149–58, 205–11.
144. SCHILDER, P. "Neuroses Following Head and Brain Injuries," in *Injuries of the Skull, Brain, and Spinal Cord,* ed. S. BROCK (Baltimore: Williams & Wilkins, 1949), pp. 298–328.
145. SCHILDER, P. "Notes on the Psychology of Metrazol Treatments of Schizophrenia," *J. Nerv. & Ment. Dis.,* 89:133, 1939.
146. SCHILDER, P. "Psychic Disturbances after Head Injuries," *Am. J. Psychiat.,* 91:155, 1934.
147. SCHILDER, P. *Studien zur Psychologie und Symptomatologie der progressiven Paralyse* (Berlin: Karger, 1930).
148. SCOTT, J. P. "Studies on the Early Development of Social Behavior in Puppies," *Am. Psychologist,* 3:239, 1948.
149. SCOTT, R. D. "The Psychology of Insulin Coma Treatment," *Brit. J. M. Psychol.,* 23:15, 1950.
150. SEARS, R. R. "Experimental Analysis of Psychoanalytic Phenomena," in *Personality and the Behavior Disorders,* ed. J. McV. HUNT, 1 (New York: Ronald Press Co., 1944), pp. 306–32.
151. SEARS, R. R. *Survey of Objective Studies of Psychoanalytic Concepts* (Social Science Research Council Bull. No. 51) (New York, 1943).
152. SHAKOW, D. *The Nature of Deterioration in Schizophrenic Conditions* (New York: Nervous and Mental Disease Publishing Co., 1946).
153. SHASKAN, D.; YARNELL, H.; *et al.* "Physical, Psychiatric, and Psychometric Studies of Post-encephalitic Parkinsonism," *J. Nerv. & Ment. Dis.,* 96:652, 1942.
154. SHERRINGTON, C. S. *Man on His Nature* (Cambridge: Cambridge University Press, 1941).
155. SHICK, A. "A Contribution to the Psychopathology of Genuine Epilepsy," *Psychoanalyt. Rev.,* 36:217, 1949.
156. SILBERMAN, I. "The Psychical Experiences during the Shocks in Shock Therapy," *Internat. J. Psycho-Analysis,* 21:179, 1940.

157. SPITZ, R. A. "Anaclitic Depression," in *The Psychoanalytic Study of the Child*, 2 (1946), 313.
158. SPITZ, R. A. "Autoerotism: Some Empirical Findings and Hypotheses on Three of Its Manifestations in the First Year of Life," in *The Psychoanalytic Study of the Child*, 3/4 (1949), 85.
159. SPITZ, R. A. "Hospitalism: An Inquiry into the Genesis of Psychiatric Conditions in Early Childhood," in *The Psychoanalytic Study of the Child*, 1 (1945), 53.
160. SPITZ, R. A. "Hospitalism: A Follow-Up Report," in *The Psychoanalytic Study of the Child*, 2 (1946), 113.
161. SPITZ, R. A. "Relevancy of Direct Infant Observation," in *The Psychoanalytic Study of the Child*, 5 (1950), 66.
162. STAINBROOK, E. J. "Shock Therapy: Psychological Theory and Research," *Psychol. Bull.*, 43:21, 1946.
163. STARR, M. A. "Cortical Lesions of the Brain," *Brain*, 1887 (ref. in G. RYLANDER, *Acta Psychiat.*, Suppl. 20, 1939).
164. STENGEL, E. "Zur Kenntnis der Triebstörungen und der Abwehrreaktionen des Ichs bei Hirnkranken," *Internat. Ztschr. f. Psychoanal.*, 21:544, 1935.
165. STENGEL, E. "Über psychische Zwangsphänomene bei Hirnkranken und ihre Bedeutung für die Lehre von der Zwangsneurose," *Jahrb. f. Psychiat. u. Neurol.*, 52:236, 1935.
166. STENGEL, E. "Studien über die Beziehungen zwischen Geistesstörung und Sprachstörung; zur Lehre von der Wortfindungsstörung und von der Paraphasie," *Monatschr. f. Psychiat. u. Neurol.*, 95:129, 1937.
167. STENGEL, E. "Weitere Beiträge zur Kenntnis des postencephalitischen Blickkrampfes," *Ztschr. f. d. ges. Neurol. u. Psychiat.*, 127:441, 1930.
168. STEKEL, W. *Compulsion and Doubt* (New York: Liveright Pub. Corp., 1949).
169. SULLIVAN, H. S. "Conceptions of Modern Psychiatry," *Psychiatry*, 3:1, 1940.
170. "Evaluation of the Results of Surgical Procedures Undertaken for the Relief of Psychoses," *Surg., Gynec. & Obst.*, 92:601, 1951.
171. TANNER, H. "Physiological and Psychological Factors in Electroshock as Criteria of Therapy," *J. Nerv. & Ment. Dis.*, 111:232, 1950.
172. THURSTONE, L. L. *Primary Mental Abilities* (Psychometric Monograph No. 1) (Chicago: University of Chicago Press, 1938).
173. VETERANS ADMINISTRATION. *Rehabilitation of Chronic Neurologic Patients* (Pamphlet No. 10-29 [May, 1949]).
174. (V.A.T.B. Rept. No. 10-46) (Washington 25, D.C., May 21, 1948) *Prefrontal Leucotomy: An Evaluation.*
175. WEIGERT, E. V. "Psychoanalytic Notes on Sleep and Convulsion Treatment in Functional Psychoses," *Psychiatry*, 3:189, 1940.
176. WEIL, A. *Textbook of Neuropathology* (2d ed.; New York: Grune & Stratton, 1945).

177. Weisner, B. P., and Sheard, N. M. *Maternal Behavior in the Rat* (Edinburgh: Oliver & Boyd, 1933).
178. Welt, L. [1887–10 cases], *Deutsches Arch. f. klin. Med.*, 4Z., 1887.
179. Wilson, Cyril. "An Individual Point of View on Shock Therapy," *Internat. J. Psycho-Analysis*, 24:59, 1943.
180. Wortis, J. "Failures with Insulin Shock Therapy," in *Failures in Psychiatric Treatment*, ed. P. H. Hoch (New York: Grune & Stratton, 1948).
181. Zubin, J., and Barrera, S. E. "Effect of Electric Convulsive Therapy on Memory," *Proc. Soc. Exper. Biol. & Med.*, 48:596, 1941.

# IX

## PSYCHODYNAMIC APPROACH TO THE STUDY OF PSYCHOSES

### John C. Whitehorn, M.D.

THE psychoses present problems of special difficulty for psychodynamics, both in application and in conception. The psychotic patient is, by practical definition, much further alienated from social contact than is the neurotic patient. It is a common experience, in the professional interview with a psychotic patient, that one gains little, if any, impression of a shared effort toward a common aim of better mental health. Even the psychotically depressed patient who bemoans his terrible condition, or the schizophrenic patient who has "insight" to the extent that a morbid condition is acknowledged, does not appear to share in a common faith with physicians or others to a sufficient extent for a ready, working partnership. Psychotic patients in general have what might be called a very high "sales resistance." They are not receptive to advice or persuasion. They appear immune to all ordinary efforts to influence them psychologically. In actual experience, that is the reason that family and friends come to believe the patient is insane. Since the very word "psychodynamic" implies a working chance for one person to exert psychological influence upon another, one might be justified in saying that the psychotic patient is the one type of person for whom psychodynamic considerations do not exist.

It is understandable that many psychiatrists whose lives have been spent in the care of psychotic patients have been incredulous or skeptical of psychodynamics.

Other psychiatrists, whose principal occupation is the psychotherapy of the psychoneuroses, may say, when one of their patients manifests distinctive evidences of a psychotic condition, "This patient is psychotic. That means, explicitly or implicitly, that he is beyond the reach of any therapy based on psychological considerations. He must be hospitalized until he is in his right mind again. Then psychotherapy can be resumed." The implication is that the psychotic patient is under the control of some physical disorder or, possibly, of psychodynamic forces so powerful or so elusive that any effort to work with the psychodynamics is futile or "quackish." For purposes of propagandistic therapy with masses of psychoneurotic patients in wartime, this attitude has at times been overstated in approximately the following form, to the neurotic patients: "Your condition is not like that of the insane. For them, of course, nothing can be done, except custodial care or surgery or electric shock treatments; but we can do a great deal for you who are neurotic by helping you understand your neurotic reactions and helping you overcome them."

Furthermore, a very considerable proportion of psychotic patients present evidence of physical disease of the brain or of biochemical disturbances affecting it. Examples are cerebral arteriosclerosis and syphilitic meningo-encephalitis or pellagra and Korsakoff psychosis. The psychotic symptoms are not the direct expression, point by point, of the cerebral damage, for comparable damage may exist without psychotic reaction. There may even be much impairment of memory, of intelligence, and of emotional sensitivity without the patient's being psychotic. A psychosis is a form of reaction, not a mere deficit or impairment, and the personality of the patient makes a significant contribution to the form of psychotic reaction; yet organic factors cannot be ignored. This is in contrast to the field of the psychoneuroses, wherein, until recently, organic factors have been generally disregarded. Speaking figuratively and approximately, "psychodynamic psychiatry" may be said to have captured the field of the neuroses, although not without some protests from neurologists and geneticists; but no one would presume to make such a claim for psychodynamics in the field of the psychoses. For those who must have it all one way or all the other way, the psychoses cannot be claimed as the exclusive territory for psychodynamics, and, since the human mind tends toward sweeping generalities, there is therefore some tendency to ignore psychodynamic considerations of any kind in the field of psychoses. The large segment sometimes called "functional psychoses"—principally schizophrenia and manic-depressive psychosis—has been claimed as "psychogenic," but such an exclusive claim is countered by the evidences of hereditary predisposition.

On the whole, then, it appears that, in the field of the psychoses, there must be worked out some mutually comprehensible and co-operative *modus vivendi* between "dynamic psychiatry" and "organic psychiatry." In the field of general medicine in recent years, respectful consideration has been given to the psychodynamics of personality as pertinent to the management of patients, even those with obvious disease of strictly organic origin. Some call this a part of "psychosomatic medicine"; others more aptly include it as a part of "comprehensive medical care." At any rate, psychiatry is being introduced into general medicine as a "basic medical science," in the sense of a psychodynamic understanding of personality functioning. Dynamic psychiatry, in this sense, should also be a working part of the traditional mental hospital specialty of psychiatry. The enlarged meaning of the term might appropriately be called "comprehensive psychiatry." It is in the perspective of this concept that the present discussion of the matter has been approached.

## Basic Implications of Psychodynamics

The most elementary implication of the term "psychodynamics" is that psychological experience does make a difference in the subsequent behavior of the human being. This proposition constitutes a fairly flat contradiction of the historically important doctrine of psychophysical parallelism, which assumed a duality of mind and body and taught that psychological processes and neural processes vary concomitantly, but without causal connection. The doctrine of psychophysical parallelism is not much mentioned in recent times, but it has exerted and still exerts much influence in shaping medical thinking, particularly toward justifying a disregard of psychological intermediary steps, on the assumption that a complete account of the neural events (never actually approached or attained, but nevertheless anticipated) would render it scientifically unnecessary to take account of the psychological. For the ordinary affairs of life, this stilted pseudo-scientific attitude is, of course, impractical. One does not try to make a living, develop a professional career, keep up one's credit with the grocer, or cultivate the arts and amenities by exclusive attention to neural processes, in disregard of sentiments, prejudices, conflicts of value-judgments, and other psychological phenomena, but it has been somehow considered permissible—indeed, scientifically appropriate—to eliminate such considerations from the study and analysis of disordered personality functioning for the sake of a spurious "scientific objectivity." At least for the meanwhile (until the physicochemically complete neural account is available and its adequacy can be tested) it is sensible and scientific to take account of whatever discernible facts appear, on the available evidence, to affect behavior disorders. Such discernible psychological facts as emotional attitudes—attitudes of the patient, of his family, and of the physician—do seem to make significant differences in the behavior, even of psychotic patients. This is the most elementary premise of dynamic psychiatry.

To gain a working command of psychodynamic principles in psychiatry requires, of course, much more than a change of logical premises or an acknowledgment of common sense. A detailed account of the cultivation, growth, and testing of a knowledge of psychodynamics has already been presented and discussed in preceding sections. Here we are more particularly concerned with the pertinence of psychodynamic considerations in the psychoses. It is a curious fact that Wilhelm Griesinger, whose publications in the latter part of the last century exerted so marked an influence in establishing the "organicist" tradition in German psychiatry, gave in his textbook (5) several well-formulated statements as to the value of what in more modern terms would be called the genetic-dynamic approach to the psychotic patient.

Some of his statements are well worth quoting here as formulations of a psychodynamic orientation:

"Theoretical hypotheses have rendered it difficult for science to recognize the results of experience.... It must be remembered that cerebral activity may be modified quite as effectually, directly and immediately by the evocation of frames of mind, emotions, and thoughts, as by diminishing the quantity of blood within the cranium, or by modifying the nutrition of the brain. ... We have, in the direct provocation of certain states of mind, a very powerful means of successfully modifying disturbances of the somatic state" (p. 327). "Nowhere is it of greater importance than in the treatment of insanity, to keep in view the individual; nowhere is the constant consciousness more necessary that it is not a disease but an individual patient that is the object of our treatment.... A penetration into the psychical individuality of the patient is here demanded, which is scarcely ever necessary in ordinary medical practice" (p. 328). "The old *ego* which in in-

sanity for a long time is not lost, but only superficially repressed, or hidden in a storm of emotion, behind which it remains
for a long time capable and ready to re-establish itself, must, as
far as possible, be recalled and strengthened. . . . The moral treatment of insanity is most successful when the *ego*, already formed,
fixed, and only temporarily repressed . . . waits the opportunity
to resume its former place" (p. 343). "The inquiry into the history of the case ought to embrace the whole of the bodily and
mental antecedents of the individual. . . . We must faithfully and
intelligently comprehend the relation of the predispositions . . .
the education and the governing inclinations of the individual. . . .
Only in this way is an insight into the true history of these diseases possible; only thus can we succeed in grasping at their beginnings those fine threads which have ultimately entwined
themselves into delirious conceptions; only thus can we . . . recognize the far-back commencement of the preparation for the
illness. . . . All of this is of the highest importance in a system of
treatment which gathers from the history of the case indications,
sometimes for the amelioration of inveterate chronic processes, at
other times for the removal of certain psychic causes, and which
requires a profound knowledge of the character of the individual
to enable us to employ all his inherent resources in support of our
active treatment" (p. 90).

These dynamic statements by Griesinger failed apparently to
exert any considerable effect upon the trend of psychiatric theory
in his day, nearly a century ago, and their quotation here and
now may be merely a futile antiquarian gesture. For this ineffec-
tiveness there may have been two principal reasons: (1) he gave
no statistical evidence of psychotherapeutic effectiveness in treating psychotic patients, and (2) he gave no detailed exposition of
psychotherapeutic tactics. It is also true that Griesinger was a
professor, and these ideas of his may have been passed over lightly by "practical" men as "of academic interest only"—a technique
of mild derision still much employed to evade having to deal with
concepts which require much intellectual effort.

Does a psychodynamic approach to the therapy of the psychoses make a statistically demonstrable difference in the rate of
recovery or social improvement of patients? An affirmative answer to this question would have great practical and theoretical
weight in influencing the opinions and practices of hospital psychiatrists. It is difficult to establish clear-cut "controls" for such

statistical comparisons. Schizophrenic patients offer a better possibility for demonstration than do manic-depressives, because the "naturally" high recovery rate of the latter leaves little room for differentials.

In the statistical evaluation of insulin treatment of schizophrenia in the New York state hospital system, the "control" series had an improvement rate of 22.1 per cent (8). A somewhat similar study in the Rhode Island state hospital (Rupp and Fletcher) indicated about 21.9 per cent improved (9). There is no reported series of schizophrenic patients on whom a specifically formulated psychodynamic therapy has been uniformly tried, but there is evidence of considerably higher recovery rates under the more intensive and individualized therapy given to schizophrenic patients in private mental hospitals. The report by Cheney and Drewry (2) indicates that nearly half (47 per cent) of a series of 500 schizophrenic cases at the Bloomingdale Hospital recovered or improved sufficiently to get along without hospitalization. The markedly higher recovery rates in the private hospital as compared to the state hospital do not prove any specific psychodynamic formulation, since they represent the general, over-all advantages of such care; but it seems highly probable that these advantages are gained by the more individualized and personalized care and treatment possible in the private hospital; and this probability does have definite psychodynamic implications. In the Henry Phipps Psychiatric Clinic, under Adolf Meyer's leadership, parergastic reactions (essentially equivalent to schizophrenic illnesses) were treated somewhat more specifically on genetic-dynamic principles and, according to Rennie's (7) follow-up studies, some twenty years after the initial admission, 61 per cent were out of hospital, only 9 per cent of whom were living at home as invalids.

In the detailed analysis and criticism of these comparative figures, many points have to be taken into account. Psychiatric skills count for something, although it is worth noting that the principal psychiatric personnel in the Phipps Clinic working most closely with these patients were young physicians on the resident staff, in training to become psychiatrists.

In comparative studies on schizophrenia it would be of considerable importance to distinguish, if possible, between the types of condition designated by Langfeldt (6) as true schizophrenia and schizophreniform reactions, but it is not now feasible to make this distinction on the case material of the reports mentioned. Perhaps, also, one should point up the indubitable fact that those schizophrenic patients who did well must have used in the recovery process assets and capacities which were of constitutional origin. Also, some whose course ran downward toward personal dilapidation may have been strongly influenced toward that course by environmentally determined psychological experiences. The case is not wholly for or against psychodynamic principles.

Without going into further analysis of these comparative results, they may be taken as at least strongly suggestive evidence that the course of schizophrenic illness is favorably influenced by a considerable amount of individualized attention. This sample, from a rather grim segment of the field of psychiatry, is offered here to call attention to the importance of psychodynamic considerations in the psychoses. There are also other reports, less statistically impressive, but giving more individual details, concerning the successful psychotherapy of schizophrenic patients, by Kempf, Sullivan, Fromm-Reichmann, Bullard, Betz, Rosen, Knight, and others.

What is the *modus operandi* of those successful psychotherapeutic efforts with schizophrenic patients? What are the reasons why such efforts are not more uniformly successful? In what respects does the "schizophrenic process" represent a personal form of reaction, susceptible to the personal dynamic influence of the therapist, and in what respects is this "process" impersonal?

These and many other questions regarding schizophrenia and other forms of psychotic reaction represent problems of special importance for the development of psychodynamic psychiatry. Yet there is a certain artificial implication of specificity implied in these questions, as in many others which are asked in psychiatry. Every patient is a person; nearly every patient has been at some time functioning in fairly gratifying fashion, with a set of personal values which bound him in a gratifying sense of morale with some other fellow-men; these human attributes are not altogether lost because he shows for a time a psychotic disturbance in his conduct of life; it is likely to happen, in the prolonged complexities of interpersonal interactions which occur during psychiatric treatment, that dormant potentialities may be activated, normal hopes and expectations may resume something of their accustomed role, and much that is still actually or potentially normal in the personality may be strengthened and encouraged. An understanding and appreciation of "human nature" may make the psychiatrist useful to a patient, even though specific morbid processes are not specifically understood or specifically combated. Psychodynamic influences in the treatment of a psychotic patient are therefore as broad as "human nature."

### BIOLOGICAL AND SOCIAL IMPLICATIONS OF PURPOSE OR MEANING IN BEHAVIOR

Among the ordinary facts of human nature which must be rated high in psychodynamic importance is the fact that the human being looks forward in time with pleasant or unpleasant anticipation, and he struggles, more or less appropriately, to master anticipated events or adapt himself to them. Human experience is not merely passive endurance of the present and desire or dread of the future; it is also active striving toward some goal. This active striving, directed toward the future as either conscious intention or unconscious impulse, is one of the primary "facts of life," distinguishing psychodynamics from the physical sciences, such as hydrodynamics.

Some students of biology, with an aversion for vitalistic conceptions and a preference for materialistic, have juggled verbally with the word "tropism," in a strenuous intellectual effort to explain, or to explain away, this disturbing biological characteristic. Whatever may be the ultimate value of "tropisms" in explanatory hypotheses, the student of human nature who wants to work with human nature without too stilted doctrinaire commitments finds it more realistic to use terms such as "impulse" and "attitude."

During the illusory "Age of Reason," stimulated by the French encyclopedists, the rationality of the human being, in relation to purposeful effort, was greatly exaggerated. In the present age we appreciate better that the futurity orientation is manifested in human experience, not just in rational planning and intention, but rather more in emotional aspects, such as drives, wishes, faith, distrust, or anxiety. In this way we express our acknowledgment of the *emotional* aspect of biological functioning not merely as an aesthetic ornament to life or a mere epiphenomenon but as part of the working organization for living. The elaborate organization of the human brain for the utilization of distance-reception (sight and hearing, with the correlated activities of *looking* and *listening*) is part of the organic preparedness for dealing with futurity—with objects or events sensed afar but not yet within range to grasp or to ward off.

The futurity-oriented nature of man's organization and way of life is manifested in complicated psychological and physiological functions for which we may use the general term "attitudes." An appreciation of attitudes is a primary necessity for a psychodynamic understanding of man.

In imitation of the parlance used in simple sorts of laboratory experiments, the word "stimulus" is often applied to an object, or a sensory cue from an object, which appears to elicit a response from a person. Even in laboratory experiments, however, it has long since been demonstrated that differences in the time, intensity, and mode of response can be produced by changing the "set" of the subject, that is, by influencing his attention and expectations. In the more vital affairs of life, as distinguished from laboratory experiments, the set or attitude of a person has a very great importance indeed in determining his reactions, to so large a degree that one's behavior is often more significantly characterized as the manifestation of an attitude, in a particular situation, than as a mere response to a particular stimulus.

One's set of patterns of preparedness for behavior constitutes one's repertoire of attitudes, some simple, some very complex. In the post-Darwinian period of the study of human nature, with increased appreciation of the biological nature of man, the term "instinct" provided a convenient and attractive concept for thinking about biological propensities as fundamental in the formation and manifestation of human behavior patterns. In so far as instinct implies a fixed, innate pattern, characteristic of a species, it is not very aptly applied to human beings, since the patterns of human behavior appear principally to be learned— socially or culturally transmitted from generation to generation rather than by innate genetic mechanisms. Yet the biological needs of man—such as sustenance, shelter, and reproduction— require in all cultures and for each generation the development and transmission of some basic cultural patterns adapted to the satisfaction of his biological needs. The great modifiability in the patterns of human behavior is one of man's greatest potential assets, but it may also render one susceptible to cultural distractions away from biological aims; hence the human being requires forceful inner impulsions to assure drive and reinforcement of his action toward biological ends. This inner impulsive force is experienced as emotion. The author has elsewhere (11) expressed the concept that there is among animals a reciprocal, or supplementary, rather than a parallel, relationship between emotion and instinct. Those species which depend largely upon fairly fixed, innate patterns of behavior have no great need for emotional incitement or prompting, whereas those species, like man, who show great capacity for the intelligent modifiability of behavior need to be incited and prompted more strongly by emotional forces to assure biologically appropriate conduct.

Although social anthropologists have built up overwhelming evidence for the cultural rather than the instinctive *patterning* of human behavior, the term "instinct" has by no means disappeared from discussions of psychodynamics. The use of the term persists for another reason—not because the *patterns* of behavior are still believed, in the face of this anthropological evidence, to be instinctive (in the sense of innate) but rather because it has been felt necessary to recognize by some term the emotional drives representing biological propensities and impelling toward the fulfilment of biological necessities. In so far as instinct implies that behavior is motivated by inner driving forces correlated with biological needs, it has retained a certain usefulness in discussions of human nature, in default of some more suitable term. Unfortunately, misunderstanding and confusion result from the failure to recognize this semantic change. Sometimes, to indicate this modified sense, the neologistic adjectival form "instinctual" is used instead of "instinctive." In this sense "instinctual" is practically synonymous with "emotional" as suggested above.

The mammalian character of the human species and the long duration of human pregnancy, infancy, and childhood impose a special biological necessity upon the human species—the need to protect and nurture the young. A tenderly protective attitude toward babies and toward mothers exists in human nature and implements mankind for fulfilling this need. Interpersonal relationships involving this biological protective propensity, such as in family life and in group solidarity, constitute one of the most characteristically human traits, and mankind is thereby provided with a sound biological foundation for altruistic interpersonal attitudes of the highest importance for individual human satisfaction and for human society. Aggressive, competitive attitudes and hostile, destructive attitudes, which also have a sound biological basis, complicate these same interpersonal relationships.

The individual person, at any particular stage of his growth, has developed, out of his innate propensities and his social experience, some organization of attitudes, more or less integrated, through which he establishes and maintains relationships with other persons. This organization of interpersonal attitudes may be designated his "personality," sometimes more elaborately called "personality structure." The manifestations of this organization of interpersonal attitudes may be designated "personality functions," and this term may also be applied to accessory and contributory functions, such as feelings, habits, thinking, fantasy, and the like, which directly subserve personal behavior.

Psychotic patients are those who are so seriously disturbed in their personality functions that, for the time being, they are socially unreliable, that is, insufficiently responsive to the needs and expectations and common sense of others. The causes of such personality disturbance, of a psychotic type and degree, may be multiple and various—cerebral lesions, intoxications, frustrations, unmanageable fusions and confusions of hostile and affectionate impulses, fixed moods of despondency, immature attitudes, psychologically traumatic experiences, etc. Indeed, it is a commonplace of psychiatric wisdom to say that the causes for a particular person's psychosis are always multiple, in the sense that any one etiological factor would not initiate or maintain a psychotic reaction if other factors did not combine to induce or to permit such a reaction. Conversely, therapeutic influences, favorable to the restoration of better personality functioning, may be found to have some efficacy in relation to any one of the etiological factors, or even in the less specific way of general support. For example, it is a common observation that the psychotic patient is not likely to be favorably moved by the usual exhortations to "snap out of it" and "get into the game"; but, if patronizing exhortations are tactfully omitted and opportunities for congenial activity are patiently and invitingly offered, many such patients may respond by participation, and the interest aroused by such activity may be of considerable dynamic importance in fostering an enjoyment of normal functioning and a resumption of socially directed and socially rewarding effort.

Whatever occurs in psychotherapeutic discussions with psychotic patients or whatever happens in their hospital living which may aid in restoring the credibility and practical faith of the patient in his normal system of attitudes and expectations may make a dynamic contribution to the therapy of such patients. In attempting to activate incentives, on this principle, the would-be therapist who did not appreciate the psychotic patient's altered sense of values and expectations could make many futile moves and egregious blunders. It would be particularly unwise to make serious plans and attempts in this direction with a particular patient, without any knowledge of that patient's former, pre-psychotic, set of values and attitudes. One treats persons, not schizophrenia or depression. On the other hand, success in therapy does not necessarily insure that one has gotten to the specific psychopathological roots of the patient's trouble. That is to say, essentially, that psychodynamics and psychopathology are not identical. One may work, psychodynamically, with what is still normal in a partially psychopathological person; and, indeed, much of the art of psychotherapy consists essentially in doing just that.

Theoretically, it is possible to consider psychodynamics in logical abstraction as something distinct from the practical clinical problem of establishing personal rapport and mutual understanding and communication. But what is theoretically possible may be practically impossible. There are physicians working in psychiatry who are strikingly deficient in the capacity for mutually meaningful communications with patients, which means more than just verbal interchange; but the author has never found any psychiatrist of this sort who showed a real comprehension of, or belief in, psychodynamics, and it is indeed difficult to see how anyone could personally validate psychodynamic principles without this capacity. In a very real sense the development and validation of psychodynamics hinge on some means of establishing rapport. The art of interviewing patients is, at least in the present stage of the development of psychiatry, inseparably involved in any successful effort to apprehend and to validate psychodynamic principles. To a considerable extent, therefore, it is necessary, for a useful discussion of the general topic, to consider the way in which psychiatrist and patient find a common ground of meaningful personal interaction. Consideration must therefore be given to the surface problem of establishing contact, as well as to the depth problem of personality structure and unconscious motivation. A more detailed statement of the author's orientation to this task may be found elsewhere

(12, 13). Here attention is directed in a more general way to the kinds of issues which emerge when psychiatrist and psychotic patient succeed in establishing mutual understanding.

## SPECIAL PSYCHODYNAMIC FEATURES IN SCHIZOPHRENIC REACTIONS

Attempts to *understand* schizophrenic behavior, rather than merely to *describe* it, have frequently taken the form of trying to apply preformed conceptions of psychopathological mechanisms, as worked out in the neuroses. It is, indeed, true that the clinical study of schizophrenic patients provides a happy hunting ground, so to speak, for those interested in the sort of material that is commonly repressed by normal and neurotic patients. The behavior and statements of schizophrenic patients exhibit such materials in rare abundance, and the patients themselves go a long way in the "interpretation" of this material. Ambivalent feelings, incestuous wishes, unrealistic impregnation fantasies, homosexual sensitivities, and much other fascinating "material," which in other patients is unconscious and strongly repressed, requiring much skill and patience to uncover, are displayed by schizophrenic patients to the student of psychopathology in embarrassing profusion—embarrassing, in a way, to the person trained in psychoanalysis of the neuroses and committed to certain expectations, because such disclosures coming from a schizophrenic patient do not seem to have the expected abreactive accompaniment or the desired therapeutic value. It has been said, half-facetiously, that schizophrenic patients were the only people who knew of Freud's discoveries before he did.

The ready disclosure of such psychoanalytically "symbolic" material may be compared to the disclosure of intimate housekeeping details by the collapse of the façade of a bombed apartment house. Many schizophrenic patients happen, by reason of their particular form of reaction, to drop the social façade maintained so meticulously by ordinary mortals. Much of the material disclosed is not inherently peculiar to schizophrenia, and it has only an indirect bearing on the schizophrenic illness. It is as if a lot of stuff is freely disclosed in the psychosis which in normal and neurotic persons has to be laboriously spied out, through a piecemeal penetration of the façade of concealment and repression. Many of these disclosures have special pertinence to a prepsychotic psychoneurotic phase in the patient's struggle for adjustment but have relatively slight direct pertinence for understanding the meaning of the schizophrenic psychosis.

In the author's opinion, much of this "symbolic" material, interesting as it is, lies a bit to one side of the main issues in schizophrenic patients. The author has found it a great advantage to approach the study of schizophrenic patients rather more broadly from the viewpoint of the psychodynamics of ordinary life. Fair success has attended attempts to comprehend the significant issues by direct dealings with such patients rather than by interpreting into another idiom.

In general, a schizophrenic reaction develops, sometimes quickly, more often gradually, as the culmination of a period of prodromal preoccupation. In the earliest stages the patient's preoccupations are usually heavily charged with anxiety, but in the midst of the psychosis (which has provided some pseudo-solution) the initial anxiety may be more or less forgotten. If one wishes to learn about such preoccupations, there is little point in asking directly. It is more profitable to inquire about the life-situation. The patient in telling about the situation—now or at an earlier time—may reveal, by the perspective in which he casts his comments, the projection of his own preoccupations. The aim of this "situational" approach is not to find the situational cause of the patient's illness but to comprehend the patient's attitudes toward his life-situation and the persons involved in it. Without such a personalized appreciation of the issues, the psychiatrist, although he may quite correctly categorize the psychosis, will have no basis for establishing personal rapport with the patient, *as the patient is experiencing the psychosis*. To every patient, his illness is a personal experience, not a category in a catalogue; and, if one wishes to establish personal rapport, for the better utilization of psychodynamic influence one needs to establish liaison through some imaginative appreciation of the patient's attitudes and experience. Rapport has to work in both directions; one may hope that the patient will establish rapport with the therapist, but the therapist can also take active steps to establish rapport with the patient, through efforts to comprehend his attitudes. There is no great advantage in pretending to agree with the patient's attitudes, but there is considerable advantage in appreciating his attitudes.

Every patient who is aware of a personal problem tends to feel that his problem is unique. In a certain sense this is true and can be promptly acknowledged. Yet the psychiatrist is greatly aided by the extent to which certain generalizations hold true.

Among schizophrenic patients, for example, one notes a very general resentment of control and a yearning for "independence." At least one can say that, in their conversations, one notes frequent use of the word "independence" or some equivalent phrase, such as "I wish they would let me alone." With regard to this yearning for "independence," the typical schizophrenic pattern of behavior is, however, passive resistance rather than an active rebellion directed toward specific concrete goals. Discussions with schizophrenic patients regarding their childhood often reveal feelings of having been obliged to be excessively good or to submit to some domineering parent who imposed a strict conventional rule. In the prodromal period the apparent lack of appreciation or affection is deeply resented, with much emphasis upon "the hollowness of it all" or some other expression implying that the game is not worth the effort. Not infrequently, then, the parents are disowned and disparaged, outspokenly or by implication. These are often difficult judgments for the independent observer to check on, but the principal psychodynamic consideration is the patient's attitude, not whether it is objectively justified or not.

An illustration may clarify this point. A schizophrenic young woman of 23, in recounting her childhood experiences, expressed much resentment against her father for what she had come to consider afterward as his unfeeling domination, and she mentioned in this connection some ill-fitting shoes provided for her by him at some time in her early childhood which she said had caused her much pain but which she had had to wear. Further discussion brought out the fact that she had not mentioned to her father the painfulness of wearing these shoes. Just how he was supposed to have known that they hurt was not at all clear; yet she blamed him bitterly for causing her this continued pain. This pattern of unreasonably blaming a parent is a very common phenomenon in schizophrenic patients' accounts of their childhood. It may also be noted that there is an additional attitudinal implication, in the account given by this schizophrenic young woman, that she may have been yearning for such a close and sympathetic attention from her father that he would have intuitively appreciated her pain and gotten her some other shoes. Such a yearning for the father's appreciation was in this case abundantly confirmed. With all due skepticism as to a patient's reportorial precision of statements about situations, the psychiatrist nevertheless does well to ponder the attitudinal implications of the patient's words. Indeed, if all statements which might be in error were discarded from consideration or merely written into the record as evidence of delusion or distortion, one would be throwing away a very large portion of the material most useful for the psychodynamic understanding of the patient's attitudes, of the conflicts within the patient, and of the issues felt to exist between the patient and others. To discard all these potentially useful cues to an insight into a patient's attitudes, on the basis of delusion or factual distortion, would be to ignore the fundamental importance of attitudes. This is perhaps the most common neglect in the hurried hospital practice of psychiatry.

In the common schizophrenic issue of "independence" one notes a certain hollowness or lack of substantiality. Such a desire is not, as it might be for others, a practical wish to have freedom to work out a definite concrete constructive ambition. Most typically, the schizophrenic patient's desire for "independence" is a resentment against influence. The influence which is resented is not purely imaginary. It is in the nature of normal social living that everyone is continuously and inescapably surrounded by a network of social influences which operate usefully to maintain socially acceptable modes of behavior. Most persons scarcely notice their "social harness" because they are gratifyingly occupied in the considerable range of freedom permitted. Perhaps it would be the same for the schizophrenic patient if he had felt significantly rewarded by the appreciation of others and the gratifying sense of personal significance. Even though in early life such a person has tried hard, through conforming to the expectations and social demands of parents and others, to gain affection and appreciation, he often feels unsuccessful and inadequate and comes to resent these demands as coercive and reacts with emotional revulsion against whichever coercive influences are felt most gallingly. Thus, at times, the most elementary social conventions are disregarded—even the primary constraints of domestication, such as bowel and bladder control. To be so "independent" as that means not freedom but futility.

When the psychiatrist attempts to exert psychotherapeutic influence upon a schizophrenic patient in a mood like this, he faces indeed a difficult task. There is required at least some period of nondirective, permissive, and appreciative contact. Yet a wholly passive attitude does not succeed. Complete passivity in the psychiatrist implies some disrespect—as if the patient were considered so weak he could not stand to have the doctor display any genuine attitudes of his own. In this connection, one must consider another rather characteristic feature of many schizophrenic patients. They appear to view the world (from the paradigm of their view of their own parents) as composed of only two possible types of persons—the strong but domineering type and the indulgent but weak type. It is useful, therefore, while avoiding any tendency toward coerciveness or domination, to provide the patient at least some glimpses of one's own capacities for decisiveness and strength, not exerted against the patient but, if possible, with and for him. With a schizophrenic patient a junior physician has often an advantage over his seniors. The patient automatically attributes a domineering attitude to the more authoritative figure, whom he sees as the "big boss." This may be entirely unjustified, but the patient reacts in this way automatically and persistently, as an expression of preformed attitudes and expectations. During insulin treatments one may note, also, that some schizophrenic patients develop an appreciation of the physician's decisive strength, acceptable because it does not seem personally coercive in this context. Conversely, any hint of nagging impatience toward a schizophrenic patient is likely to arouse a massive, though often passive, resistance. As an expression of the sensitivity to whatever is felt as social coercion, even in the later stages of a patient's recovery from a schizophrenic reaction, any special emphasis upon meeting conventional expectations, as a basis for appreciating the patient's success, is likely to be deeply resented and may precipitate a relapse. The personal appreciation of the therapist appears to be most helpful to the social and economic rehabilitation of the schizophrenic patient when it can be based on the patient's attractive personal qualities and individual talents rather than on correct behavior or success in business.

The foregoing comments are offered as illustrative of the general sensitivity of schizophrenic patients to coercive influences. If one deals with the schizophrenic patient in a pattern suggested by these considerations, the possibilities of useful rapport are considerably enhanced. From the therapeutic standpoint, this is gratifying; from the scientific standpoint, it constitutes a certain measure of experimental verification of the psychodynamic importance of the independence motif. For one who is primarily interested in achieving valid formulations, a particular caution should be borne in mind: do not *press* the patient for direct verbal confirmation of this underlying attitude, for the patient is likely to react antagonistically to this form of social pressure also. Some highly intelligent schizophrenic patients may spontaneously offer abstract formulations of this independence motif, but far more commonly the expression of this motif takes the form of "negativism" or of "ideas of reference," or even less sharply pointed, vague resistiveness.

The characteristic schizophrenic "independence," or reaction-against-influence, is manifested in relation to sex in a variety of subtly similar but apparently contrasting ways, such as in ascetic withdrawal, homosexual panic, or autistic love affairs. Freud's classical paper on the Schreber case (4) has especially highlighted the preoccupation with the homosexual problem as an important feature of paranoid schizophrenia, of which there has been much clinical confirmation—also much misunderstanding.

The schizophrenic reaction-against-influence can extend so far as to make him feel an unwilling victim of sexual impulses—coerced, so to speak, from within. "You can't get away from biology," was the pathetic, resigned comment of one paranoid schizophrenic man, about to return home to his wife. He was a poetical, impractical, but intellectually brilliant schoolmaster, married to a practical-minded, forceful, lusty wife. In his "sickest" periods he had spent rapturous weeks and months in contemplation of the Virgin Mary—poetical visions of femininity devoid of crude sexual drive, in which he had experienced a glorious sense of "freedom from biology." For a fellow such as this, many of the features of social life—feminine dress, dancing parties, polite manners, cosmetics—may appear in effect as aphrodisiac accessories in a combined social and biological conspiracy to seduce one, willy-nilly, into sexual and matrimonial subjection.

It is true that for many men with attitudes somewhat similar to those of this schoolmaster society also provides conventional defenses against emotional entrapment by females, only to leave them unexpectedly susceptible to, and unguarded against, the arousal of sexual feeling by another male, since the biological constitution of mankind is rather nonspecific in this respect—as with other anthropoids—and leaves one open to such homosexual arousals. It is the author's clinical impression that many paranoid schizophrenic reactions—in the form of both panic and delusional defenses—represent reactions against homosexual impulses in this sense, not because of any specially pathological "homosexuality" but because the patient feels influenced in an unwelcome way, at an unguarded point, and becomes intensively preoccupied in improvising defenses. Back of it all, for the schizophrenic, lies the reluctance to be caught up in any influences which might sweep him into the dangerous current of life.

A paranoid schizophrenic girl had manifested in the prodromal phase a pattern of behavior which might be called intensive nymphomania—an extravagant succession of affairs in which she exposed herself to overt sexual experience with men in what might be described as a desperate pursuit of a kind of emotional immunity—seeking an unattainable "independence of spirit" by making light of the physical sexual relationships. She did not succeed—her spirit was repeatedly bruised by these experiences—but that only increased the desperateness of this curious search for "spiritual freedom." She was, naturally enough, preoccupied about the condemnation by her parents and by the church and by society in general, out of which preoccupations she evolved the conviction of a conspiracy to make a prostitute out of her—or rather, more precisely expressed, "to make her out a prostitute" by the misinterpretation of her own spontaneous, "idealistically motivated" behavior.

The autistic love affair, so prominent a feature of many hebephrenic patients, may appear superficially, like the above example, to express a strong sex desire, but its very silliness—the absence of practical social steps toward effective sexual mating—hints at something amiss, and in some of these cases, too, one can come to understand and appreciate the dynamics better by taking account of the independence motif. The one-sided romance has for the schizophrenic a certain charm. One may have much of the poetical and romantic pleasure, while free of conventional responsibilities and the blunt sexual demands of others or crude sexual impulses in one's self. Such fairy-like, spiritual freedom does not seem a very substantial desideratum to ordinary men and women, but it is in the general vein of the schizophrenic aversion to "social harness."

The foregoing diversified comments regarding the issues involved in schizophrenic reactions and the attitudes of schizophrenic patients may be pulled together in the following generalized formulation: Schizophrenic patients are by no means completely different from the rest of mankind. They share in the broad, basic psychodynamically important characteristics of human living—anticipatory striving at conscious and unconscious levels toward what is desired and against what is dreaded, in patterns of behavior which are shaped by social experience but which derive their important biological meanings from the fact that they fulfil biological needs. Schizophrenic patients, being human in this way, may be influenced, favorably or unfavorably, by somewhat the same interpersonal influences that have universal human significance. But the schizophrenic is characteristically "independent" in a special sense: he has special resistances against being coerced by conventionality, special antipathies toward being influenced or "victimized" to serve another's ends—even a very generalized reaction-against-influence. He is therefore rather resistive to authoritarian or rationalistic efforts at psychotherapy. Schizophrenic patients are not, however, beyond the possible psychotherapeutic reach of interpersonal dynamic forces, provided that there is a generous expression of personal, individual consideration and appreciation by an interested person, strong enough to rely upon but not domineering.

## Special Psychodynamic Features of Psychotic-depressive Reactions

For the consideration of psychodynamics, the term "psychotic-depressive reaction" covers a broader territory than just the cases reported in the usual state hospital statistics as manic-depressive psychosis and involutional melancholia. A considerable proportion of the toxic and organic psychoses of middle life and late life—such as arteriosclerotic, general paretic, pellagrous, and others—manifest the clinical characteristics of depression, although, of course, otherwise catalogued in the statistical report. The depressive form of reaction in such conditions appears to be determined by the personality in considerable measure. Treatment aimed wholly at organic factors may leave the patient in a depressed state which requires a grasp of the personal dynamics for its adequate understanding and best treatment. There is a current tendency to categorize as "depression" almost any abnormal mental state of sadness or grief, but the author considers this unsound. "Depression" is used here in the more restricted sense of a definite curtailment of personal and organic function-ing—retardation or agitation or extreme moody preoccupation which seriously limits one's ability to carry on. Psychoneurotic depressive reactions are not considered here because they are dealt with elsewhere. The territory remaining under the heading of "psychotic-depressive reactions" is still very large and hetero-geneous.

From the standpoint of personal meanings and emotional atti-tudes, what does it mean to be depressed? From patients' own remarks, two general themes stand out prominently—the feeling of guilt and inadequacy (mental, moral, and physical) and the lack of personal meaning: "Everything is changed"; "I feel dead"; "Nothing seems real." For descriptive categorization the psychiatrist may classify these and similar depressive comments as "feelings of unreality," "depersonalization," or even "nihilistic delusion"; but what is their reactive significance for the patient? In most general abstract terms these appear to be expressions of diminished vitality, dependent upon self-inhibition.

Disturbances of oral and anal functions (loss of appetite and constipation) and evidences of unconscious anal preoccupations in depressive reactions point up for special consideration issues which characterize a very early stage in personality development, as worked out by Abraham (1). The prominence of obsessive character traits or frank obsessive-compulsive symptomatology in the prepsychotic life of depressed patients further emphasizes the link with the toilet-training period of life. Caricatured scrupulosity and grossly unreasonable explanations of guilt feel-ings bear witness to an exaggerated sense of responsibility regard-ing self-control.

In searching clinically for a basis of mutual understanding with depressed patients—some way of appreciating the patient's expe-rience of his psychosis and of establishing communication—an appreciation that the patient has demanded of himself and of others a very extreme degree of self-control has frequently provided the key to otherwise unintelligible self-accusations and self-recriminations. Many of these patients demand of themselves a control of themselves or of events amounting almost to omnipotence, failing which they feel guilty and insecure. When one perceives this point and comments upon it, these patients do not usually agree—they do not usually quite agree with anything one says—but subsequent conversations are often less inhibited, as if the patient, although constrained not to agree, feels relieved that the other fellow is looking into that aspect of the guilt feeling.

Indeed, in a fair proportion of depressed self-accusatory patients, one finds many little evidences of self-justifying countercurrents, manifested sometimes in subtle derogation of others who might be accusing them; sometimes in somewhat paranoid formulations, whereby others are blamed as unfair; and very often manifested in self-accusatory statements of such excessive absurdity as to elicit direct contradiction or at least disbelief in the listener. Not infrequently the current of self-accusation and the countercurrent of self-justification strongly suggest to the listener that a patient is trying hard, but unsuccessfully, to achieve a state of penitence, and the protracted duration of the condition may represent the continual inability to feel as penitent as he thinks he should.

The psychiatrist with any considerable breadth of human experience and sympathy has been acquainted with grief and sorrow as the common lot of mankind and knows of the responsiveness of many grief-stricken persons to appreciative and sympathetic counsel. Against such a background of comparison, the psychopathologically depressed patients exhibit a striking contrast in their stiff-necked resistance. One senses, in many, a great bitterness and hatefulness. The perception of this component of hostility or resentment is a point on which one may note much disagreement among psychiatrists. As a point of systematic psychiatric formulation, it has become an article of dispute. Some psychiatrists assume an element of hostility in all depressive psychotics, as a part of "the mechanism"; others admit its presence only on overwhelming testimony in the form of a clearly stated acknowledgment by the patient; still others (of whom the author is one) perceive evidence of hostile feeling in many depressed patients and acknowledge its importance in the dynamic formulation of those patients, without assuming its universality in depressions.

Those instances in which it proves possible for the psychiatrist to comment to the patient with equanimity and without partisan bias upon the personal issues underlying such partially manifested hostility have been, not infrequently, instances in which recovery begins rather promptly thereafter. If, however, the psychiatrist, on only partial evidence, "takes sides" against that person against whom the patient feels hostile, then patient and doctor are likely to get much entangled in prolonged misunderstandings. One must be circumspect and just; with few types of patients is it so necessary to be just—and yet there is a strong temptation, arising out of sympathy for the patient, to try to relieve his or her guilt feeling by hastily taking sides. This constitutes one of the commonest stumbling blocks for the inexperienced and un-wary therapist.

One of the current psychiatric problems of great importance is to establish a rational understanding of the well-demonstrated efficacy of electro-convulsive treatment for relieving the depres-sive state. This treatment can be most reliably depended upon to relieve the self-accusatory, agitated depression in which the pa-tient seems to be asking for punishment. It is somewhat too simple to suppose that E.C.T. works just by fulfilling the request for punishment; yet this conception seems to have some perti-nence. The behavior of such patients before and after shock re-minds one strongly at times of the small boy who has worked himself into a hostile, tense, rebellious mood, quite recalcitrant to threats, yet whose whole attitude may be changed abruptly, by prompt corporal punishment, into a mood of relaxed and friend-ly rapport. Also, to continue the analogy with the small boy, such treatment does not of itself solve any fundamental problems, but it may be a great help in establishing a preparedness for some thoughtful, freer discussion. To push the analogy one step further, the patient, as well as the small boy, may need further help in finding a face-saving and personally dignified and grati-fying way of feeling significant and powerful without having to make such a tremendous issue of complete self-determination or self-control. Since there are many depressed patients whose way of life had become unbearably obsessive and self-demanding in their prepsychotic maladjustment, lasting improvement often de-pends upon the amelioration of that underlying neurotic attitude. This means reaching some working compromise on the omnipo-tence issue.

Many mothers in middle age have to change the pattern of their devoted interest in the family and give up some fondly nur-tured ambitions for their children because the children mature, marry, and, if normal, become preoccupied with their own lives and new families. Fathers may have somewhat similar experiences but are rather more likely to be troubled about getting brushed aside and losing status in their business or professional career. Such situations, frustrating to long-ingrained habits and patterns of striving, may provide occasions for psychotic reactions of either paranoid or depressive type, or mixed. Perhaps one is fortunate, though unhappy, not to be wholly self-righteous at such a time. Self-disparaging ruminations, in which one recounts and magnifies one's own mistakes, errors, and inadequacies and directs the disgruntled resentment against one's self, are distinctly unpleasant but not so malignant as the paranoid expression of self-righteous resentment against others. When these reactions are mingled in the same patient, success in relieving guilt feelings may have the unfortunate effect of releasing paranoid trends, more difficult to work with.

The clinical distinction between endogenous depressions and reactive depressions offers interesting psychodynamic implications. The distinction is not so sharp as the textbook case material would indicate, and often hinges upon the perspicacity of the psychiatrist in comprehending (or failing to comprehend) the sometimes intricate bearing of the patient's attitudes and expectations upon the life-situation. For example, one nice old gentleman had suffered, over two decades, a series of depressions, considered to be of the classical endogenous type until it became apparent that each depression had occurred after some brilliant success of his remarkably gifted oldest son. The series was climaxed at last by a prompt and successful suicidal attempt immediately following the receipt of news that the son had received an important appointment in the government service in a field where the father had long prided himself upon his superior knowledge and understanding.

In perceiving, evaluating, and dealing with suppressed jealousies, resentments, rivalries, and other morally condemnable feelings in depressed patients, one runs considerable risk of shattering the patient's morale either by condemnatory or by overprotective attitudes. Skill and care in finding and using acceptable words for the discussion of these touchy matters may spare psychiatrist and patient much distress. There is a subtle but important distinction between fine sentiments and mawkish sentimentality. There are nice distinctions between feeling hurt, resentful, hostile, or vindictive—distinctions sometimes slurred over by a hasty psychiatrist but important to the patient because of differences in moral gravity. Our language is rich in substantially synonymous forms of expression, carrying, however, differing weights of social approval or disapproval, and the depressed patient may be quite fastidious about these moralistic connotations.

Despite these special sensitivities as to terms implying guilt, it has been notable in the author's experience, however, that patients who have depressive reactions show, in general, a rather limited appreciation of the subtleties of language as compared with some who have schizophrenic reactions. The schizophrenic seems to realize that there are many matters not precisely expressible in words, and his language tends to be allusory, metaphorical, and indirect, even when he has a highly developed verbal skill and is fairly well motivated to communicate, whereas the depressive patient tends to expect of himself and of others that one should be able to state flatly exactly what one means and mean exactly what one says. The depressive type abhors metaphor and subtlety and requests direct, blunt, even harsh speech, although characteristically inclined to add a qualifying "but . . ." aimed at a rather pedantic accuracy. The schizophrenic is more approachable through polite circumlocution and is a bit revolted at pedantic, schoolmaster-like efforts to pin things down in one-two-three formulations. These considerations have much psychodynamic importance, since the psychiatrist ordinarily has to depend on interviews in which speech plays a large role, both for obtaining the clinical material for psychodynamic formulations and for exerting psychodynamic influence. Skill in adapting verbal means of communication to the special characteristics of the patient has much pertinence for one's success or failure in these tasks. There are nonverbal means of communication which also have much psychodynamic importance, but nonverbal phenomena are more difficult to record and to utilize in the formulation of dynamics. Interesting and significant observations and interpretations on posture during interviews have been reported by Felix Deutsch (3).

The manic type of reaction has a close relationship to the depressive. In most manic patients the depressive features may be detected without great difficulty by close and continuous observation. The manic behavior constitutes an exaggerated pattern of self-expression, covering personal uneasiness—a sort of self-administered antidote to depression, not quite effective. Psychodynamically, there is a close resemblance to whistling in the graveyard. The manic patient, like the more frankly depressive, manifests by implication a high evaluation of self-control and self-determination. It is expressed by the manic as an overwhelming insistence on self-determination amounting to an obsessive obligation to do as one pleases, rather than in self-condemnation for one's failure to control. For the recovering manic, as for the recovering depressed patient (they may be one and the same person), there is a like need to reach a working compromise on the omnipotence issue. A suddenly deflated manic runs a grave risk of suicide. Self-termination is the ultimate, and quite final, expression of the self-determination mania.

Considered from the psychiatrically important viewpoint of regaining a sense of rapport with one's fellows, the manic patient's expressiveness provides better chances than does the depressive patient's subdued aggressiveness. The hospitalized manic, in his impudence against authority-figures, can nearly always find an appreciative audience, not merely among other patients but also among employees and staff. Silly as it may be in its inception, rapport so begun may grow into something constructive.

In the foregoing discussion of psychotic depressive reactions, the central theme has been the patient's high evaluation of self-control or self-determination (the omnipotence theme), with the various subordinate themes which grow out of this attitude, which may be rather arbitrarily listed as follows: (1) the struggle to inhibit hostile impulses; (2) self-condemnation for inadequacy or guilt; (3) the struggle to achieve penitence and its self-justifying countercurrents, (4) the general inhibitory tying-up of psychological and some physiological functions, or (5) the effort to cut this Gordian knot by excessively self-assertive behavior. There are helpful analogies with the experiences of the young child in the phase of early toilet training and in life's early struggles to achieve mastery, but in combination with social approval. To speak frankly, however, one is not always able to fit all depressive reactions into one paradigm.

As in dealing with schizophrenic reactions, so also in dealing with psychotic depressive reactions, the avenues of therapeutic approach to psychodynamic influence lie along the lines of the general dynamics of human nature, seeking to activate and to utilize the resources of the patient and to help him thereby to work out a more satisfying way of life with a less circumscribed emphasis upon these special issues.

## REALITY AND PSYCHOSIS

In attempts to define psychosis, the point has often been made, descriptively, that psychotic thinking is unrealistic. Since reality is itself a concept difficult to define and to use with precision, the descriptive value of this statement is dubious. The discriminative value of the statement is also diminished by the observation that nonpsychotic persons also foster many illusions and carry on a large part of their mental operations with the use of prejudiced attitudes and folk beliefs which could scarcely be called realistic or even logical. A more useful criterion than reality is the consensus of the group. It is descriptively valid to point out that the psychotic person's beliefs and thought processes diverge in considerable degree from the cultural norm. Whether this divergence be temporary or permanent, during its existence it seriously hinders the psychotic person in enterprises requiring social collaboration—and there are few enterprises in our culture which do not in some way involve social interaction.

In addition to the descriptive purpose, the "reality" criterion is often used in a dynamic sense, in the familiar cliché that the schizophrenic patient has withdrawn from reality. Certainly, there is much in the schizophrenic reaction for which "withdraw" seems an appropriate verb; but, rather than say oracularly that he has withdrawn from reality, it makes more sense to say that he has withdrawn from other persons. Because it is largely through emotional association with other persons that one keeps sensible—as illustrated by the communicative or consensual implication of the term "common sense"—withdrawal from such association is a step toward strange and bizarre forms of folly. Even in its folly the human mind is not often altogether original. Because of the special independence motif of the schizophrenic reaction, with its revulsion against conventionally coercive influences, there is often an otherworldly or quasi-spiritual quality which may link the schizophrenic, at least in his own feelings and formulations, with spiritual or religious characters.

In Storch's monograph (10) of 1922 an attempt was made to equate certain schizophrenic statements and modes of thought to "primitive, pre-logical" modes of thought, as formulated by Lévy-Bruhl, and also to point up similarity or identity with presumed archaic prelogical stages in the culture of the patient. Storch's aim was primarily phenomenological, but he sought to develop his theme along lines of genetic psychology. Rather than depend upon questionable theories as to primitive and archaic psychology and their similarities with the schizophrenic, the writer has found it more useful, and apparently sounder practice, to trace out, in individual schizophrenic patients, the emotional antagonisms to common sense and to the personal representatives of common sense.

To many physicians, psychologists, and social workers whose personal knowledge of schizophrenic persons has been tangential rather than familiar, the phrase "withdrawn from reality" and the correlated phrase "reality testing" have had a special appeal, because these terms have gained a certain familiar ring from discussions of psychoanalytic theories of the ego and its role in the subordination of the pleasure principle to the reality principle. For those working within the psychoanalytic frame of doctrines, it is of pressing importance to develop a more adequate psychoanalytic conception of the ego and its disturbances, particularly for the dynamic understanding of the psychoses. The great practical importance of a period of "reality testing" in the treatment of the schizophrenic patient has been stressed by Zilboorg (14).

When the schizophrenic patient resumes trustful relationships with others, tentatively accepting the physician as the representative of the consensus, the growth of confidence is a slow stepwise process. This relationship is tested repeatedly. Through its usefulness in holding out the possibilities for endurable and gratifying relationships with other significant persons, the schizophrenic tendency to withdraw may be counteracted.

Storch, in his lengthy discussion of Strindberg's schizophrenic illness, refers to the latter's "fear of dependence on another, the dread of being placed under some influence." Storch says: "His fear of being influenced reminds one very forcibly of the fear of the primitive that a spell will be cast on him; and can be best understood by a comparison with this primitive apprehension." There is no need to refer this to primitive cultures or to archaic times or to some withdrawal from "reality." The dynamics are clearer if one sticks to the point that the schizophrenic withdrawal is primarily a withdrawal from certain personal relationships.

## General Comment

The preceding discussions of schizophrenic and depressive psychoses, including some references to paranoid reactions, have been shaped up to illustrate the possibilities and advantages of approaching the study and treatment of psychotic patients with respectful consideration for the psychodynamic forces in human nature. Little emphasis has been put on highly specific mechanisms. The general principles are not confined to the so-called "functional psychoses," but have pertinence for many patients for whom organic disease and toxic conditions are also significant factors in the etiology of a psychotic reaction. It is assumed that attention to psychodynamics should not inhibit the proper clinical study of each patient for all practical possibilities of correcting or ameliorating any organic factors.

## BIBLIOGRAPHY

1. ABRAHAM, K. "Notes on the Psycho-analytical Investigation and Treatment of Manic-depressive Insanity and Allied Conditions," in *Selected Papers* (London: Hogarth Press, 1927), chap. vi.
2. CHENEY, C. O., and DREWRY, P. H. "Results of Non-specific Treatment in Dementia Praecox," *Am. J. Psychiat.*, 95:203, 1938.
3. DEUTSCH, F. "Analysis of Postural Behavior," *Psychoanalyt. Quart.*, 16:195, 1947.
4. FREUD, S. "Psycho-analytic Notes upon an Autobiographical Account of a Case of Paranoia (Dementia Paranoides)," in *Collected Papers*, Vol. 3 (London: Hogarth Press, 1946), Case No. 2.
5. GRIESINGER, W. *Mental Pathology and Therapeutics*, translated from the German (2d ed.) by C. LOCKHART ROBERTSON and JAMES RUTHERFORD (New York: William Wood & Co., 1882).
6. LANGFELDT, G. *The Schizophreniform States: A Katemnestic Study Based on Individual Re-examinations, with Special Reference to Diagnostic and Prognostic Clues and with a View to Presenting a Standard Material for Comparison with the Remissions Effected by Shock Treatment* (London: Humphrey Milford, for Oxford University Press, 1939).
7. RENNIE, T. A. C. "Follow-Up Study of Five Hundred Patients with Schizophrenia Admitted to the Hospital from 1913 to 1923," *Arch. Neurol. & Psychiat.*, 42:877, 1939.
8. ROSS, J. R., et al. "The Pharmacological Shock Treatment of Schizophrenia: A Two-Year Follow-Up Study from the New York State Hospitals with Some Recommendations for the Future," *Am. J. Psychiat.*, 97:1007, 1941.
9. RUPP, C., and FLETCHER, E. K. "A Five to Ten Year Follow-Up Study of 641 Schizophrenic Cases," *Am. J. Psychiat.*, 96:877, 1940.
10. STORCH, A. *The Primitive Archaic Forms of Inner Experiences and Thought in Schizophrenia: A Genetic and Clinical Study of Schizophrenia*, translated by CLARA WILLARD (Nervous and Mental Disease

Monograph Series," No. 36) (New York: Nervous and Mental Disease Publishing Co., 1924).

11. WHITEHORN, J. C. "Concerning Emotion as Impulsion and Instinct as Orientation," *Am. J. Psychiat.*, 88:1093, 1932.

12. WHITEHORN, J. C. "Guide to Interviewing and Clinical Personality Study," *Arch. Neurol. & Psychiat.*, 52:197, 1944.

13. WHITEHORN, J. C. "The Material in the Hands of the Biochemist," *Am. J. Psychiat.*, 92:315, 1935.

14. ZILBOORG, G. "Affective Reintegration in the Schizophrenias," *Arch. Neurol. & Psychiat.*, 24:335, 1930.

# X

## CONTRIBUTIONS OF PSYCHOANALYSIS TO THE STUDY OF THE PSYCHOSES

### Henry W. Brosin, M.D.

THERE is considerable psychoanalytic literature concerning the major psychoses, even though this has not been the primary working area for most psychoanalysts. With the wider dissemination of psychoanalytic training, especially in closed mental hospitals, we may hope for a much more intensive research-therapeutic program which will justify current assumptions that a large causative component of the psychotic process is psychological. It is notable that some of the leading analysts—Freud, Abraham, Schilder, Sullivan, and Alexander—do not subscribe to a total psychogenic etiology as an adequate explanation for ego weakness (11, 37, 62, 79, 95, 96). This was the situation in 1902–14 when Freudian concepts were first given a home in a closed hospital at Burghölzli in Zurich, Switzerland, by Bleuler, Jung, Ricklin, and Abraham, at a time when both neurosis and psychosis were generally regarded as without psychological meaning, since they were thought to be due to organic conditions such as anemias, infections, or irritations. The story of these early days when the psychodynamics of psychoses were eagerly studied has been told in part by Jung (70) and Brill (20). The productivity of this period is evident in the writings of this group in the *Jahrbuch für Psychoanalyse*, Vols. 1–6 (1909–14), which includes important essays by Bleuler, Bjerre, Grebelskaja, and Maeder. Unfortunately, this interest was not sustained. Sporadic essays and histories of cases continued to appear, however, with the result that most contemporary psychiatrists assume that the psychotic process is intelligible, even though they are uncertain about the etiology.

With the appearance of Freud's *Three Contributions to the Theory of Sex* (1905) (52) to reinforce the earlier writings, especially *Studies in Hysteria* (1895) (19), "Further Remarks on the Defence Neuro-psychoses" (1896) (45), and *The Interpre-*

*tation of Dreams* (1900) (46), students had enough evidence to permit them to grasp some of the psychotic mechanisms, especially in the spheres of reality testing, hallucinations, delusions, and illusions. The evidence for the existence of an active "unconscious," the logic of the emotions, the nature of repression and substitutive mechanisms, the purposefulness of psychotic behavior, and the direct relation of current symptom pictures to the genetic-dynamic development of the patient in the family setting became living concepts which stimulated workers to new efforts. This attitude was revolutionary, for, even though few patients showed marked improvement and an understanding of the etiology of psychosis remained incomplete, there was new hope that this psychological method would lead to better understanding and consequently to more effective therapy of the psychologic conflicts in the patient. Psychoanalysis furnished an instrument for the study of the underlying dynamics in the family organization in hospital policies and practices, and in the psychological meaning of physical and chemical therapies. The unfolding of these possibilities has been slow, but their potentiality remains large. Freud's papers on the Schreber case (1911) (51), "On Narcissism" (1914) (49), "A Case of Paranoia Running Counter to the Psychoanalytical Theory of the Disease" (1915) (44), "Mourning and Melancholia" (1917) (48), "Neurosis and Psychosis" (1924) (50), and "The Loss of Reality in Neurosis and Psychosis" (1924) (47) are perhaps his most important essays on the psychoses; but many of his other writings reinforce the general concepts which are useful in interpretation of psychotic behavior.

Though few in number, the contributions of Karl Abraham to this subject deserve special attention. Beginning in 1907–8 at Burghölzli with "The Psycho-sexual Differences between Hysteria and Dementia Praecox" (1908) (3), he continued with "Notes on the Psychoanalytical Investigation and Treatment of Manic-depressive Insanity and Allied Conditions" (1911) (2), establishing beyond doubt that some cyclic mood disorders could be favorably influenced by psychoanalytic therapy and could be understood in terms of the Freudian models for the neuroses. His major contribution, "A Short Study of the Development of the Libido, Viewed in the Light of Mental Disorders" (1924) (5), presents one of the few important psychoanalytic concepts not originating with Freud.

While still an enthusiastic Freudian, Jung wrote about twenty-five papers between 1902 and 1910, the most important of which deal with his association experiments and schizophrenia (1907) (70). He gives a 51-page report of a partial analysis of a paranoid woman which illustrates the Freudian approach. This account is more impressive than his efforts in the first half of the monograph to distinguish between hysteria and dementia praecox.

One of the most brilliant case histories in the literature on this subject is Victor Tausk's "On the Origin of the 'Influencing Machine' in Schizophrenia" (1919) (130). Here we find a step-by-step reconstruction of the probable phases of the development of a delusion from its primitive beginnings in childlike psychotic thinking to an organized pattern. It is assumed that these patterns enable a patient to maintain a precarious emotional balance with his distorted interpersonal relations and help him defend himself against a more regressive state. As in the lively descriptions of the horse phobia in "Little Hans" (43) and the delusions of multiple deities in Schreber (51), we are privileged in Tausk's presentation to see the origin, growth, and readaptation of these defensive idea-systems unfold as in a moving picture.

Storch (128), Ferenczi (38, 39), and Groddeck (59) are among those who opened up further potentialities for the comprehension of psychotic mechanisms during the second period of psychoanalytic development (1914–24), as described by Rickman (95). The observations that every man during some period of his early development has the potentialities for behaving, thinking, and acting in patterns much like those utilized by a schizophrenic, manic, obsessive, or phobic patient alter considerably the attitude of the investigator toward the phenomena of bizarre behavior.

## HALLUCINATIONS

Gradually, by means of repeated observations, it was demonstrated that hallucinatory behavior, which seems so foreign to the well-integrated man, was not uncommon in various psychogenic, as well as in toxic or organic, deliria. A simple example is that of the desert prospector who, thoroughly dehydrated, hallucinates drinking water when he has only sand. Less severe is the projection of wishes into a mirage, so that the traveler thinks he sees an oasis but is only translating the heat waves into a desired picture. This illusion has the same goal as a hallucination, although less reality distortion is involved. Delusions and illusions are means of protecting the ego from dealing with painful perceptions. That the hallucinations could be fitted into a meaningful mosaic if one studied the current and past setting was another step forward in the understanding of psychosis. This was buttressed by Storch's and Freud's conclusions (and later from child psychiatry) that, in the early days of ego formation before the boundaries of the "me" and the "not-me" are firmly established, the infant is capable of gratifying his wishes by means of hallucinatory activity (128). As the ability of the ego to distinguish sharply between external and internal realities is weakened by toxic or emotional factors, there follows increased distortion of the external realities because of the intense personal needs. External realities which are unacceptable are falsified into something less threatening to the individual. Bleuler (14, 15), following Freud, was among the first to see that this propensity was present in the dreams of normal adults as well as in schizophrenics. Child psychiatrists furnish many examples of the similarities between infantile thinking and adult dreaming. In fact, hallucinatory wish-fulfilment may be thought of as an early crude form of abstract thinking which is later progressively modulated into daydreaming, imaginative construction of future events, and, at best, scientific thinking, utilizing abstract symbols (92). Fatigue, fear, or toxicity may cause regression in normal persons from the level of abstract thinking to that of the prelogical emotional thinking which employs concrete pictures as its vehicle rather than abstract symbols or words.

One aspect of this hallucinatory wish-fulfilment is the ability to deny unpleasant realities such as have been described in cases of general paresis, aphasia, severe tuberculosis, and lobotomy. Anna Freud has called this type of denial a "pre-stage of defense" (42). S. Freud believed that, when ego integrity is well developed through long practice in reality testing, regression to such complete falsification is not possible, but it is obvious from the examples given that the potentiality remains. In this connection there should be mentioned the selective hysterical hallucinations explained by Freud as "perceptions at the time of the repression" and differentiated from psychotic hallucinations (46, 50). Psychotic hallucinations are a category of primitive defense mechanisms which occur under many circumstances in different patients. One cannot make dogmatic assertions about their origin and purposefulness because of the multiplicity of determinants, although it is simple to define them as "substitutes for perceptions after the loss or damage of objective reality testing" (46, 47, 50) or "outward projection of inner feelings" (20). The experimental psychologists and physiologists must help determine the essential conditions which call for the Freudian mechanisms. Furthermore, the complexity of the content which is often anxious, self-accusatory, or guilty, but seldom concomitant with pleasure, needs much more careful study.

Herman Rorschach (99) attempts a description of the relation of the sense organ involved with the character structure and the age of the patient. He found in his series that only patients with a high capacity for "introversiveness" had somatic hallucinations and that these hallucinations decreased with age. Patients with visual hallucinations had an intermediate capacity for "introversiveness," and these diminished with time, to be replaced by auditory hallucinations, which also deteriorated with time. That the latter were by far the most common fits in with the fact that most persons have a relatively limited "introversiveness." Persons with a relatively empty "type of experience," that is, having neither strong introversive or extratensive qualities, had little or no capacity for hallucination. Rorschach further remarks that this is of interest in connection with the fact that some poets have marked color and sense-organ preference at various stages of their life. In examining an extensive analysis of the imagery of Goethe and Schiller, he finds that they follow the general pattern outlined above (99).

Hallucinations, like dreams, are intricate mental defense patterns occurring when the perceptive functions of the individual, owing to internal or external pressures, are under severe or disruptive stress. While some hallucinations are relatively simple attempts at creating acceptable substitute realities, many of them are representations of the repudiated forces of the id and the superego and are the projected expression of failure in repression of ego-alien material.

## DELUSIONS, PROJECTIONS, AND PARANOIA

Delusions are based on ideas, not on sense-perceptions; these may contain elements of wish-fulfilment, anger, pain, fear, guilt, or reproach, just as in dreams. Reality is distorted in condensed symbolic fashion in order to satisfy the strong inner need to project painful inner ego-alien forces having their origin in both the id and the superego. They may be simple or extremely complex and are sometimes highly integrated into a tight, orderly system. They, too, have many component ideas which vary in their organization, as illustrated in Freud's Schreber case and in Tausk's "Influencing Machine." Delusions such as Schreber's were conceived by Freud as having a twofold purpose: (1) to serve as a defense against unacceptable homosexuality and (2) to provide a restitution (71, 72). Their fluid dynamic character can be seen in shifts from a phobic defense to a more primitive delusion, as in patients who alter their fear of contamination by dirt or bacteria to the fixed idea that they have been infected or poisoned. A dirt phobia may become obsessive when increasing pressure compels acting out avoidance patterns in a rigid way, but these remain on the "as if" basis, e.g., "I am compelled to act as if this were the case." When the patient actually believes that the sugar bowl or saltcellar contains poison, then the defense is delusional. Hypochondriacal delusions in psychoses are said to occur when the special investment of energy is attached to organ representations in the regressive process. These defenses along with others, such as literal cannibalistic fantasies, the belief in utter unworthiness and of being hated by everyone, commonly found in severe depressions, are transitional stages on the road to full-blown persecutory delusions.

Persecutory delusions may be seen in all stages of development from nondelusional delicate suspiciousness, with a tendency to interpret most events egocentrically, to the most bizarre constellations of deities. All these have the common property of projection of the conflictful elements from within upon the environment. "Not I, but *you*, are responsible" is a common formula. An overly severe conscience often makes the patient blame some significant person for his unconscious hostility or homosexuality. Often the hypersensitive person is keenly alert in his unconscious to the minute quantities of ambivalent or hostile feelings in others and blames them for his own reaction. Sachs's excellent metaphor, which is quoted by Freud at the end of *The Interpretation of Dreams*, is of special pertinence here: "What a dream has told us of our relations to the present (reality) we will then seek also in our consciousness, and we must not be surprised if we discover that the monster we saw under the magnifying glass of the analysis is a tiny little infusorian" (46). The paranoid magnifies his awareness of his own and other persons' drives out of context in an exaggerated fashion. Characteristics of one's own attitudes, usually from a punishing conscience, may be blamed upon the persecutor. Organs which are sources of conflict may be externalized as inventions. Freud was the first, in the Schreber case, to describe the development of a delusional system through the phases of denial, distortion, and projection from its roots, as in Schreber's ambivalent relation to his father and father-surrogates (doctor, God), and his castration fears. The progressive system of delusions was Schreber's attempt to deny his passive homosexuality, which stands developmentally between infantile self-love and genital love. He used the now familiar formulae:

1. I do not love him, I hate him     (denial).
2. He hates me     (projection).
3. I hate him because he persecutes me   (rationalization).

In the family of projections there are also ideas of reference and ideas of being influenced, usually in a severe, hypercritical manner, just as if the patient were being scolded by his conscience. It is probable that the patient's feeling that people are looking at him is a part of his wish to have relationships with them. Other types of projection are illustrated by the litiginous paranoid, who fights against a hated father; the person with delusions of jealousy, who used denial and displacement in the Freudian formula of "I do not love him, for she loves him" (when there is no justification in reality but because the patient is really interested in the third person).

Erotomania can be caused, according to Freud, by the logic of "I do not love him—I love her." Since there is the same need for projection, there is another step added to support the first thesis, namely, "I notice that she loves me," which enables the completion of the final proposition "I do not love him—I love her, because she loves me" (51, p. 449).

## SCHIZOPHRENIC MECHANISMS

So far we have discussed mechanisms which might be described as attempts of an ineffective or damaged ego to defend itself against its own turbulent drives or against a harsh conscience. These are the commonly seen efforts at healing or restitution. There are schizophrenic phenomena which have been called "direct expressions" of this degradation of the damaged ego, now weakened through the loss of object relationships. It is a matter of interpretation which processes should be included in the category of direct expressions of the damaged ego, but fantasies of world destruction, somatic sensations, depersonalization, and confusion probably belong here. Archaic language, bizarre motility, delusions of grandeur, probably more complex, are better understood in the light of the ego, which under stress permits regression to the archaic processes of the first and second years of life.

There remains a number of technical difficulties involved in understanding the formation and relationships of the various paranoid ideas. Waelder finds that earlier theories (delusions resulting from a withdrawal of libido from the outer world and being concentrated on the narcissistic ego; delusions as products of projection; delusions as denial; delusions as attempted restitution; delusions as containing a historical truth and with those representing the return of the repressed) offer the possibility of an integrated theory.

There are three possible solutions to the conflicts between individual instinctual equipment and reality; an equilibrium can be established by changing reality (alloplasticism) or by changing the instinct (autoplasticism) or by changing neither but denying one or the other. These methods lead, wherever successful, to various types of normality, i.e., a dominating type, a submissive type, and a type with a rich phantasy life. When unsuccessful, they provide the breeding ground for psychopathy, psychoneurosis, and paranoia respectively.

Furthermore, it is suggested that if warded-off instinctual drives make their come-back, the return has the same form as the defence mechanism had; they return, as it were, through the same door through which they were ousted (ismorphism). If the defence mechanism had the form of denial, the return must have the form of an assertion. One type of paranoid idea at least, the delusion of persecution, may be the result of an (incomplete) return of a denied instinct [132, p. 176].

Freud (51) stressed the relationship between various levels of development, such as auto-erotism (severe loss of object love), narcissism (megalomania), to the various types of psychosis. He believed dementia praecox to be more regressive than paranoia and proposed for the former group the more general name of "paraphrenia." With weakened and abandoned object relationships, the patient exhibits extreme isolation and separation from the world, which is translated into such images as "world destruction," in which the patient himself or significant persons are dead or altered in the direction of being shadows, fleeting, strange, or unreal. These images and ideas may be more or less severe, depending on the economic emotional balance of the individual, but may progress to the more severe stages of depersonalization, body sensations, and catatonic stuperous withdrawal. Hypochondriacal complaints, according to Tausk, usually precede the more severe sensations of body or organ estrangement or the somatic delusions, which may be bizarre, such as "insects under the skin" or "tigers in the stomach" (130). Most patients make periodic, intense, though short-lived, attempts to establish either erotic or hostile object relationships, but their clumsiness usually prevents a durable positive benefit.

The familiar feelings of expansiveness, power, special abilities, and grandeur are akin to manic states and spiritual exaltation. There is a recapturing of the infantile omnipotence which denies injury to the prestige of the self-system and an attempt at correction by overcompensation. Those individuals who can tolerate social isolation may defend themselves with a towering, portentous aloofness which enables the patient to retain an extraordinary opinion of himself and his mission, such as saving the world, knowing the secrets of electricity, cosmic forces, or nuclear energy. This enables many of them to maintain a façade of integrity, in contrast to the glaring regressive phenomena of hebephrenia and catatonia. In this connection the work of Shakow (111) on the nature of the deterioration in schizophrenic states will help the student grasp the difficulties inherent in the concept of deterioration.

More modulated patterns of affect withdrawal have been described as the "hollow men" or the "as if" persons, who seem on early acquaintance to be intelligent, social, and adaptive but are later found to have severe emotional handicaps (24). On the other hand, French and Kasanin (41) have reported two cases of psychosis in which unconscious learning apparently took place unobtrusively behind the mask of conspicuous and disturbing psychotic manifestations.

Psychoanalysts are also contributing to the experimentation with group therapy, but in the absence of a definitive summary, only single references can be given. Slavson (113), Powdermaker and Frank (86), Grotjahn (60), Stanton and Schwartz (123, 124, 125), and Ezriel (28) are among those who have presented theories about group dynamics according to psychoanalytic principles, but most of the work is with children and neurotics. Stanton and Schwartz have carefully observed and recorded the dynamics of a hospital ward as a social organization.

Space prevents further exposition of the dynamics of automatic obedience, echolalia, echopraxia, negativism, catatonic mutism, furor, confusion, excitement, and stereotypy, but the references given will help the student's search for their meaning (37, 62, 95, 96, 103).

In summary we can state that, by the application and extension of knowledge gained from the psychoanalytic study of dreams and neuroses, the content and behavior of schizophrenics become intelligible, even though the etiology to a great extent remains unknown. It is inferred that the reality-testing functions are defective in schizophrenics and that this makes them more vulnerable to injury. This defective ego may be caused in part by poor interpersonal relationships during the early years of life. Multiple identifications with reasonably warm, stable adults, necessary to emotional health, are lacking, so that the patterns of behavior developed to meet life's needs are fragile and uncertain. Preventive psychiatry and psychiatric therapy have the task of building up such patterns, in order that the person may achieve satisfactions in a healthy fashion. This problem involves utilizing numerous methods for helping the person through both conscious guidance and "uncovering" techniques of the unconscious conflicts to integrate more adequately his means for dealing with internal and external demands. By means of examples from daily living, the patient is shown superior means of managing his affairs. The books by Bettelheim (13), Erikson (27), Levy (75), Redl (93), and Spock (122) contain excellent expositions and examples. Various studies on the separation of mothers from their babies also furnish dramatic examples of the importance of good relationships between parents and children (18, 107–9, 115–21).

## MANIC-DEPRESSIVE MECHANISMS

The psychoanalytic method of interpreting the emotional content of psychotic behavior has not produced valuable differentiations between various categories of mental disorder. This is not to deny profound differences in the clinical picture, dynamics, prognosis, or treatability among the multiple manifestations of the schizophrenics and the cyclic mood disorders or their subgroups. These differences are seen to be significant phases in a complex total organization in which the symptomatology is dependent upon the economic balance of the emotional forces at play. The classic discussion at lengthy ward rounds regarding the diagnosis of dementia praecox versus a manic-depressive disorder loses much of its meaning when the genetic-dynamic development is disclosed and the current balance of power between the destructive and the restitutive powers determined. Such discussion has even less meaning when a group of experienced analysts carefully review the world literature on manic-depressive disease in the light of their own experience in numerous detailed case reviews, only to find that manic-depressive disease is probably not a sound unitary concept. History shows that Kraepelin had shrewd critics during the years he developed his diagnostic dichotomy, but their voices were lost in loud, if premature, applause from other sources. Teachers like Pappenheim, Ernest Meyer, Korsakoff, Serbski, Sommer, Bianchi, and Adolf Meyer pointed out the fallacies in diagnosing by prognosis or by ruthlessly refusing to admit that schizophrenic patients might not be treated more effectively (138).

The papers which give the basic psychoanalytic knowledge about the cyclic mood disorders are probably Abraham's "Notes on the Psychoanalytical Investigation and Treatment of Manic-depressive Insanity and Allied Conditions" (1911) (2); "The First Pregenital Stage of the Libido" (1916) (1); "A Short Study of the Development of the Libido Viewed in the Light of Mental Disorders" (1924) (5); Freud's "Mourning and Melancholia" (1917) (48); and Radó's "The Problem of Melancholia" (1927) (89). The first two stress these points: that the psychotic has nearly equal ambivalent emotions toward himself and toward others and that this is a barrier to therapy; that the ambivalence originates early in personality development (pregenital); that oral demands and conflicts expressed directly and indirectly tend to increase; and that the hatred for the self represents a turning-inward of hostility which was formerly directed outward. Freud described the "pathognomic introjection" occasioned by the loss of a love object, causing a representation of this object to become part of the superego. The ensuing battle between the ego and the superego reproduces the former fight between the ego and the lost love object.

Abraham advanced several other theories in his 1924 paper (5), as well as substantiating Freud's views. Here is outlined the familiar developmental scale of oral and anal levels of organization, each with its own problems of integration and corresponding expression of failure to maintain equilibrium. In much greater detail he pictures the interplay between the ego and the superego and the mutual recrimination which must be worked out in the depressive process. He also elaborates on the dynamics of mania as oral hunger for objects, "increased mental metabolism," which is aided by a paralysis of the superego functions, thus enabling the patient to seek gratification without inhibition and so gain a heightened sense of well-being and prestige. Conscience values are so weakened that the instinctual forces can seek direct gratification via the ego functions, and the manic can express his self-love in an unbounded fashion in contrast to the depressive, who cannot openly admit any regard for the self. The manic somehow regains his feelings of infantile omnipotence where there were no reality barriers against pleasure and no objects to fear. Abraham also offers shrewd guesses about early life-experiences which predispose the individual to depressions, stressing the probable early depressions in childhood.

Radó (89) interprets self-accusation as a means whereby the ego placates the strict superego and its ambivalent introjected object. The refinements of his explanation of the introjection of the object in both the ego and the superego, showing the multiple functions of the ego, help one to comprehend these states.

Lewin's work on cyclic mood disorders, *The Psychoanalysis of Elation* (78), studies the defenses expressed as euphoria or hypomania. In a systematic manner he presents the beginning phases of empirical analytic thinking and practice which underlie current theories. The Freud-Abraham view of mania as a triumph and such intimately related subjects as the mourning rites of savages described by Roheim (1923) (97, 98), the Radó (1928, 1926) (88, 90) observations on drug addiction, the Alexander studies on neurotic characters (1927, 1929, 1930) (7, 8, 9), emphasizing the bribery of the superego by ego suffering, are given lucid exposition. Space does not permit more than mention of the importance of the denial mechanism (Lewin, 76, 77; Deutsch, 25); the depressive position in the first year of life (Klein, 74); anaclitic depression (Spitz, 120); disappointment in infancy (Gerö, 56, 57; Jacobson, 68, 69). Lewin's own contributions on the types of denial—diffuse denial, hypomanic neurotic characters, identifications, "technical elation" as a screen affect and as resistance—the relation of mania to the sleep system, the "blank dream," and his extensions to the theory of oral eroticism and the sense of reality are important additions to the comprehension of personality patterns.

While earlier psychiatrists described reactive or situational depressions occasioned by loss of some cherished relationship through death or separation, it remained for Freud to show that the internal psychological work done in depressions was akin to the process of mourning; for in both circumstances the person is unwilling to admit the need to give up the lost object and to reinvest, so to speak, his emotional capital in some other desirable person or enterprise. The separation process becomes more complicated when the mourner has active feelings of affection and dislike simultaneously for the lost one. In fact, the mourner may for a time hate the object of his concern for deserting him, even though the latter is not responsible. Under such circumstances the mourner does not feel free to express his mixed feelings but is compelled by his conscience to turn the aggression inward to punish himself. Often the repression of hostility is incomplete, so that the mourner may impulsively exhibit his rage in active ways: he may kill the deserter and then commit suicide in order to obliterate the object incorporated within himself. Some of the fantasy material of the depressive concerns oral incorporative destruction (devouring) of the ambivalently loved object. Since the love object is represented as a part of his personality through introjection, the depressive must needs hurt himself when he attacks the introjected object. With such attacks upon loved ones comes guilt, which, in turn, demands punishment to maintain psychic equilibrium (2, 48).

As analysts became familiar with these interpretations, it was apparent that the major cyclic mood disturbances are not always adamant reactions which run a predestined course, possibly because of a genetic, endocrine, or metabolic basis. The usual textbook curves describing the course of the disease were abstractions taken from hundreds of records; but examination and the therapeutic success of many an individual case revealed that the onset was related to a psychogenic factor and that the development of the disorder had psychological coherence. It remains for more controlled studies to show what varieties of mood disorders can be so influenced.

### Psychoneuroses and Psychoses

Some differences between psychoses and neuroses become apparent from our survey, even though both have similar historical development and dynamic defenses.

1. In the psychotic, the ego functions are severely damaged in one or more spheres, especially in the loss or diminution of object relationships. The ego cannot cope with the environment, so it falsifies or distorts the data in order to maintain mastery. The neurotic tries to work out his conflicts within himself and only secondarily "acts out" his conflict.

2. The psychotic seeks infantile pleasures of rudimentary, often undisguised, type, such as narcissistic, autoerotic, symbolic, objectless pleasure.

3. The psychotic exhibits behavior of infantile origin which may be regressive (archaic language and motility, delusions of grandeur, somatic symptoms, depersonalization, and destructive fantasies about the self, other people, or the world) or restitutive (hallucinations, delusions).

4. The psychotic expresses many emotions, especially hostility, more openly than the neurotic does. He has less need for sado-masochistic refinements or ambivalence. Projection is more commonly employed by the psychotic than repression.

5. Anxiety is not so tightly organized in the psychotic, except in delusions, as compared with the neurotic. The psychotic shows much less guilt, shame, and sensitivity about his own and other persons' performance.

6. The integrative functions of the psychotic's ego are so disorganized that he seeks the satisfaction of isolated drives, and his personality is so impaired that his life may be in danger.

7. Modulated expression of personal needs compatible with conventional practices is lacking in the psychotic, who therefore is often in danger of injury or arrest.

8. Incomplete repression often causes the psychotic to be plagued with primitive thoughts and desires which cannot be controlled. When these are allied to "magic," the distress is even more acute.

9. Under stress the psychotic may resort to gross flight and massive withdrawal rather than to defensive symptom formation, as in the case of the neurotic.

## CURRENT PSYCHOTHERAPEUTIC TECHNIQUES

Although many psychiatrists and psychoanalysts have treated psychotic patients without the use of physical methods, this area has not had strong continuity of interest. It is instructive to know of the early work at Ward's Island, New York, and Burghölzli before 1914 and the repeated efforts, with some success, at St. Elizabeth's Hospital, the Phipps Clinic, the New York State Psychiatric Hospital, Worcester State Hospital, and others (Nunberg, Kardiner, Kempf, Oberndorff, W. A. White, Paul Federn); but more concentrated attention upon psychotherapy came with the demonstration by H. S. Sullivan (1925) that psychotherapy could be carried out more effectively if human relations, as well as physical and administrative practices, were expressly designed to meet the patient's needs. To this end he selected hospital aides and nurses who had a special capacity for understanding schizophrenic patients because they themselves were sensitive, shy, and able to feel the reality of internal conflicts. With training to regard patients as hurt human beings instead of hopeless threats, the attendants became unusually skilful in their work and had corresponding success. Even after Sullivan left the Sheppard and Enoch Pratt Hospital, the attendants were able to carry on successfully. Later, in collaboration with Frieda Fromm-Reichmann, systematic long-term treatment methods were developed which have been utilized elsewhere. The active exchange of opinions regarding many techniques for treating psychotics augurs well for the future in this difficult field. At present the enormous importance of the transference-countertransference aspect of therapy is receiving increased scrutiny, for it may be one of the crucial factors in treatment (34, 29–31, 80, 110, 112). Perhaps one will learn which kinds of therapists can work with the various reaction types and then train these persons painstakingly in the arduous task of convincing the withdrawn, frightened person that ordinary living can be gratifying and worth while.

The reports by J. N. Rosen (100–102) that vigorous, direct interpretations of unconscious material carried on intensively enabled patients to improve more quickly has also stimulated wider experimentation. Until the case studies treated in this manner are brought under more rigorous control, however, it is not possible to evaluate either the methods used or the results (26, 135).

Most workers follow the methods of Federn, Sullivan, and Fromm-Reichmann.

We can hope that intensive work in many places will establish better treatment methods (135). It is certain that such studies will also make possible better collaboration with experimental psychologists, neurophysiologists, biochemists, and endocrinologists, who will reveal new aspects of the functions of the central nervous system when under stress.

## BIBLIOGRAPHY

1.  ABRAHAM, K. "The First Pregenital Stage of the Libido (1916), in *Selected Papers* (London: Hogarth Press, 1926), pp. 248–79.
2.  ABRAHAM, K. "Notes on the Psycho-analytical Investigation and Treatment of Manic-depressive Insanity and Allied Conditions (1911)," in *Selected Papers* (London: Hogarth Press, 1927), pp. 137–56.
3.  ABRAHAM, K. "The Psycho-sexual Differences between Hysteria and Dementia Praecox (1908)," in *Selected Papers* (London: Hogarth Press, 1927), pp. 64–79.
4.  ABRAHAM, K. *Selected Papers* (London: Hogarth Press, 1927).
5.  ABRAHAM, K. "A Short Study of the Development of the Libido, Viewed in the Light of Mental Disorders (1924)," in *Selected Papers* (London: Hogarth Press, 1927), pp. 418–501.
6.  ACTH CLINICAL CONFERENCE. *Proceedings of the First Conference*, ed. J. R. MOTE (New York: Blakiston Co., 1950).
7.  ALEXANDER, F. "The Neurotic Character," *Internat. J. Psycho-Analysis*, 11:292, 1930.
8.  ALEXANDER, F. *Psychoanalysis of the Total Personality* (New York: Nervous and Mental Disease Publishing Co., 1929).
9.  ALEXANDER, F. "Zur Theorie der Zwangsneurosen und der Phobien," *Internat. Ztschr. f. Psychoanal.*, 13:20, 1927.
10.  ALEXANDER, F., and FRENCH, T. M. *Psychoanalytic Therapy: Principles and Applications* (New York: Ronald Press Co., 1946).
11.  BELLAK, L. *Dementia Praecox: The Past Decade's Work and Present Status, a Review and Evaluation* (New York: Grune & Stratton, 1948).
12.  BELLAK, L. "A Multiple-Factor Psychosomatic Theory of Schizophrenia," *Psychiat. Quart.*, 23:738, 1949.
13.  BETTELHEIM, B. *Love Is Not Enough: The Treatment of Emotionally Disturbed Children* (Glencoe, Ill.: Free Press, 1950).
14.  BLEULER, E. "Autistic Thinking" and "Autistic-undisciplined Thinking," in D. RAPAPORT (ed.), *Organization and Pathology of Thought: Selected Sources* (New York: Columbia University Press, 1951), pp. 399–450.
15.  BLEULER, E. "The Basic Symptoms of Schizophrenia," in D. RAPAPORT (ed.), *Organization and Pathology of Thought: Selected*

*Sources* (New York: Columbia University Press, 1951), pp. 581–645.

16. BLEULER, M. "Forschungen zur Schizophreniefrage," *Wien. Ztschr. f. Nervenh.*, 1:129, 1948.

17. Boss, M. "Psychopathologie des Traumes bei schizophrenen und organischen Psychosen," *Ztschr. f. d. ges. Neurol. u. Psychiat.*, 162:459, 1938.

18. BOWLBY, J. *Maternal Care and Mental Health* (Geneva: World Health Organization, 1951).

19. BREUER, J., and FREUD, S. *Studies in Hysteria* (New York: Nervous and Mental Disease Publishing Co., 1936).

20. BRILL, A. A. *Introduction in the Basic Writings of Sigmund Freud* (New York: Modern Library, 1938), pp. 3–32.

21. CLARK, L. P. "Some Practical Remarks upon the Use of Modified Psychoanalysis in the Treatment of Borderland Neuroses and Psychoses," *Psychoanalyt. Rev.*, 6:306, 1919.

22. CLARK, L. P. "The Treatment of Narcissistic Neuroses and Psychoses," *Psychoanalyt. Rev.*, 20:304, 1933.

23. DEUTSCH, H. "Homosexuality in Women," *Internat. J. Psycho-Analysis*, 14:34, 1933.

24. DEUTSCH, H. "Some Forms of Emotional Disturbances and Their Relationship to Schizophrenia," *Psychoanalyt. Quart.*, 11:301, 1942.

25. DEUTSCH, H. "Zur Psychologie der manisch-depressiven Zustände, insbesondere der chronischen Hypomanie," *Internat. Ztschr. f. Psychoanal.*, 19:358, 1933.

26. EISSLER, K. "Remarks on the Psychoanalysis of Schizophrenia," *Internat. J. Psycho-Analysis*, 31:139, 1951.

27. ERIKSON, E. *Childhood and Society* (New York: W. W. Norton & Co., 1950).

28. EZRIEL, H. "A Psycho-analytic Approach to Group Treatment," *Brit. J. M. Psychol.*, 23:59, 1950.

29. FEDERN, P. "Bibliography," available in *Internat. J. Psycho-Analysis*, 32:242, 1951.

30. FEDERN, P. "Panel Discussion on Countertransferences and Attitudes of the Analyst in the Therapeutic Process," *Bull. Am. Psychoanal. Assoc.*, 5:46, 1949.

31. FEDERN, P. "Panel Discussion on the Theory and Treatment of Schizophrenia," *Bull. Am. Psychoanal. Assoc.*, 4:15, 1948.

32. FEDERN, P. "Psychoanalysis of Psychoses: Errors and How To Avoid Them," *Psychiat. Quart.*, 17:3, 1943.

33. FEDERN, P. "Psychoanalysis of Psychoses: The Psychoanalytic Process," *Psychiat. Quart.*, 17:470, 1943.

34. FEDERN, P. "Psychoanalysis of Psychoses: Transference," *Psychiat. Quart.*, 17:246, 1943.

35. FEIGENBAUM, D. "The Paranoid Criminal: A Casuistic Study," *M. Rev. of Rev.*, 36:222, 1930.

36. FELDMANN, S. "Über Erkrankungsanlässe bei Psychosen," *Internat. Ztschr. f. Psychoanal.*, 7:203, 1921.

37. FENICHEL, O. *The Psychoanalytic Theory of Neurosis* (New York: W. W. Norton & Co., 1945).

38. FERENCZI, S. *Further Contributions to the Theory and Technique of Psychoanalysis* (London: Hogarth Press, 1926).

39. FERENCZI, S. *Sex in Psychoanalysis* (Boston: Gorham Press, 1916).

40. FERENCZI, S. "Stages in the Development of the Sense of Reality," in *Sex in Psychoanalysis: Contributions to Psychoanalysis* (New York: Brunner, 1950), pp. 213–39).

41. FRENCH, T. M., and KASANIN, J. "A Psychodynamic Study of the Recovery of Two Schizophrenic Cases," *Psychoanalyt. Quart.*, 10:1, 1941.

42. FREUD, A. *The Ego and the Mechanisms of Defence* (New York: International Universities Press, 1946).

43. FREUD, S. "Analysis of a Phobia in a Five-Year-Old Boy (1909)," in *Collected Papers*, 3 (London: Hogarth Press, 1946), 149–289.

44. FREUD, S. "A Case of Paranoia Running Counter to the Psycho-analytical Theory of the Disease (1915)," in *Collected Papers*, 2 (London: Hogarth Press, 1946), 150–61.

45. FREUD, S. "Further Remarks on the Defence Neuro-psychoses (1896)," in *Collected Papers*, 1 (London: Hogarth Press, 1946), 155–82.

46. FREUD, S. *The Interpretations of Dreams* (New York: Macmillan Co., 1942).

47. FREUD, S. "The Loss of Reality in Neurosis and Psychosis (1924)," in *Collected Papers*, 2 (London: Hogarth Press, 1946), 277–82.

48. FREUD, S. "Mourning and Melancholia (1917)," in *Collected Papers*, 4 (London: Hogarth Press, 1946), 152–70.

49. FREUD, S. "On Narcissism: An Introduction," in *Collected Papers*, 4 (London: Hogarth Press, 1946), 30–59.

50. FREUD, S. "Neurosis and Psychosis (1924)," in *Collected Papers*, 2 (London: Hogarth Press, 1946), 250–54.

51. FREUD, S. "Psycho-analytic Notes upon an Autobiographical Account of a Case of Paranoia (Dementia Paranoides) (1911)," in *Collected Papers*, 3 (London: Hogarth Press, 1946), 387–470.

52. FREUD, S. *Three Contributions to the Theory of Sex* (4th ed.; New York: Nervous and Mental Disease Publishing Co., 1930).

53. FROMM-REICHMANN, F. *Principles of Intensive Psychotherapy* (Chicago: University of Chicago Press, 1950).

54. FROMM-REICHMANN, F. "Transference Problems in Schizophrenics," *Psychoanalyt. Quart.*, 8:412, 1939.

55. GARMA, A. "Psychoanalytic Investigations in Melancholias and Other Types of Depressions," in *Yearbook of Psychoanalysis*, 3:75, 1947.

56. GERÖ, G. "Der Aufbau der Depression," *Internat. Ztschr. f. Psychoanal.*, 22:379, 1936; also "The Construction of Depression," *Internat. J. Psycho-Analysis*, 17:423, 1936.

57. GERÖ, G. "Zum Problem der oralen Fixierung," *Internat. Ztschr. f. Psychoanal. u. Imago*, 24:239, 1939.

58. GRODDECK, G. *The Book of the It: Psychoanalytic Letters to a Friend* (London: Daniel Co., 1935).

59. GRODDECK, G. *Die psychische Bedingtheit und psychoanalytische Behandlung organischer Krankheiten* (Berlin: S. Hirzel, 1917).

60. GROTJAHN, M. "The Process of Maturation in Group Psychotherapy and in the Group Therapist," *Psychiatry*, 13:63, 1950.

61. GROTJAHN, M., and FRENCH, T. M. "Akinesia after Ventriculography: A Contribution to Ego Psychology and the Problem of Sleep," *Psychoanalyt. Quart.*, 7:319, 1938.

62. HENDRICK, I. "Contributions of Psychoanalysis to Study of Psychosis," *J.A.M.A.*, 113:918, 1939.

63. HENDRICK, I. "Ego Development and Certain Character Problems," *Psychoanalyt. Quart.*, 5:320, 1936.

64. HENDRICK, I. "The Ego and the Defense Mechanisms: A Review and Discussion," *Psychoanalyt. Rev.*, 25:476, 1938.

65. HINSIE, L. E. "Schizophrenias," in S. LORAND (ed.), *Psycho-analysis Today* (New York: International Universities Press, 1944), pp. 274–86.

66. HOCH, A. "The Psychogenic Factors in Some Paranoic Conditions, with Suggestions for Prophylaxis and Treatment," *J. Nerv. & Ment. Dis.*, 34:668, 1907.

67. HOLLOS, S. *Hinter der gelben Mauer* (Stuttgart: Hippokrates, 1928).

68. JACOBSON, E. "Depression: The Oedipus Complex in the Development of Depressive Mechanisms," *Psychoanalyt. Quart.*, 12:541, 1943.

69. JACOBSON, E. "The Effect of Disappointment on Ego and Super-ego Formation in Normal and Depressive Development," *Psychoanalyt. Rev.*, 33:129, 1946.

70. JUNG, C. G. *The Psychology of Dementia Praecox* (New York: Nervous and Mental Disease Publishing Co., 1936).

71. KATAN, M. "Schreber's Delusion of the End of the World," *Psychoanalyt. Quart.*, 18:60, 1949.

72. KATAN, M. "Schreber's Hallucinations about the 'Little Men,'" *Internat. J. Psycho-Analysis*, 31:32, 1950.

73. KIMURA, H. "Psychoanalytic Investigations of Delusions in Paranoia; Delusions of Grandeur," *Beitr. z. Psychoanal. (u. Sendai Japan)*, Vol. 1, No. 2, 1932.

74. KLEIN, M. "Contribution to Psychogenesis of Manic-depressive States," *Internat. J. Psycho-Analysis*, 16:145, 1935.

74a. KLEIN, M. "Zur Psychogenese der manischdepressiven Zustände," *Internat. Ztschr. f. Psychoanal.*, 23:275, 1937.

75. LEVY, D. M. *Maternal Overprotection* (New York: Columbia University Press, 1943).

76. LEWIN, B. D. "Anal Eroticism and Mechanism of Undoing," *Psychoanalyt. Quart.*, 1:343, 1932.

77. LEWIN, B. D. "Analysis and Structure of a Transient Hypomania," *Psychoanalyt. Quart.*, 1:43, 1932.

78. LEWIN, B. D. *The Psychoanalysis of Elation* (New York: W. W. Norton & Co., 1950).

79. LEWIS, N. D. C. *Research in Dementia Praecox (Past Attainments, Present Trends, and Future Possibilities)* (New York: National Committee on Mental Hygiene, 1936).

80. Mann, J.; Menzer, D.; *et al.* "Psychotherapy of Psychoses: Some Attitudes in the Therapist Influencing the Course of Treatment," *Psychiatry*, 13:432, 1950.

81. Mullahy, P. (ed.). *A Study of Interpersonal Relations: New Contributions to Psychiatry* (New York: Hermitage House, 1949).

82. Nunberg, H. "On the Catatonic Episode," *Internat. Ztschr. f. Psychoanal.*, 6:25, 1920.

83. Nunberg, H. "Die synthetische Funktion des Ich," *Internat. Ztschr. f. Psychoanal.*, 16:301, 1930; also, *Internat. J. Psycho-Analysis*, 12:123, 1931.

84. Nunberg, H. "Über Depersonalizationszustände im Lichte der Libidotheorie," *Internat. Ztschr. f. Psychoanal.*, 10:17, 1924.

85. Piaget, J. *The Language and Thought of the Child* (New York: Harcourt, Brace & Co., 1926).

86. Powdermaker, F., and Frank, J. D. "Group Psychotherapy with Neurotics," *Am. J. Psychiat.*, 105:449, 1948.

87. Radó, S. "An Anxious Mother: A Contribution to the Analysis of the Ego," *Internat. J. Psycho-Analysis*, 9:219, 1928.

88. Radó, S. "The Physical Effects of Intoxication: Attempt at a Psychoanalytical Theory of Drug-Addiction," *Internat. J. Psycho-Analysis*, 9:301, 1928.

89. Radó, S. "The Problem of Melancholia," *Internat. J. Psycho-Analysis*, 9:420, 1928.

90. Radó, S. "The Psychic Effects of Intoxicants: An Attempt To Evolve a Psycho-analytical Theory of Morbid Cravings," *Internat. J. Psycho-Analysis*, 7:396, 1926.

91. Rapaport, D. (ed.). *Organization and Pathology of Thought: Selected Sources* (New York: Columbia University Press, 1951), p. 401.

92. Rapaport, D. "On the Psychoanalytic Theory of Thinking," *Internat. J. Psycho-Analysis*, 31:161, 1950.

93. Redl, F. *Mental Hygiene in Teaching* (New York: Harcourt, Brace & Co., 1951).

94. Rickman, J. "The Application of Psychoanalytical Principles to Hospital In-patients," *J. Ment. Sc.*, 94:764, 1948.

95. Rickman, J. "Development of Psycho-analytical Theory of Psychoses, 1894–1926," *Internat. J. Psycho-Analysis*, Suppl. No. 2, pp. 1–106, 1928.

96. Rickman, J. *Index Psychoanalyticus, 1893–1926* (London: Hogarth Press, 1928).

97. Roheim, G. "Heiliges Geld in Melanesien," *Internat. Ztschr. f. Psychoanal.*, 9:384, 1923.

98. Roheim, G. "Nach dem Tode des Urvaters" (Abstract), *Internat. J. Psycho-Analysis*, 4:368, 1923.

99. Rorschach, H. *Psychodiagnostics* (Bern: H. Huber, 1942).

100. Rosen, J. N. "A Method of Resolving Acute Catatonic Excitement," *Psychiat. Quart.*, 20:183, 1946.

101. Rosen, J. N. "The Survival Function of Schizophrenia," *Bull. Menninger Clin.*, 14:81, 1950.

102. ROSEN, J. N. "The Treatment of Schizophrenic Psychosis by Direct Analytic Therapy," *Psychiat. Quart.*, 21:3, 1947.

103. ROSENFELD, H. "A Note on the Psychopathology of Confusional States in Chronic Schizophrenics," *Internat. J. Psycho-Analysis*, 31:132, 1950.

104. SCHILDER, P. *Introduction to a Psychoanalytic Psychiatry* (New York: Nervous and Mental Disease Publishing Co., 1928).

105. SCHILDER, P. "Neuroses and Psychoses," in S. LORAND (ed.), *Psychoanalysis Today* (New York: International Universities Press, 1944), pp. 249–60.

106. SCHILDER, P. *Psychotherapy* (New York: W. W. Norton & Co., 1951).

107. SCOTT, J. P. "Genetic Differences in Social Behavior of Dogs," *Am. Psychologist*, 5:261, 1950.

108. SCOTT, J. P. "Genetics as a Tool in Experimental Psychological Research," *Am. Psychologist*, 4:526, 1949.

109. SCOTT, J. P. "Studies on the Early Development of Social Behavior in Puppies," *Am. Psychologist*, 3:239, 1948.

110. SEGAL, H. "Some Aspects of the Analysis of a Schizophrenic," *Internat. J. Psycho-Analysis*, 31:268, 1950.

111. SHAKOW, D. *The Nature of Deterioration in Schizophrenic Conditions* (New York: Nervous and Mental Disease Publishing Co., 1946).

112. SILVERBERG, W. V. "The Concept of Transference," *Psychoanalyt. Quart.*, 17:303, 1948.

113. SLAVSON, S. R. *Analytic Group Psychotherapy with Children, Adolescents, and Adults* (New York: Columbia University Press, 1950).

114. SOLOMON, H. D. "Newer Developments in Psychiatry," *Digest Neurol. & Psychiat.*, 18:58, 1950.

115. SPITZ, R. A. "Emotional Growth in the First Year," *Child Study*, spring, 1947, p. 68.

116. SPITZ, R. A. "Hospitalism: A Follow-Up Report on Investigation Described in Volume I, 1945," in *The Psychoanalytic Study of the Child*, 2 (New York: International Universities Press, 1946), 113–17.

117. SPITZ, R. A. "Hospitalism: An Inquiry into the Genesis of Psychiatric Conditions in Early Childhood," in *The Psychoanalytic Study of the Child*, 1 (New York: International Universities Press, 1945), 53–74.

118. SPITZ, R. A. "The Importance of Mother-Child Relationship during the First Year of Life," *Ment. Health Today*, 1948.

119. SPITZ, R. A. "The Smiling Response: A Contribution to the Otogenesis of Social Relations," *Genet. Psychol. Monogr.*, 34:57, 1946.

120. SPITZ, R. A., and WOLF, K. M. "Anaclitic Depression: An Inquiry into the Genesis of Psychiatric Conditions in Early Childhood," in *The Psychoanalytic Study of the Child*, 2 (New York: International Universities Press, 1946), 313–42.

121. SPITZ, R. A., and WOLF, K. M. "The Role of Ecological Factors in Emotional Development in Infancy," *Child Development*, 1949.

122. Spock, B. *The Pocket Book of Baby and Child Care* (New York: Pocket Books, 1946).

123. Stanton, A. H., and Schwartz, M. S. "The Management of a Type of Institutional Participation in Mental Illness," *Psychiatry*, 12:13, 1949.

124. Stanton, A. H., and Schwartz, M. S. "Medical Opinion and the Social Context in the Mental Hospital," *Psychiatry*, 12:243, 1949.

125. Stanton, A. H., and Schwartz, M. S. "Observations on Dissociation as Social Participation," *Psychiatry*, 12:339, 1949.

126. Stärcke, A. "The Reversal of the Libido-Sign in Delusions of Persecution," *Internat. J. Psycho-Analysis*, 1:231, 1920.

127. Stengel, E. "The Application of Psychoanalytical Principles to the Hospital In-patient," *J. Ment. Sc.*, 94:773, 1948.

128. Storch, A. *The Primitive Archaic Forms of Inner Experiences and Thought in Schizophrenia: A Genetic and Clinical Study of Schizophrenia* (New York: Nervous and Mental Disease Publishing Co., 1924).

129. Sullivan, H. S. "Conceptions of Modern Psychiatry," *Psychiatry*, 3:1, 1940.

130. Tausk, V. "On the Origin of the 'Influencing Machine' in Schizophrenia," *Psychoanalyt. Quart.*, 3:137, 1934.

131. Thompson, C. *Psychoanalysis: Evolution and Development* (New York: Hermitage House, 1950).

132. Waelder, R. "The Structure of Paranoid Ideas: A Critical Survey of Various Theories," *Internat. J. Psycho-Analysis*, 32:167, 1951.

133. Waelder, R. "The Principle of Multiple Function: Observations on Over-determination," *Psychoanalyt. Quart.*, 5:45, 1936.

134. Weiss, Edoardo. *Principles of Psychodynamics* (New York: Grune & Stratton, 1950).

135. Whitehorn, J. C. "Psychotherapy," in N. G. Harris (ed.), *Modern Trends in Psychological Medicine* (New York: Paul B. Hoeber, Inc., 1948), pp. 219–36.

136. Wholey, C. C. "A Psychosis Presenting Schizophrenic and Freudian Mechanisms, with Schematic Clearness," *Am. J. Psychiat.*, 73:583, 1917.

137. Wilson, C. P., and Cormen, H. H. "A Preliminary Study of the Hypnotizability of Psychotic Patients," *Psychiat. Quart.*, 23:657, 1949.

138. Zilboorg, G. *A History of Medical Psychology* (New York: W. W. Norton & Co., 1941).

139. Zilboorg, G. "Manic-depressive Psychoses," in S. Lorand (ed.), *Psycho-analysis Today* (New York: International Universities Press, 1944), pp. 261–73.

# XI

## PRINCIPLES OF PSYCHIATRIC TREATMENT

### Maurice Levine, M.D.

A DISCUSSION of psychiatric treatment can have as its starting point some of the well-established principles of all medical practice. One precept has stood the test of time above all others. It can be phrased in this way: treatment which is based on adequate diagnosis is superior to treatment which is focused simply on the relief of symptoms.

The clearest demonstration of the value of this principle is to be seen in the treatment of a patient who has abdominal pain. In such a case it surely is not good practice to be satisfied merely with the giving of medicine to alleviate the pain. It is imperative that the treatment of such a patient be based, whenever possible, on a definite diagnosis. For example, the diagnostic conclusion that the symptom of abdominal pain of a particular patient is part of an acute salpingitis leads to treatment which is much more likely to be specific and safe and effective.

In a similar fashion the treatment of a patient who has edema is more likely to be effective if the treatment is based on a diagnosis of cardiac decompensation than if the treatment is directed merely toward the elimination of fluid. And, again, the treatment of a patient who has insomnia can be more specific and safe and effective if, in a particular case, the insomnia is recognized as one aspect of a depression. The treatment then can be based on the implications of the diagnosis of depression rather than based merely on the relief of the symptom of insomnia.

The second principle of good medical practice is, in a sense, a corollary of the first. It is that diagnostic understanding should, whenever possible, include an understanding of etiologic factors. It is not enough to make a diagnosis of salpingitis or of cardiac decompensation or of depression. It is of greater value to establish the fact that the salpingitis is due to gonorrhea, that the cardiac decompensation is based on beriberi, and that the depression is based on emotional conflict centering around feelings of guilt.

Such etiologic understanding adds still greater specificity and safety and effectiveness to the therapeutic procedures.

This emphasis on the role of diagnostic and etiologic understanding as the basis of treatment permits the comment that many of the preceding chapters of this book, which discuss various problems of diagnosis and etiology, are in a broader sense chapters on treatment as well.

But a note of warning must be sounded at this point. This emphasis on the superiority of treatment which is based on diagnostic understanding over treatment which is focused on direct dealing with symptoms should not be construed as a recommendation for a coldly scientific approach. In all fields of medical practice it is essential that the physician be interested in his patient as a person, that he somehow transmit to his patient the fact that his primary goal is to be helpful, and that his interest is not limited to the abstract intellectual process of making a diagnosis or of discovering etiologic factors. In such a therapeutic attitude he must be deeply interested in the patient's symptoms, must want them to be gone, must be able, within limits, to feel with the patient, in his discomfort, pain, and unhappiness. But his warm human interest in alleviating the patient's symptoms is not enough. It is characteristic of the work of the physician that he has a double orientation, often difficult to achieve, of having not only a therapeutic attitude of human helpfulness but also a concomitant attitude of working beyond the symptoms to an understanding of diagnosis and etiology, which then can be used for a more effective therapy.

A third principle of good medical practice is that treatment should be individualized, be adapted to and governed by the specific needs of the particular patient. Such an approach makes medical practice difficult and time-consuming, but there can be no doubt that it adds immeasurably to therapeutic effectiveness. In medicine and surgery some routinization of treatment procedures is possible and time-saving. Many broken arms can be treated in a similar fashion. Routine dosages of medication may be used in similar infections. But better medical and surgical practice takes into consideration such individually variable factors as drug-sensitivity, resistance, immunity, and recuperative strength. And the best medical and surgical practice recognizes the individual personality variables, factors such as patterns of reaction to pain and suffering, attitudes toward the physician, anxiety about sickness, and neurotic patterns which might interfere with co-operativeness in medical procedures, such as the wearing of a cast.

In psychiatry, routine procedures have little value. Human beings, in their emotions, in their interpersonal relations, in their patterns and trends, differ from one another more than one broken bone differs from another. Consequently, in psychiatry, individualization in treatment is even more urgent than in the other fields of medical practice.

It follows from the above discussion that therapy in medical practice, and especially therapy in psychiatry, must be based on a clear understanding of the problems of the patient under treatment and that, to an extraordinary degree, the prescription for treatment is written by the understanding of the problem rather than by a set of therapeutic rules. It follows, further, that a chapter on psychiatric treatment must pay more attention to the interdependence of understanding and therapy than to a description of therapeutic techniques. Consequently, a discussion of specific methods of treatment will be deferred to the end of the chapter.

To clarify further the logic of the rather unusual sequence of topics in this chapter, a parallel may be drawn with the teaching of surgical treatment. In surgery a description of the techniques of various breast operations can become much more meaningful when the student first has been given a clear conception of the ways in which various specific pathologic processes and physiologic patterns (e.g., lymphatic drainage) determine the operative procedures.

Such a formulation of the principles of treatment is not so easy to teach or to learn as one which would emphasize simple rules and routine and technical procedures. Therefore, it is of high value to have a frame of reference to use in this approach to the treatment of psychiatric patients, an approach that emphasizes diagnostic and etiologic understanding, individualization, and the basic dependence of therapy on understanding the patient as a person. One frame of reference that has proved to be of value is that of basing therapy on the following six considerations:

A. Clinical diagnosis      D. Transference
B. Dynamic diagnosis     E. Countertransference
C. Genetic diagnosis      F. Treatment possibilities

Such a frame of reference is useful in actual work with an individual patient. It provides an architecture for the formulation of the data about the patient that will permit the psychiatrist to have a broad and solid basis for his therapeutic work. And such a listing can provide the architecture for the general discussion of the problems of psychiatric treatment in this chapter. With such a framework, the discussion can be related intimately to the material of the previous chapters, rearranged and rephrased in such a fashion as to indicate its immediate pertinence to therapy.

## A. Clinical Diagnosis

By "clinical diagnosis" is meant the shorthand formulation of the broad general category in which the patient's reaction belongs, such as paresis, schizophrenia, delirium, hysteria, neurotic character.

In all medicine the concept of clinical diagnosis is a complex one, with many inconsistencies in the classification systems of clinical diagnosis. Some clinical diagnostic terms are essentially descriptive, e.g., petit mal; some refer to pathology, e.g., appendicitis; and some to etiology, e.g., syphilis. In psychiatry the usage of clinical diagnosis is even more problematic. Not only is there a comparable inconsistency in the criteria of classification, but also there is an even greater variation of cases within any diagnostic category, and the points of greatest diagnostic and therapeutic importance lie in the dynamic interplay of environmental forces and personal reactions in the individual patient. In psychiatry, perhaps even more than in medicine in general, systematic diagnostic terminology is in a transitional state.

But, even with the present unsatisfactory state of clinical diagnostic formulations and the dominant importance in present-day psychiatric treatment of dynamic and genetic considerations (to be outlined below), there remains some value in a partial preservation of attempts at clinical diagnosis. A total elimination of clinical diagnosis ignores the value of reliable or partly reliable generalizations that have precipitated out of centuries of experience. Without such clinical evaluation, treatment is less soundly based and runs the risk of serious error.

The dependence of therapy on clinical diagnosis can be seen from the following examples: Depressed patients will be treated differently if their depression is part of paresis or of a deep-going depression that may be called "manic-depressive" or of a neurotic depression. The treatment of patients with manifest anxiety will in part depend on whether the anxiety is part of a typical anxiety neurosis, or is part of a traumatic neurosis, or is part of the picture of the breakdown of previous defenses during the development of a psychosis. Asthma with important emotional factors in its etiology must be treated in one way if the patient is schizophrenic and in another if the patient is a compulsive character. Psychotherapy of psychogenic headache must depend on a consideration of whether the headache is part of the general picture of conversion hysteria, of hypochondriasis, of migraine, or of anxiety neurosis.

Under this category, of clinical diagnosis, is included the diagnosis of any specific physical disorder to be found by the general practitioner or specialist with whom the psychiatrist is collaborating in the study of the patient. Such a diagnosis must be based on adequate medical history-taking, physical examination, and laboratory studies. Treatment that is soundly based must include both somatic and psychologic investigations, since errors may arise in both directions. A disorder predominantly emotional in origin may give the impression of being a disorder primarily anatomic or physiologic in origin, e.g., abdominal pain which is a hysteric conversion symptom may simulate appendicitis. In the other direction, primarily structural and physiologic disorders may simulate those primarily emotional; e.g., a brain tumor may have compulsive manifestations as presenting symptoms; a pancreatic tumor may give the clinical picture of an anxiety neurosis. Further, when both psychologic and somatic etiologic factors are of importance, psychotherapy may have to be associated with simultaneous treatment of a somatic nature. A patient who has coronary artery disease, whose attacks of pain are precipitated by conflict and anxiety, should be treated simultaneously by psychotherapeutic and somato-therapeutic measures.

In general, it is best that the relevant physical studies be made before treatment is begun or during the exploratory period. In this fashion, if the disorder is primarily psychogenic, the therapist can feel confident of his orientation and can withstand the pressure of many patients during treatment to return again and again to the defense of attributing their problems to physical disease.

Further, it must be mentioned that the psychiatrist can play a role in the evaluation of the patient's physical status. The internist must make a diagnosis of "neurosis" largely by a process of exclusion; if he finds no adequate somatic cause for the symptoms, he concludes that the disorder must be largely psychogenic. But diagnosis by exclusion is not adequate; the psychiatrist (or the psychiatrically oriented internist) must attempt to find pertinent positive factors in the psychologic sphere to account for the disorder. For example, in a case of a gross tremor of one hand, negative physical studies may, by exclusion, lead to a probable diagnosis of conversion hysteria. But a convincing diagnosis of conversion hysteria can be achieved only by the discovery of life-experiences, conflicts, anxiety, purposes, or motives which seem to have etiologic significance and can be linked with the tremor in terms of the "logic of the emotions."

Parenthetically, in connection with the problem of finding pertinent positive factors, it must be mentioned that many psychogenic manifestations are not of themselves directly meaningful. Some are; for instance, hysteric blindness may be directly understandable as a defense against unacceptable peeping tendencies. Some are not; for example, a diarrhea at times may not have psychologic meaning of itself, but may be the physiologic concomitant of anxiety, which is meaningful; a hypertension of itself is not symbolic or defensive, but the physiologic concomitant of suppressed rage, which is meaningful.

To return to the relevance of clinical diagnosis to therapy, the generalization can be made that the clinical diagnosis may serve to prevent mistakes and may give leads as to the variety and depth of treatment. When it is probable that the patient's reaction is largely schizophrenic, psychotherapy should avoid direct interpretations productive of anxiety, although this statement may have to be modified if the recent work of Rosen (39) and others is found to be generally applicable. Further, if the clinical diagnosis is that of a panic state, the psychotherapy may have to be much more emphatically supportive than if the clinical diagnosis is that of a somewhat similar anxiety state. If the clinical diagnosis is that of hypertension with episodes of hypertensive encephalopathy, the psychotherapy must be different from that of a patient with hypertension without encephalopathy. If the clinical diagnosis is of hypochondriasis, psychotherapeutic attempts must be far more cautious and circumspect than if the clinical diagnosis is of hysteria.

## B. Dynamic Diagnosis

Therapeutic attitudes, responses, maneuvers, and techniques are dependent not only on the clinical diagnosis, as indicated above, but even more so on the dynamic diagnosis. This term refers to the understanding of the forces that currently are operative in the production of the patient's difficulty, the environmental pressures and internal pressures (drives, purposes, motives, anxiety) that account for symptoms, for character problems, and for disturbed interpersonal relations. For the sake of clarity, the term "dynamic diagnosis" is contrasted with "genetic diagnosis," which refers to the understanding of the genesis and origin and development of those forces which currently are at work. In a broad sense such genetic factors are "dynamic" also, as forces and stresses which molded the personality; but it is of practical value to consider the two groups of forces separately.

In the category of dynamic diagnosis are included (*a*) the environmental forces which are of importance either in precipitating the reaction or in keeping it active, such factors as the loss of love objects, the danger of death and mutilation (as in combat reactions), and the effect of current neurotic attitudes of a parent on a child; (*b*) the internal restrictive, permissive, punitive, and standard-setting forces of the personality, which go by the shorthand term of the "superego"; (*c*) the instinct derivatives, the drives, impulses, unacceptable attitudes, and fantasies of the patient, which are spoken of as the "id" (including sexual, hostile, narcissistic, passive, and other drives); and (*d*) the integrating, synthesizing, compromising, solution-forming, defense-creating aspects of the personality, called the "ego," which is in contact with the environment (through external perception and control of motility) and in contact with id and superego through a kind of internal perception and influence. In a sense, the ego serves three masters—id, superego, and external world—and at the same time attempts to be their master. As indicated in other chapters of this book, most of the forces involved in such psychodynamics are unconscious.

It must be stated, with emphasis, that such a formulation of dynamic forces in terms of id, superego, and ego is not to be understood as indicating that there are three separate and distinct compartments, or three little men fighting for control. The terminology is used only as a convenient shorthand, as a way of indicating that there are three sets of forces and functions, blending and interacting, each one being many-sided and complex, partly organized and partly unorganized. Understood in this fashion, this terminology provides a useful tool for clear thinking.

Essentially, the dynamic diagnosis in an individual case is the understanding of the forces of the above four groups (id, ego, superego, and external world) as they operate and interact in the specific person and situation under consideration. It is the formulation of the ways in which certain environmental and internal (id and superego) forces in conflict produce anxiety, which, in turn, leads to specific defensive attempts by the ego to lessen the anxiety and to provide some solution of the conflict.

Unfortunately, it is difficult to outline such a condensed formulation of the essence of psychodynamic thinking without seducing many students into using a too theoretical formulation of the problems of individual patients and a too theoretical approach in therapy. Perhaps such a tendency can be counterbalanced by emphasizing the fact that it is far more important for the student to observe or to sense correctly one single dynamic force, e.g., that the patient, underneath his amiable attitude, really hates his boss, than for the student to be able abstractly and without immediate feeling to write a five-page theoretical discussion of id and superego. The student should use theoretical learning only as a way of general orientation to the field and later as a way of cross-checking his thinking about a specific patient against known theoretical concepts. While he is in the interview room with the patient, he need not try deliberately to think of general or theoretical constructs. In such an exploratory or psychotherapeutic interview he should essentially be an understanding, thinking, feeling, responding sample of humanity in direct contact with another sample of humanity in trouble.

The above comment, on the attitude of the therapist during interviews, leads to another, on the processes occurring in the therapist in his interviews with patients. Essentially, two processes occur, as part of the therapist's attempts to understand the forces operative in the patient and to understand the ways in which the patient might be helped. They are: (*a*) the "intellectual" process and (*b*) the "empathic" process. (Again, such terminology is not to be taken too literally or rigidly. It is quite possible that the intellectual approach is, in the last analysis, based on empathic processes involved in any process of perception. The terminology is used simply to characterize the two rather different processes by which one human being comes to understand another.)

The intellectual process involved is that the therapist uses his perception and logic and reason to figure out what is wrong with the patient and what forces are at work. He collects pertinent evidence and correlates it. He puts together past history and significant recent events, notices chronologic sequences, observes discrepancies. For example, he notices that a patient becomes flushed and tense when he mentions his boss, even though the patient says that the relationship is all that it should be. The therapist's reason tells him that such a discrepancy must mean that conflicting forces are active. Or the therapist notices that the patient talks a great deal about his father, his siblings, and his associates but never mentions his mother, even though the patient might be expected spontaneously to make some comment about her. The therapist must suspect that such an omission may be meaningful. Or the therapist, knowing from the relatives or referring doctor or from the patient himself about some of the patient's demanding and controlling attitudes and observing now that the patient is anxious and bewildered after some frustrating experience, may intellectually construct the hypothesis (to be verified) that the patient has a pattern of becoming anxious and bewildered whenever he cannot succeed in dominating or controlling his environment or his problems.

The second process involved in interviewing which leads to an understanding of the dynamic diagnosis may be called "empathic," a process essentially of limited and temporary identification with the patient. What happens in empathy may be phrased in this way: "How would I feel under the same circumstances?" "If I were in his shoes and behaved that way, how might I really be feeling?" Another phrasing may be used, which in part involves empathic and in part intellectual processes: "How would a child feel under the circumstances?" The latter phrasing occasionally is very effective in giving the therapist some conception of the patient's hidden reactions, since a child under the same circumstances would be less likely to keep his feelings hidden from others or from himself and would be less likely to have complicated his direct feelings by evasions, subtleties, and complex patterns. As an example: Suppose that a patient, who has always been very independent and self-sufficient, tells, without appealing for pity or sympathy, of the many jobs he now has to do and at the point of going on to some other comments sighs fairly deeply without noticing it and has a momentary slump in his body attitude. The therapist at that moment, out of his "free-floating attention" and "unconscious speaking to unconscious," identifies himself with the patient momentarily and then says to himself: "Under those circumstances I'd certainly want to sigh many times; I'd feel very tired; I'd like someone to help me out while I relax; a child in such circumstances might feel overwhelmed and very eager for someone to take over and help and protect; I wonder if this man doesn't have some dependency needs that he is unable to express or to satisfy."

The process of empathy is, of course, facilitated if the therapist has had comparable experiences. One internist, after a discussion of the material of the preceding paragraphs, remarked that his understanding of the problems of his patients during the experience of illness was tremendously improved after he, for the first time, had had a serious illness. Another stated that he had had no tolerance for the complaints of patients with backache until he himself had a slipped intervertebral disk. It is to be hoped that neither became too sympathetic!

But empathy is possible without actual comparable experience. All human beings have similar impulses, conflicts, and anxieties; and usually an inner awareness of the therapist's own human problems, combined with an ability to feel for and with others, provides an adequate basis for the necessary understanding of the experiences or feelings of the patient.

Parenthetically, the danger of excessive identification must be mentioned, as leading to too great an agreement with the patient's rationalizations, to too much sympathy with the patient's attempts to "blame" others, to too great participation in the patient's anxiety, to too little expectation of better adjustment, to too strong an attitude of permissiveness for the satisfaction of neurotic needs, to the loss of the independent leadership necessary for a good therapeutic relationship. But, with all its dangers, the process of identification is crucial in psychodynamic understanding and therapeutic progress. If it is handled correctly, it can lead to a type of immediate comprehension of the patient's problems that in many ways is superior to the intellectual variety of understanding. The insight gained through empathy is, of course, to be checked intellectually, with the added accumulation and correlation of pertinent evidence.

From the above comments on the empathic and intellectual processes in interviewing, it should be obvious that a question-and-answer type of interview is far less likely to produce valid and pertinent information than an interview in which spontaneity, free flow of thinking and feeling, relaxation, and undirected recounting of events and ideas and feelings are fostered.

Out of such intellectual and empathic processes the therapist comes to have an understanding of some of the forces at work in specific cases, to arrive at some of the elements of the dynamic diagnosis. For example, he might conclude that basic in some cases of prolonged convalescence is such a motivation as a desire for attention, for protection, or for control of the situation; that basic in some cases of constipation is the force of fear of a loss of security and possessions; and that in some cases of handwashing compulsion the basic force is guilt over masturbation and masturbation fantasies.

And through such intellectual and empathic processes the therapist comes to understand the interrelation between current situational or precipitating forces and the internal drives which are mobilized. For example, in one case he may conclude that a child's overeating and obesity are based on the child's attempt to compensate for his rejection by his mother. In another case the therapist may come to recognize that a certain patient's emotional upheaval is based on the fact that the marriage of his motherly older sister put an end to their usual relationship and mobilized in him intense ungratified needs for dependence and security.

The interrelation of understanding and therapy—the guiding concept of this chapter—is most evident in connection with the material of this section on dynamic diagnosis. The therapeutic work of the psychiatrist in any particular case is pre-eminently based on his dynamic diagnosis; and the chief purpose of supervised training in psychotherapy is to increase the student's ability to understand the dynamic problems of his patients and to base his therapy on dynamic understanding.

As a sample of the close dependence of psychotherapy on dynamic understanding, the following may be cited: The study of the psychodynamics of a number of patients with duodenal ulcer indicates that the ulcers are primarily the end-result of physiologic patterns set up by strong dependency needs which could never be expressed or satisfied because of the force of the patients' internal condemnation of their dependent wishes, a condemnation based on the narcissistic attitude that to be dependent is to be inferior, second-best, infantile, or feminine. In any specific patient whose patterns may approximate this formulation, psychotherapy must, first of all, be based on the decision that, qualitatively, these two forces—his dependency drives and his narcissistic drives—are actually the important ones in his personality problems. Further, the psychotherapy must be based on a quantitative estimate of the force of these drives. As one component of the therapy based on such evaluations, the patient must be given some satisfaction of his dependency needs. If they are not too great, the gratification provided by the therapeutic relationship may lead to a diminution of gastric symptoms. If his narcissism is very strong, however, the satisfaction of the dependency needs cannot be direct and open (until later in treatment) and must be presented as a medical necessity, e.g., the need for close nursing care, frequent feedings, and medication. If a workable therapeutic relationship is developed, incidental comments can then be made which indicate that even mature adults can have strong dependent wishes and legitimate dependent satisfactions, without considering themselves weak, and without hurt pride. Further, the patient can be given the living experience that in the relationship with the therapist he can have a moderately dependent role, without having the experience of being treated as second-best or inferior. In some cases more extensive "insight" into the interplay of dependency needs and pride may be given. From these comments, which indicate some of the possible therapeutic procedures, it is clear that in such a case psychotherapy must include specific attitudes, specific actions, and specific comments on the part of the therapist which are related directly to an understanding of the dynamic diagnosis. (The foregoing is by no means a complete statement of the psychotherapeutic possibilities in such cases; therapy may include responses to genetic factors as well, i.e., to the sources of the dependency and narcissism.)

A second example of the dependence of therapy on dynamic diagnosis: if a patient gives evidence of having a "hypertrophied" superego, of internal restrictions and prohibitions that are excessive and rigid and overly strict (e.g., if it is obvious that he can permit himself no pleasure without great guilt; that he must overwork to satisfy his conscience; that he cannot even have a hostile or sexual or imperfect thought), the therapist must respond with a permissive attitude and must attempt, by his attitude and comments, to indicate that normal adults may permit far more than the patient permits himself and that he can identify with someone who has a more tolerant attitude toward himself. Involved in this is the fact that in therapy the patient may come to see that he may have impulses toward the therapist of a sort which he previously had regarded as intolerable but which the therapist obviously now regards as unimportant. The end-result may be that the patient may come to be less self-critical and self-punitive and may eventually integrate some of the therapist's attitudes into his own superego.

If the therapist has come to understand that the patient's strictness toward himself was based on his fear that, without such excessive internal prohibitions, he might become uncontrolled and unlimited in his drives toward satisfaction, it is part of the therapist's function to indicate by attitude, comment, and living experience the fact that new and strong limits can be set which are healthier and more mature, in the therapeutic relationship and in life.

In another case the therapist may come to see that the patient has never developed adequate internal limiting forces—that, in contrast to the previously mentioned patients, this one has developed proficient techniques of bribing or cajoling or side-stepping his too permissive conscience. In such a situation the therapeutic responses may have to be much more in the direction of the setting of limits, of a clarification of the ways in which undue permissiveness toward one's self may actually block an intelligent self-interest, of providing a new parent-figure (the therapist) who combines realistic permissiveness with a realistic acceptance of limitations.

The dependence of therapy on dynamics is even more apparent when it is recognized that one of the general functions of psychotherapy (in many cases) consists in the giving of insight, the development of a conscious awareness and understanding of previously unrecognized trends, impulses, and fantasies. The therapist cannot use the technique of insight unless he previously has made a diagnosis of the existence of specific pathogenic forces, which he now will attempt to clarify.

Further, the dependence of therapy on dynamic diagnosis is shown in the fact that the therapist (in many cases) hopes to point out to the patient the differences between his distorted expectations in human relations, now clearly reflected in his attitudes toward the therapist (expectations based on his dynamic patterns and his unfortunate previous experiences or fantasies), and the actualities of his relationship with the therapist. Such a contrast, clearly explained by the therapist, may have great value in bringing home to the patient a real awareness of his patterns of distorted expectations in human relations, which may have played a role of high importance in his symptom formation and life-problems. The patient may thereby develop a profound conviction that human beings actually are far different from his expectations, and on that basis his own patterns and anxieties may diminish. This process has been called the "corrective emotional experience" (3). To be able to point out such a contrast between the patient's expectations and the realities of the therapist's attitude, the therapist must previously have come to a diagnostic understanding of the patient's relationship with others and the part which the patient's distortions played in disturbing those relationships.

A final example of the dependence of therapy on dynamic diagnosis is evident in the rational use of environmental manipulation. For example, if adequate study of the problems of an overly aggressive, "predelinquent" boy indicates that the neurotic pressures emanating from his parents are predominant, one essential therapeutic move may consist in the removal of the boy from his home environment.

The above discussion of the ways in which therapeutic maneuvers or responses are prescribed by the dynamics of the person or of the situation to be treated is focused on the correlation of specific psychotherapeutic responses with specific dynamic configurations. There is, however, a more fundamental issue which must be presented in this section on the interrelationship of dynamics and therapy.

This basic issue can be formulated in this way: that fundamental to all therapy is a sound "therapeutic attitude," to which various specific types of therapeutic activity may be added. Essentially, the sound therapeutic attitude is simply one of human decency and respect for other human beings, of helpfulness and understanding. Such an attitude sounds simple and easy to achieve and to maintain, but it is not. Patients often present a surface that is unpleasant and illogical and provocative, and the therapist often has immature tendencies of his own, ready to be called into action in a way that would be at variance with a therapeutic attitude.

The most effective way of achieving a persistent therapeutic attitude is by having extensive psychotherapeutic experience, under adequate supervision, with a stringent scrutiny and discussion of the student's deviations from a therapeutic attitude. Such supervision and self-scrutiny (and, in some instances, psychotherapy) offer a far-reaching stabilization of therapeutic attitude. No study of textbooks can substitute for such experience, and the following paragraphs are not intended as a substitute. Rather they are an attempt to clarify the basic meaning and purpose of a correct therapeutic attitude. To do this, some of the material on dynamic diagnosis given above can be reformulated and simplified. If one wants to have a label, the following paragraphs may be entitled the "three-layer approach" to dynamic understanding and psychotherapy.

The starting point for such an approach is the fairly well-established central fact that a large part of human problems may be understood in terms of the simple concept of anxiety and defenses against anxiety. (This excludes those difficulties which are the direct result of hereditary factors, e.g., some types of feeble-mindedness; or which are the direct result of brain damage, e.g., the memory defects in organic psychoses; or which are the direct result of intoxication, e.g., the disorientation in a bromide psychosis. But even in some of these conditions, basically not to be understood as defensive reactions against anxiety, the anxiety-defense concept is of value. In a bromide delirium, for example, the brain malfunction may lead to a loss of the usual activity of the forces of repression, and auditory hallucinations may appear, e.g., hallucinated voices which speak of the death of a relative toward whom the patient for some time had had obvious but repressed death wishes. With the breakdown of the usual defense of repression, anxiety appears, and a different defense is called into play in the emergency—the defense of projection, which permits the patient again to "disown" the hostility by having its content attributed to a source, a voice, outside himself.)

The concept of defenses against anxiety is a fundamentally simple one, as simple and as clarifying as the concept of homeostasis in the field of physiology. In fact, the defense-against-anxiety concept can be considered as an extension into the field of personality reactions of the physiologic principle of homeostasis. Essentially, the concept of homeostasis is that the organism must adapt not only to the environment in which it lives, to its external milieu, but also to an internal milieu, to the changes within itself. In this adaptation, patterns of response have been developed, some healthy and some not, to meet the changes in the internal milieu and to avoid the internal danger that would arise if the threatening forces, e.g., an excessive retention of water, were not stabilized or balanced or brought into equilibrium.

In the field of personality problems such a concept stresses the fact that there are internal as well as external personal dangers which threaten the organism. External dangers (fire, wild animals, robbers, etc.) produce the danger signal of fear, to which the individual responds with defenses, such as flight or fight or calling for the fire department or the police. Internal dangers (unacceptable impulses, severe pangs of conscience, etc.) produce a type of fear also, which usually goes by the term of "anxiety." Against such internal dangers, defenses are developed as well, defenses which appear as adequate adaptations, as psychiatric symptoms, as character traits, and as disturbed human relations.

Examples could be given that would cover an enormous part of the field of human psychology and psychiatry. A few will suffice to indicate the extraordinarily clarifying value of this concept which stems largely from Freud. A boy in the throes of a masturbation conflict, who believes that masturbation is making him into a weakling and that he will become psychotic or impotent, develops severe anxiety and responds to that anxiety with the defense of trying to show his great strength, of becoming aggressive and domineering, defiant, afraid of nothing, sneering, contemptuous, and bullying toward smaller children. A mother, unconsciously having antagonistic rejecting impulses toward her child, develops anxiety and becomes oversolicitous and overprotective and prevents the child from having those pleasures which entail average risks. A man has a coronary occlusion, develops anxiety of desperate intensity, and tries to protect himself against the anxiety by an emergency defense of using those techniques which in his childhood were effective in alleviating what seemed overwhelming anxiety, such techniques as feeling and behaving in a helpless fashion, making excessive demands, becoming whining and domineering. A patient developing a Korsakoff psychosis, unable to remember events of the immediate past, develops anxiety about disintegration, loss of ability to deal with life, loss of one of man's most prized functions, his memory; and then develops the second Korsakoff symptom, confabulation, which acts as an effective defense against his anxiety, by a total concealment, from himself, of his defective functioning. A child who has had repeated convulsions in school, who thereby has aroused anxiety in the other children which has led them to reject and stigmatize him, develops anxiety and then defends himself by the development of patterns which play a part in what at times is called the "epileptic personality": patterns of egocentricity (of self-aggrandizement, as a defense against this anxiety of feeling rejected), of suspiciousness (an exaggerated defensive alertness against the possibility of further slights or hurts), and of unpleasant aggressiveness (based on the attitude that attack is the best defense).

In some instances the anxiety is so great or the defensive capacity so diminished that the anxiety appears on the surface, either in acute anxiety attacks or in chronic psychologic or physiologic expressions of anxiety.

It is to be noted that in the above examples many of the defenses were unpleasant, e.g., demanding attitudes, suspiciousness, overprotectiveness, bullying. In the face of such defenses, a therapeutic attitude is not always easy to maintain.

The concept of defenses against anxiety can be formulated, schematically, as involving two layers—the outermost layer, the defenses; and an immediately subjacent layer, the anxiety. Here one must add that anxiety and defenses do not occur in a vacuum, that there is a third, a deeper, portion (or layer) of the personality, which, for simplicity, can be called the "basic layer." And to this must be added the fact that experience with human beings points strongly to the conclusion that the unpleasant aspects of their personalities inhere essentially in the first layer—the defenses—and that the third layer often includes many unexpected assets of warm humanity, of decency and worth-whileness. Psychiatric experience indicates that, fundamentally, human beings have many potentialities and positive qualities, when one looks beyond and beneath the defenses forced upon them by their anxiety.

Again a note of warning must be sounded about the possible misuse of such a schematic mode of phrasing. This "three-layer" formulation is intended again as shorthand, as a clear way of expressing some simple and vital relations of groups of forces and functions. It is not to be regarded in the same manner as a geographic or geologic description or an anatomic dissection. At times many sequences are involved, all of which could be called "layers." Some defenses lead to further anxiety and thus to further defenses. For example, the defense of becoming unaggressive and noncompetitive may lead to the anxiety of being beaten and hurt; this, in turn, may lead to a defensive urge to show strength by fighting; this, in turn, to anxiety; and this to a defense of being obsequious and sycophantish. The concept of three layers is one of the useful concepts in which the designation is far from exact; there often are many more layers than three, and actually there are no layers at all in the dictionary sense.

This three-layer concept of defenses against anxiety helps to clarify the problems of psychodynamics, but more important is the fact that it also clarifies the problem of therapeutic attitude and atmosphere. An adequate therapeutic attitude must be based on the needs of each of the three layers. The very existence of defenses, of anxiety, and of the basic layer of personality calls for a therapeutic attitude that has at least three facets.

The therapist must respond to the first layer—the defenses—with a nonjudgmental, noncondemning attitude, a feeling of human tolerance, and a conviction that they are merely defenses. He must have the feeling that the defenses, even though they are in part unpleasant or unacceptable, could not lead him to a rejection of the patient as a human being. Out of this must grow the recognition that an attitude of contempt or punishment is not only wrong therapeutically but also wrong in terms of fact and logic and that the response called for is a response to the total person, not just to his defenses. Fundamentally, the therapist must be guided by a full awareness of the fact that beneath the defenses are two other, more significant, layers. Perhaps this point may be underlined by such expressions as "a misbehaving child is almost always somehow a frightened child" (even the spoiled child, in large part, continues his self-centered behavior out of anxiety) and that "the irritating qualities of human beings are fundamentally the result of anxiety which the patient could not handle otherwise."

But such a tolerant, permissive, understanding attitude is not the only component in the therapeutic response to the defenses.

The tolerant attitude must be combined with a varying amount of firmness, of an expectation of better adjustment, and of setting limits to the acting-out of unacceptable defenses. A certain amount of such firmness must be pervasive in the therapeutic attitude generally, as it must be in the leadership attitude which all parents must have during the normal development of their children. And, in certain instances, firmness must be the dominant note in the therapist's attitude (although the understanding and fellow-feeling attitude must always persist strongly as well). Absolute firmness is necessary in the presence of great anxiety or of panic or when there is actual danger to the patient or to others; a depressed patient may be made to feel more guilty when tolerance and acceptance are accentuated and less guilty when strict firmness is emphasized; a dependent patient may need emphatic firmness as a prerequisite for a therapeutic relationship; a patient afraid of his own inability to control his unacceptable defenses may require great firmness as an essential aspect of the therapist's attitude.

Along with the above tolerance-and-firmness combination as the response to the layer of defenses, the therapist must respond to the layer of anxiety. Again his response must be generally the same, with individual variations in specific situations. In general, his response must be one of human friendship and warmth and reassurance, of providing a certain security and feeling of acceptance, which often acts as a force to lessen anxiety. The therapist must somehow put across to the patient the fact that he now provides a new potential source of strength. He must transmit to the patient the vital reassurance that an adult of some strength and experience will now try to help him solve some of the problems that have led to anxiety and that the therapist believes the patient to be capable of learning how to meet his conflicts and anxiety more adequately than before. When it is true, he must give the patient the feeling that the situation, external or internal, does not call for the amount of anxiety which he now has. Often the therapist, by his detachment and objectivity and by his emphasis on talking of hidden problems, creates in the patient a greater objectivity, with the feeling that the anxiety is not so threatening as it seemed to be. Still another factor in lessening the patient's anxiety is that the therapist does not join in the patient's anxiety, even when the patient has told him of a condition or situation which has evoked great anxiety in the patient himself.

In addition to such general security-giving aspects of the therapeutic attitude, the therapist tries in more specific ways, whenever he can, to lessen or undercut or eliminate the anxiety. If the therapist knows the nature of the specific anxiety which has led to the defenses, his reassurance can be more pointed, and he gives specific information or clarification or interpretation. If he knows that the aggressively hostile boy is defending himself against anxiety based on distorted ideas about the effects of masturbation, he can give emphatic reassurance. If he does not know the specific anxiety, a large part of his therapeutic work will consist of attempts to discover the dynamic conflicts which are operative in the anxiety (if such exploration is not contraindicated in the particular case); he then works directly to alleviate the anxiety by comments or explanations or attitudes which will change the dynamic picture. It is to be emphasized that in such a dynamic exploration and therapy there is implicit the fact that the therapist believes the individual patient to be strong enough to use the insight—a fact which in itself tends to alleviate anxiety. In summary, the therapeutic attitude toward the second layer—the anxiety—consists of offering a certain general security and affection and help and reassurance, and a specific reassurance when specific anxieties are evident or uncovered.

Along with the response to the "upper" two layers, the therapist must have a healthy positive attitude toward the third layer—the basic personality. This is not difficult with patients whose anxiety and defenses have not prevented the obvious development of many trends toward maturity and strength and achievement. But, even with other, less fortunate patients, he must somehow sense, with conviction, that, underneath the defenses and the anxiety which are so disturbing to the patients or to others, there exist important aspects of the personality which are worthy of respect. The therapist must know that with many of his most neurotic patients he is dealing with persons who fundamentally are likable and worth while and who have potentialities for self-development which have been blocked by unfortunate external or internal forces. With some of his patients, in whom he finds layer after layer of defensive distortions, he must know that beneath all these distortions is the inborn capacity for healthy development. He must have a genuine regard for his patients as human beings and know that they are, or could be, worthy of warmth, of respect, and of acceptance. If the therapist has such a conviction of his patients' fundamental acceptability, the patients will know it, even though it remains unspoken. And it is probable that no psychotherapy of lasting value can be done unless the therapeutic atmosphere includes such a response to the basic personality.

In connection with the above material about the three-layer concept as it relates to therapeutic attitude, the following should be added: Mistakes in psychotherapy are often based on an overemphasis on one or another of the three layers. An overemphasis on the anxiety layer may lead the therapist to have too sympathetic and permissive an attitude, which can have a noxious, rather than a therapeutic, effect. A strongly permissive attitude should be the result of the fact that the patient requires such an attitude for therapeutic reasons (e.g., because his parents were too punitive and prohibiting); a strongly permissive attitude should not be the result of the therapist's being too impressed by the patient's anxiety. Further, an overemphasis on the layer of defenses may lead to an underestimation of the need to respond to the other two layers as well, so that the therapist's approach becomes superficial and often punishing or rejecting or controlling. The essential point is that the therapeutic attitude must include responses to all three layers of the patient's personality and that the modifications in therapeutic emphasis must be based on the dynamics of the problem at hand, not on an inadequate orientation to the general problem of therapy or on the countertransference problems of the therapist.

## C. Genetic Diagnosis

Whenever possible, psychiatric therapy should be based not only on clinical and dynamic diagnoses but also on genetic diagnosis. This last term refers to an understanding of the origin and development of the patient's personality and current conflicts and to an appraisal of the situations, experiences, and reactions which led to the development of the current dynamic constellation.

A passing comment on terminology must be made. Students trained in biology occasionally infer that the term "genetic diagnosis" connotes heredity or constitution, since in biology the term "genetic" is the adjective referring to the genes and chromosomes. In psychiatry the term "genetic diagnosis" refers to the totality of those forces involved in the genesis and origin of

current forces; such genetic forces are hereditary or constitutional in small part but are predominantly a matter of early
life-experience and individual reactions.

As typical examples of the genetic factors which are to be
considered in individual cases seen in psychotherapy, the following can be cited: prolonged contact of the patient as a child with
an adult whose personality or behavior provided material for
unhealthy identification; cruelty, deprivation, overindulgence,
overstimulation, excessive gratification, intimidation, or inconsistency, in infancy; problems of weaning and toilet training;
problems of infantile sexuality; development of attitudes of fear
and envy and feelings of inadequacy in connection with sexuality
(e.g., the little girl's envy of the penis and the little boy's anxiety
about castration); a pervasive disturbing atmosphere in childhood (e.g., emanating from a sadistic father) which was productive of early anxiety; specific traumatic experiences, e.g., a circumcision for which the child was not prepared, at a time when
he expected drastic punishment for his activity or wishes; only-
child or oldest-child or youngest-child or middle-child experiences. These and a host of other life-experiences which, occurring with undue intensity or at a vulnerable period in the life of
the child or in a particular sequence or configuration, may have
led to the development of the unhealthy aspects of the child's
personality, to those forces which currently are operative in producing the patient's disorder.

The genetic factors leading to strength (such as identification
with an emotionally healthy older sibling) must also be included
in the evaluation, since the sources of relative maturity provide
therapeutic leads, as do the sources of unhealthy development.

It must be stressed that genetic diagnosis must include an
understanding not only of the environmental forces which im-
pinged on the patient earlier in life, for better or for worse, but
also the patient's reactions to those forces, his impulse stirrings,
his anxiety, his defenses, and his fantasy distortions of the environment, either at the time or in retrospect.

To illustrate the content of a genetic diagnosis, the group of
patients with peptic ulcer referred to above may be considered
again. The predominant elements in the dynamic diagnosis were
their strong unconscious dependent trends and their narcissistic
rejection of dependency as weakness. The genetic diagnosis
would then be the statement of the origin of both the dependen-

cy pattern and the excessively high standards. For example, the genetic diagnosis might include the fact that in childhood such a patient was seriously unwanted, unloved, and rejected, leading, on the one hand, to a lifelong hunger for love and protective care, i.e., for dependent satisfactions, and, on the other hand, to the attitude that never again will he permit himself to be in a position of weak dependency when he might be hurt or humiliated. Or in another case the dependent attitude might have had its origin as a regression, as a flight from the fears connected with genital sexuality, and the excessive rejection of dependent roles might be based on a fantasy of the bodily dangers related to passive dependent homosexual impulses.

Therapeutic decisions and procedures are, in various ways, based on an understanding of such genetic factors. If dependency trends and excessively high standards have their genesis in the childhood experience of serious rejection, the therapist must know that the therapy will involve a long period of the patient's testing him out to see if the therapist will reject him. He will know that he must have unending patience and acceptance and must refuse to be provoked into a rejecting attitude. But he must set realistic limits (e.g., not permit the patient to phone him at all hours), even though the patient may construe the setting of limits as a rejection. If such limits are not set, the patient may develop a too dependent attitude. And, more important, if such realistic limits are not in force, the patient may fail to have the necessary living experience that there can be patterns of adjustment other than his usual dichotomy of either being totally dependent or being rejected.

In the above example it is apparent that the genetic diagnosis determines some of the therapist's attitudes and behavior. If, in addition, insight therapy along genetic lines is to be used, it is obvious that the interpretive comments made to the patient must be based on an understanding of the genetic diagnosis.

One essential aspect of genetic diagnosis in relation to therapy is the attempt to establish the relative importance of fixation and of regression. In an impotent man it is of importance to know whether his impotence is essentially based on regressive patterns— i.e., is based on childhood experiences and reactions which led him to have and to retain a fear of masculine sexuality and its supposed dangers—and whether such experiences then led him to regress to the attitude of wanting to be a protected baby instead of a man. In such a case the impotence then would have at least two sources: his fear of sexual activity itself (and what it symbolizes) and, second, his fear that sexual activity, as a sign of being a man, would jeopardize his hoped-for role of being a protected baby. In another patient the impotence may be much more a product of fixation. Then the impotence would not be related to childhood experiences that led to fear of masculine sexuality or to a regression to the role of being protected but, instead, would be based primarily on experiences that led to fixation at a level before the development of strong masculine impulses or fantasies. Overindulgence or its opposite, severe rejection, in the first two years of life is an example of the type of experience which can lead to an enormous accentuation of the need passively to be loved, to be protected, to be treated as a baby. In such a case the later impotence would not be the expression of a fear of masculinity or of the loss of the dependent position assumed in flight but fundamentally would be the direct continuation of a very early pattern, that nothing must be allowed to jeopardize the possibility of receiving a baby's type of love. There the impotence would be the result of a fixation on oral dependency, and masculine potency is to be avoided as representing maturity, responsibility, and a giving attitude, which would be at variance with the lifelong orientation toward passivity. Further, such an oral fixation may lead to marked feelings of inadequacy and inferiority, since the patient comes to feel weak and childlike. In the face of adult situations to be met, the patient may feel totally inadequate and afraid, emotions which, in turn, can interfere with his masculine performance. (Again, a warning against regarding such a teaching formulation as complete, e.g., most patients with impotence also have serious problems in the area of hostile aggressiveness.)

The pertinence to therapy of genetic formulations which include the problem of "regression versus fixation" can be phrased in this way (and usually it is not an "either-or" decision but one of relative emphasis): If the emphasis, genetically, is on regression, it must be recognized that the patient had previously made some strong developmental thrusts toward maturity, which may be repeated in the treatment with greater chance of success, and hence the prognosis is better. Often, if the emphasis is on regression, the patient has greater ego strength, is more able to make use of the therapist's help and more able to go along with a more rapid therapy. If the emphasis is on regression from anxiety about something (e.g., masculine sexuality) which is fundamentally acceptable to the adult ego, the efforts of the therapist receive assistance from the adult strivings of the patient and from the added increment of pleasure which the patient knows improvement will bring. If the emphasis is on fixation, however, the therapist is in a sense asking the patient to give up a pleasure, or a hoped-for pleasure (dependency), around which his whole life has been oriented and to substitute for it a pleasure toward which he has developed little or no drive, which is for him rather hypothetical. More directly, the implications for therapy in this problem are these: Emphasis on regression permits more active therapy, emphasis on fixation calls for slower, more cautiously dosed attempts at therapy. Emphasis on regression permits a greater implication of the need to face and conquer anxiety and a greater chance that, in the setting of the therapeutic situation, life can be met more directly and effectively, and successful life-experiences can add their curative value. Emphasis on fixation calls for the expectation of a much more protracted therapy (if it can be done at all), in which a prolonged process of gradual identification with the therapist may be the most effective tool of modification. In addition, in the patients in whom fixation is more important than regression the therapist must concentrate his attention, his attitudes, and his comments on the pregenital problems, in the hope that through the patient-physician experience and through insight some resolution of the fixation may take place; in the patients in whom regression is more important the therapist may concentrate his attention on the patient's hidden anxiety about masculinity and maturity, anxiety toward the therapist, toward current situations in the patient's life, and toward the important figures of his childhood.

Another aspect of the relevance of genetic understanding to therapy: If the therapist becomes convinced that the patient's childhood was permanently and basically disfiguring to his personality, he may decide that little can be done and that he must limit his therapy to superficial techniques, such as environmental manipulation or some supportive contact. Even in such superficial psychotherapy, genetic understanding is of value; if the therapist recognizes that the patient, in childhood, had a good relationship only with an elderly aunt, he may try to arrange for a therapeutic contact with a social case worker who is older than the patient.

The last statement—on the choice of a woman therapist—deserves some amplification, since the whole problem of the choice of a therapist offers a good example of the use of genetic data in therapeutic work. If, for example, it is clear that in childhood a man patient had an extremely conflictful relation with his father and other men figures but fairly good relations with his mother and sisters, it probably would be best to arrange for a woman therapist; otherwise, the transference distortions with a man therapist may be too great to permit perspective and the growth of insight. If the patient then matures in therapy, a period of therapeutic work with a man therapist may be advisable. On the other hand, the opposite decision as to male or female therapist may be made in another case if the childhood conflict was not quite so intense and the patient is more mature and evinces greater strength. If, for example, a male patient, with a relatively strong adjustment capacity, had a childhood characterized by slight problems with his mother and moderate problems with his father, the decision might well be to have him treated from the beginning by a male therapist. Usually such a patient will not develop too great distortions in his transference attitudes. Further, it will be of high value in the therapy to have him confronted with the need for an adjustment with a new father-figure, to have his problems with fathers mobilized by the situation, to have the corrective emotional experience of a good relationship with a father-figure, and (if insight therapy is used) to develop insight into his own problems in relation to authoritative male figures.

The above type of application of genetic understanding to therapeutic work has its greatest sphere of usefulness in psychoanalytic therapy. But it is applicable in less deep-going contacts. A man internist may decide to treat a patient himself or refer the patient to a woman internist or psychiatric case worker (granting that all are qualified for the type of therapy they are attempting) on the basis of genetic considerations such as those given above.

## D. Transference

It will be apparent that a good part of the material of the following two sections (on transference and countertransference) could logically be included as part of the preceding sections. But an emphasis on transference and countertransference is so vital to the student's orientation and understanding and so important in work with individual patients that it seems best to present them as independent topics.

Until the development of psychoanalytic therapy by Freud, little attention was paid to the physician-patient relationship, other than to make use of the passive dependent attitudes of patients for the purpose of authoritarian orders or suggestions. Other attitudes of patients were taken personally and were regarded as lack of co-operation, as stubbornness, as disturbing attachments, as situations to escape, or as adulation which was pleasing to the physician's pride and competitive strivings. Fortunately, Freud's use of the technique of relaxed free association and his close attention to the nuances of meaning of the patients' talk and attitudes and behavior led him to see the essential importance of the patient-physician relationship, which now plays a crucial role in dynamic psychotherapy.

Freud saw that patients often reacted to the therapist in many ways that were not logical or appropriate to the actual situation of patient and doctor. With no provocation on the part of the physician, patients may develop fear, hostility, suspicion, resentment, defiance, undue dependence, excessive compliance, love, idolatry, contempt, etc. For these spontaneous, excessive, illogical, and inappropriate reactions he suggested the term "transference," to indicate that the dynamic meaning of such responses was that the patient was reacting to the therapist not in terms of reality but in terms of transferring to the therapist feelings and reactions which he had had to other important figures in his life, particularly his parents.

The term "transference" actually has a somewhat broader meaning than is indicated by the concept of "transferring" from one to another. It refers to all the patient's illogical reactions to the therapist, including his stereotyped and patterned responses applied when they are not appropriate, his various automatically applied defenses, his attempts to satisfy ungratified wishes, and his projection of his own conscience attitudes.

Such transference reactions exist alongside the more appropriate reactions to the physician, of a realistic acceptance of him as someone who is trying to help and to cure, as an experienced, trained person in whom the patient can have a reasonable trust and confidence.

In psychotherapy, the attitudes of the patient to the therapist must be of profound importance, since psychotherapy consists largely of the transmission from patient to therapist and from therapist to patient of words, of attitudes, of interpersonal contacts. The tools of interpersonal communication (and so of psychotherapy) are language, intonation, gestures, facial expressions, and behavior. Such communication between therapist and patient is dependent on the development of a workable relationship. The transference distortions of the patient may seriously interfere with such communication and therefore with the therapeutic process. Consequently, one of the basic problems of some aspects of psychotherapy is to by-pass or to minimize or to eliminate the transference distortions.

In other aspects of psychotherapy, however, the therapist, instead of trying to by-pass the transference problems, puts them in the foreground as the focus of therapy. The rationale of such a procedure can be phrased in this fashion: Emotional problems are largely based on interpersonal difficulties and frequently are expressed as interpersonal difficulties. Consequently, it is of value to have such problems under direct observation in a controlled interpersonal situation. The contact of therapist and patient offers, in a sense, a laboratory setting of a standardized procedure. If the therapist's reactions are not distorted, the distortions which arise may clearly be understood as originating from the patient. His reactions then become significant samples of his behavior and motivation, and the therapy can work directly with the transference manifestations as a reliable sampling of the patient's personality problems. The hope then is that modification of the patient's patterns in this significant situation will lead to a modification of patterns in other aspects of his life-adjustment.

From this it is clear that transference attitudes must be of great pertinence to therapy. In documenting this pertinence, one simple but fundamental point should first be made, viz., that good therapy must be based on a knowledge of the inevitability of transference manifestations. A good therapeutic attitude cannot be based on the naïve assumption that all patients will be logically co-operative, eminently reasonable, properly grateful, and so considerate that they will have illogical reactions to others but not to the therapist. If the therapist expects transference problems, he is not shocked or surprised or taken in when they appear, and he may then preserve a good therapeutic relationship. For example, if a therapist has done a good job and yet the patient becomes openly hostile and critical toward him, the therapist can recognize such a reaction as transference and deal with it objectively, without regarding the patient as an ungrateful wretch. He can avoid being angry and can thus prevent a situation in which his own resentment would block his usefulness to the patient. Or, for example, if a patient is high in his praise of the therapist and regards him as the embodiment of perfection, the therapist must avoid the temptation to be flattered and must recognize the patient's attitude as a transference distortion.

In a variety of ways specific therapeutic decisions and responses should be based on observation of the transference. In the exploratory period the transference reactions of the patient give important clues in the three categories of diagnostic thinking listed above, and so are helpful in determining the type of therapy to be used. For example, an atmosphere of coldness, of withdrawn separateness, in the attitude of the patient to the therapist may help in the making of a clinical diagnosis of schizophrenia, with the therapeutic implications of that diagnosis. If, in the introductory interviews, a depressed patient is unable to make a workable positive contact with the physician and has a transference attitude of exclusion and impenetrable self-absorption, the advisability of shock therapy concomitant with, or followed by, psychotherapy is suggested; if a depressed patient turns more rationally for help or has a transference attitude of seeking dependence and forgiveness, the possibility of further attempts at psychotherapy is suggested.

With regard to dynamic diagnosis, the transference attitudes are even more important and significant for therapy. Transference attitudes often are indicative of the patient's predominant trends, the defenses and current forces at work which are the most important to deal with in treatment. Often a patient presents a psychodynamic picture that is complicated and even chaotic; he may show, in his life-patterns and relations, various problems of dependence, aggression, sexuality, narcissism, guilt, and a variety of defenses, all apparently of significance. A rather reliable guide in estimating the immediate importance of a trend is the transference; if narcissistic attitudes toward the therapist appear with some frequency or intensity, he can be certain that such attitudes are a vital part of the current dynamic problems of the patient. As a corollary, in therapy it may be difficult to decide where "the abscess is pointing," where therapeutic work is most promising, if one relies solely on dynamic study of the patient's reactions in life. In such a case it may be extremely helpful to center the therapy about those problems which appear in the transference.

Another angle of the value of transference manifestations in dynamic diagnosis should be mentioned. If the dynamic diagnosis is based on data about the patient's relations with his family and friends, the diagnosis may at times be uncertain. The relatives or friends often have their own distortions. It may be difficult to decide whether the patient's reaction is distorted and, if so, to what degree. For example, if a woman complains repeatedly of mistreatment by her husband, one may conclude, on the basis of what she says and how she says it and on the basis of similar attitudes in the past, that she is masochistic and is exaggerating the mistreatment by her husband, or perhaps provoking it. But in some cases the conclusion will still be under question. If, then, she attempts to provoke the therapist or if she interprets his objectivity as coldness and his comments as attempts to hurt her and insult her, the doubt of the dynamic diagnosis disappears completely. In such fashion, diagnostic thinking becomes certain, and therapy more soundly based. The therapist then knows that he must avoid being provoked and must maintain a steady, firm leadership. Still further, if insight therapy is to be used, he then will have incontrovertible data for interpretation. If he were able to interpret her masochism only by referring to her relations with her husband, she might be unconvinced, saying that the therapist would agree with her if he knew her husband. If, however, he can interpret her masochism on the basis of her attitudes toward himself, he can be much more convincing.

With regard to genetic diagnosis, the transference manifestations are of high value and again give leads for treatment. If a patient regards the therapist as a father-figure and constantly seems to expect rejection, the conjecture is called for that the patient was rejected by his father, or felt rejected by his father, or had impulses toward the father (and now toward the therapist) which made him feel, out of guilt or anxiety, that he should be rejected by his father.

In such fashion, transference manifestations contribute to diagnostic decisions, clinical, dynamic, and genetic, which have therapeutic pertinence of the type described in previous portions of this chapter.

To illustrate the value of transference manifestations in dynamic understanding and therapy, a portion of the treatment of a specific case of essential hypertension can be given. In some such cases the clue to the understanding of the chronic elevation of blood pressure may be found in the transference. The patient in question was one whose life, as far as could be seen, was free of emotional conflict and problems. So far as he and his family could tell, he got along well with everyone, was liked by everyone, let nothing disturb his equilibrium. At first glance, there was nothing to suggest that there were emotional tensions in his life that might be causing a high tension in his blood pressure. In his relation with the psychiatrist he was cordial and agreeable, and it soon was obvious that he was much too amiable, too agreeable, too pleasant, too submissive. Shakespeare, long before Freud, might have said, "methinks the gentleman doth protest too much." Shakespeare, like Freud, would have been benevolently skeptical about this patient's degree of amiability and imperturbable docility. If the telephone bell interrupted an interview, he would be obviously tense and flushed, as if in anger; but he denied being angry and said that the interruptions were of no consequence, that the psychiatrist was a very busy man who must take his calls, and that he, the patient, did not mind it in the least. From many sequences such as this in his behavior with the psychiatrist, the inference became highly probable that beneath his calm exterior there existed intense reactions of anger, which are known to be associated with a rise of blood pressure. This dynamic diagnosis of an underlying unexpressed hostility was verified when, during treatment, he repeatedly had dreams of obvious hostility, such as shooting an enormous fountain-pen-full of muddy black ink over the face of a man he did not recognize, who had a small mustache, who was partly bald, who wore steel-rimmed glasses, and whose business seemed to consist of trying to look through a skull with X-ray eyes. The patient did not recognize his victim in the dream, but from the description it was obvious that it was the therapist, whose work as a psychiatrist might be lampooned as an attempt to look into heads with X-ray eyes. In essence, a study of the patient's transference revealed the dynamic picture of a façade of excessive amiability concealing intense unexpressed hostility, which may have been associated with his hypertension.

Such dynamic understanding, of which the transference data

are an essential part, has clear-cut implications for therapy. In such a case the therapist must not be too appreciative of the patient's considerateness and amiability and docility. He will know that the patient will agree with any interpretation that the therapist makes, in order to be agreeable and friendly, even if he is unconvinced or if he disagrees. The therapist must know that hostility which is so denied and so concealed by totally opposite behavior must provoke serious anxiety in the patient and, consequently, that "bull-in-the-china-shop" early interpretations must be avoided. The therapist must work for the creation and development of a relationship in which the patient will feel safe enough to have some hostility, to express it slightly, and eventually to recognize and not be concerned about the fact that he has certain hostile tendencies. Then, if genetic material is to be worked through in a psychoanalysis, the patient can eventually come to understand and to modify some of the sources of his excessive hostility or of his superego strictness which would not countenance even a trace of hostility.

Another point to indicate the importance of transference in therapeutic procedures is this: By emphasizing transference problems, the therapist is dealing with actual current living experiences which are vividly meaningful to the patient, and the therapy may have an immediacy and aliveness that otherwise may be difficult to achieve. Interpretation of past events and reactions often has a distant and unconvincing quality that may disappear completely when they are seen from a fresh point of view, arising out of an understanding of the immediate living relationship with the therapist.

Further, in psychotherapy a lessening of transference problems may clear the way for acceptance of insight along other lines; if the patient has an unresolved attitude of being mistreated by the therapist, it will be difficult for him to accept as helpful any comments made by the therapist about the other aspects of his life-adjustment. Consequently, in psychotherapy with some patients (particularly those who are likely to develop negative transference attitudes) a clarification of transference distortions becomes the first essential of the therapy.

Another item: for various reasons, the patient often resists the efforts of the therapist to help him. The whole problem of such "resistance" in psychotherapy often can best be handled through the transference, since many types of resistance tend to focus on the relationship between patient and therapist. The resistance based on anxiety over becoming aware of unconscious trends, the resistance based on the urge to avoid the narcissistic blows of having to admit mistakes or of being helped by someone else, the resistance based on fear of being dominated by another person, the resistance based on the urge not to give up infantile pleasures, all lead to defenses directed toward the therapist and can best be dealt with by attention to transference problems.

In essence, then, treatment which is based on adequate understanding of transference manifestations has many advantages: clinical, dynamic, and genetic diagnoses are made more clear and reliable; leads become apparent for the focusing of attempts at therapy; and insight and corrective emotional experiences are made far more productive.

### E. Countertransference

It seems probable, although there is no statistical evidence to support the conclusion, that countertransference accounts for a large percentage of mistakes and failures in psychiatric treatment. For example, shock treatment may be used inappropriately because the psychiatrist is unwilling to use more time-consuming methods or because he is unduly aggressive or because he is unable to withstand the family's urging that he do something drastic immediately. Another example: Psychotherapy, in a modifiable patient, may fail because the therapist is unable to resist being hostile and rejecting when the patient is provocative. Consequently, it is urgent that all therapists have a vivid understanding of countertransference problems and of their implication for therapy.

In the previous section, the debt of psychiatry to Freud for the concept of transference was indicated. But Freud did not stop with the understanding of the transference. He realized that all human relations are two-way streets, that the patient is not the only fallible human being in the interaction of patient and physician. In fact, in all of the contacts of two human beings, it must be recognized that both may be responding illogically as well as logically. When a husband complains that his wife is behaving irrationally toward him, the psychiatrist who hears the story must wonder if the husband also does not behave irrationally

toward his wife and perhaps provoke some of her illogical behavior. When a mother complains that her child reacts with defiance and antagonism to her, the psychiatrist must wonder if the
mother also is not reacting illogically to the child. And so Freud
put the question, What of the medical two-way street, what of
the physician's reactions to the patient? And, observing himself,
with his customary courage and honesty, Freud discovered certain
tendencies in himself that were inappropriate and tended to interfere with his successful work with patients. Subsequently, he
made the same observation in supervising the work of the physicians he was training in the use of his new techniques. For this
phenomenon—the distorted reactions of physicians to patients—
Freud suggested the technical term of "countertransference."

Some examples, taken from the general practice of medicine,
can be given to indicate typical mistakes based on countertransference. A physician who is too sympathetic with sick people
may pamper his patients, may make them realize too vividly that
sickness has its pleasures, and so prolong his patients' convalescence. On the other hand, a physician who is overdemanding
that his patients be strong and mature and self-reliant may do
injury by holding up to his patients an impossible ideal. Patients
of such a physician may become excessively critical of their own
human limitations, may ignore their actual need for rest, for leisure, and for recuperation, and may struggle too strenuously to
be as strong as the physician expects them to be.

Every physician must resist the importunities of some of his
patients for more and more medicine. If the physician has the
personality characteristic of being unable to say "No," of being
too amiable and agreeable, he is very likely to give too much
medicine to demanding patients or to patients who play on his
sympathy. And, of course, the excessive use of medicine has its
dangers, of drug addiction or of undue dependence on medicine
or of some accumulated physical effects of the medicine itself.

Another type of mistake is based on what can be called excessive therapeutic ambition. All physicians must have some therapeutic ambition, must want to help their patients, must try in
part to build their security and prestige by being successful, by
curing their patients as quickly as possible. Such therapeutic ambition is of real value to the doctor and to the patient. But therapeutic ambition may be excessive and defeat its own ends. If the

physician is very insecure and has too great a need for fame and fortune, he may then have too great a need for cured cases, for the kind of case he can boast about or expect others to boast about for him. He may then become impatient with those who do not respond or may, in an open or concealed fashion, be angry and resentful toward them. Some medical problems are complicated and difficult to solve, requiring patient consideration of a number of diagnostic possibilities and the use of one after another of therapeutic attempts until the problem is solved. The emotions of anger and resentment that arise in the doctor when excessive therapeutic ambition is thwarted are not conducive to clear thinking or to the gradual working-through of a difficult medical problem. Furthermore, a patient may sense the physician's impatience and resentment and become anxious or resentful or self-critical, so that a secondary neurotic problem is superimposed on the primary problem, which is still unsolved.

Another example of countertransference has to do with the unnecessary stimulation of anxiety in patients by a physician who likes to be totally safe in his diagnoses, who has an excessive fear that some other physician who may later examine the patient will find something that the first physician has missed. In moderate degree such concern for one's reputation is valid and appropriate and one of the safeguards of medical practice, tending to assure adequate and careful examinations. But, like all good things, such concern can be overdone. The physician who is excessively afraid of the opinions of others may try to protect himself by avoiding definite diagnoses, may try to straddle the fence so that, no matter what happens later, he cannot be said to have missed a point. If such a physician examines a patient who thinks he may have heart disease, does a thorough job plus whatever special examinations are called for, and finds absolutely nothing except an almost surely functional murmur, the physician may then be unable to give the necessary reassurance. He may damage the patient and help to produce a cardiac neurosis by remarking that the examination is essentially negative but that there is a little murmur that might be watched or that the patient's heart is in fine shape but that it might be better not to take quite so much exercise as before. Such excessively conservative statements produce anxiety which is totally unnecessary. They may protect the physician from criticism in an occasional case, but at the expense of the well-being of some of his patients.

The above examples were chosen from the general practice of medicine, to indicate that countertransference is a problem not only of psychiatry but of all attempts at human helpfulness.

The specific countertransference mistakes indicated in these examples, e.g., excessive therapeutic ambition, are, of course, problems of psychiatric therapy as well. In fact, countertransference problems are more frequent in psychiatry than in general medical practice, in part because psychotherapy makes greater use of the patient-physician relationship and in part because the psychiatric atmosphere is to some degree permissive and the patient is more likely to express feelings or attitudes that may stir counterreactions on the part of the psychiatrist. Further, countertransference problems are important in psychiatry because the psychiatrist so frequently tries to modify the patient's adjustment, an attempt that often arouses resistive defenses on the part of the patient, which, in turn, may lead to inappropriate responses on the part of the psychiatrist. If the patient uses the defense against the treatment of appealing for sympathy, the psychiatrist may become too sympathetic or may have an attitude of contempt for one who seeks sympathy. If the patient defends himself against change or against unpleasant insight by attacking the psychiatrist as a threat, the psychiatrist, in turn, may counterattack or become frightened and appeasing. Another patient may defend himself against the arousal of guilt feelings by the time-honored technique of feeling less guilty if one can make someone else feel guilty. In such a defense he may try to make the psychiatrist feel guilty over having done something, over not having done something, or over not having achieved a cure. The psychiatrist, even though he has done his best, may easily make the mistake of feeling guilty. Obviously, such countertransference reactions may give the patient momentary satisfaction, but they have no therapeutic value and may delay the patient's recovery.

In psychiatric practice, countertransference reactions may appear even when they are not mobilized by specific reactions on the part of the patient, as in the above examples. A therapist may be afraid of older women and so with older women patients may have an attitude of anxiety or of defensive aloofness or of aggressive domination. Or a man therapist may have excessive competitive attitudes toward men of his own age, and with such patients may have a need to show that he is brighter, quicker, more successful, and better adjusted. In such circumstances he unconsciously may be averse to having the patient improve and thereby become a stronger potential competitor. Or the therapist may have a lifelong defense of his own of overintellectualization, and so his contact with patients becomes a sterile intellectual game instead of an interpersonal process that includes feeling tones, warm human contact, and understanding empathy.

Countertransference problems may lead psychiatrists to an incorrect evaluation of their patients' conflicts. One psychiatrist may be unable to see some of the important problems of his patients because they are problems which he does not want to see in himself. His defense is trying to ignore the existence of such problems altogether, and so he cannot see them in his patients even when they are of central importance. Another psychiatrist may see too much instead of too little, may believe that some of his patients have certain conflicts which actually are not present or are of little consequence. His mistake is based on a defense which is different from that used by the other psychiatrist. He attempts to alleviate his anxiety over some conflict of his own by imputing that conflict to others in an even greater degree, so that his own seems unimportant by comparison. With such a defense, he may come to believe that some insignificant problems of his patients are of high importance in their psychodynamic picture.

The implications of the countertransference for therapy need hardly be detailed, since they are obvious, once the problem is stated. Some of the implications are these: The therapist need not be shocked if he has countertransference problems, since they are universal; but he must not permit himself to act out his tendencies to the detriment of the patient. If his distorted reactions are mild and under control, he need not be concerned about them. If they are intense or out of control, he needs psychotherapy for himself. If he finds that he has difficulty with one type of patient, he should refer such patients to other therapists until he has lessened his own problem.

In general, the safeguards against the interference of countertransference with therapy consist of intensive supervision over an adequate period of time with an adequate variety of patients, stringently honest self-scrutiny, and psychotherapy of the therapist.

It is apparent, then, that treatment in psychiatry has a much greater chance of success if the countertransference is minimal and undisturbing. In such circumstance, mistakes in diagnosis and therapy can be lessened, the transference reactions are more significant and more reliable tools of treatment, the patient has a far greater chance to correct his mistaken expectations in interpersonal relations, and the therapist's responses and comments are far more likely to be suited to the actual needs of the therapy.

## F. Treatment Possibilities

The treatment of an individual patient is dependent on the points of understanding outlined in the preceding five sections. In addition, the following must be taken into consideration in reaching decisions about therapy: (1) the specific techniques of treatment which may be suitable; (2) the training and skill of the therapist in the use of specific techniques; and (3) the practical aspects of treatment. The remainder of this chapter will consist of an elaboration of these points.

### 1. TECHNIQUES OF PSYCHIATRIC TREATMENT

The following groups of therapeutic procedures for the amelioration or cure of psychiatric difficulties may be listed:

*a*) Procedures intended essentially for the protection, safety, and general care of the patient, his family, and society. They include hospitalization (at times commitment) of seriously disturbed patients; prevention of aggressive acting-out (suicide, antisocial behavior); custodial care of those unable to care for themselves, e.g., the feeble-minded; specific procedures of general care, e.g., feeding of patients who refuse to eat, hydrotherapy in states of excitement. In the use of such procedures, their psychotherapeutic implications must be considered as well as their more obvious purposes. For example, hospitalization may provide a valuable temporary satisfaction of dependent needs but, like all such satisfactions, runs the risk of stimulating regressive tendencies. Another example: Individuals who are near panic because of their anxiety that some unacceptable unconscious impulses may break through may find the restrictions of hospital life a welcome auxiliary source of control.

*b*) Procedures aimed at a correction of structural pathologic processes, e.g., surgical removal of a brain tumor or evacuation of a subdural hematoma.

*c*) Procedures aimed at a correction of pathophysiologic processes, e.g., medicinal and other treatment of delirium tremens and bromide delirium; medicinal and fever treatment of paresis; thyroid medication in cretinism.

*d*) Medicinal or surgical treatment to ameliorate some of the physiologic concomitants of emotion, e.g., the limited use of sedatives and antispasmodics in anxiety-tension states; the use of stimulants in certain depressive states; the use of hypnotics when insomnia is troublesome; vagotomy in some cases of peptic ulcer. In such circumstance, when the problem is essentially psychogenic, it is often wise to be direct with the patient about the role of the medicinal treatment and to state clearly to him that the medicine is not intended to be a cure but rather to give symptomatic relief and that some variety of more direct dealing with his personality problems is in order.

*e*) The use in selected cases of such physical methods of therapy as electric shock treatment and insulin coma (see also chap. x). A variety of modifications and combinations of physical methods of therapy have been developed in recent years, and the student is referred to the pertinent literature for a statement of techniques and procedures (5, 23, 24, 41). The chief current procedures are those of electro-convulsive therapy and insulin coma therapy, in which patients are in the one instance subjected to an electric current through the brain substance, with the production of a convulsion, and in the other are given enough insulin to produce a response of several hours of hypoglycemic coma. The electro-convulsive procedure is usually repeated some five to fifteen times over a period of several weeks. The insulin coma procedure is usually repeated some twenty to sixty times over a period of several months. Electro-convulsive therapy seems to have its greatest sphere of usefulness in severe depressions which usually are labeled "manic-depressive" and "involutional melancholia," and in many instances when psychotherapy is unpromising it is the treatment of choice. It may be of value in certain other cases, in bringing about an increased interpersonal contact which is basic for psychotherapy. Insulin coma therapy seems to be of value in the treatment of some cases of early schizophrenia. It seems probable that in most instances shock therapy should be combined with appropriate psychotherapy.

The rationale of these physical methods of treatment is far from established. Many physiologic explanations have been offered, but none is accepted generally. Various attempts at a psychodynamic formulation of the influence of such treatment have also been offered. It has been suggested that the treatment arouses a fear of death, which leads to a defensive attempt at a re-establishment of contact with the world of reality. It has been suggested that the treatment offers a punishment which is avidly seized on by the guilt-laden patient as a way of doing penance and receiving absolution and thus rendering unnecessary any further self-punishment, which had been the motivating force in some of his previous symptoms; this would apply particularly to the self-destructive tendencies of the depressed patient. It has also been suggested that the treatment may work especially in patients whose resistance to interpersonal influence had blocked any attempt at psychotherapy or workable personal contact but who now in shock therapy are up against overwhelming physical forces which cannot be resisted, with the end-result that the patient gives up his pattern of resistance and begins to conform.

Other physical methods of treatment are now being investigated: lobotomy, which involves a surgical interruption of pathways between frontal cortex and subcortical structures, and topectomy, which involves a surgical removal of small areas of cortical substance.

*f*) Psychotherapy, which may be roughly defined as the carrying-through of a planned program for modifying the emotional life and adjustment of the patient, through new life-experiences and psychologic processes which can influence the patient in the direction of health. Most often this occurs in the setting of an interpersonal relationship between one patient and one therapist.

In a textbook of dynamic psychiatry, it is this form of psychiatric treatment which should receive greatest attention. In the following pages, the most useful modes of psychotherapy are summarized.

One general comment is necessary before embarking on a discussion of the techniques of psychotherapy. In line with the persistent emphasis in this chapter on the fact that psychotherapy must be based on adequate diagnostic understanding, it is clear that any type of psychotherapeutic approach must be preceded by an exploratory period of one to ten interviews with the patient. Such an exploratory period will provide an opportunity for the accumulation of significant clinical, dynamic, and genetic material, so that decisions can be made as to the variety of psychotherapy to be considered. In such an exploratory period the explorer must have an adequate therapeutic attitude, in order to avoid doing damage. And occasionally a good therapeutic attitude during the exploratory period will lead to an amelioration of the presenting symptoms.

In this connection it must be stressed that even a single consultation interview or examination must be thought of in therapeutic as well as diagnostic terms. With such an emphasis, it is possible to avoid having the experience be traumatic or antitherapeutic. With such a therapeutic attitude, a therapeutic gain is possible even from a single contact. And if the consultation leads to the recommendation that treatment is indicated, acceptance of the recommendation will be facilitated if the consultation itself had a therapeutic orientation. In brief, a diagnostic consultation must not concentrate so intently on the eliciting of information of diagnostic value that the therapeutic implications of the consultation are forgotten.

To return for a moment to the exploratory period and the understanding which is its goal. From the preceding sections of this chapter the student may have the impression that in all cases the exploratory period must lead to a rather thorough understanding of clinical, dynamic, and genetic diagnosis, of transference and countertransference. Thoroughness is of value in many instances, but unnecessary in others. For example, in the study of a patient who may have delirium tremens, the clinical diagnosis is at first the important consideration, for the determination of the immediate treatment regime. The other facets of the study are at that time of only secondary value. Later, during the treatment of the delirium, an understanding of some of the other aspects of the case may occasionally be useful. For example, the patient's attitude to his parents and his customary modes of dealing with authority may give leads that can be of value in the management of his reactions on the ward. Still later, when the delirium is over and the question of psychotherapy in the treatment of the patient's chronic alcoholism becomes the central issue, the other aspects of psychiatric study, e.g., dynamic and genetic appraisal, become crucial. In other words, the psychiatric study must be oriented around the pertinent goals of therapy at the time that the study is made.

Psychotherapeutic procedures, rather artificially, may be subdivided in the following fashion:

*a*) *Indirect psychotherapy.*—Indirect psychotherapy consists of procedures which influence the patient indirectly through having a direct effect on his surroundings. One example is environmental manipulation, i.e., a modification of the external living conditions to lessen noxious pressures or to provide a more beneficial type of influence. A simple example of this is the placement of a child in a well-chosen foster-home. Another type of indirect psychotherapy is the treatment of a parent to produce changes in his attitudes toward the child who was the original patient. In this type of indirect psychotherapy, the emphasis is on the improvement of some key person in the child's surroundings rather than on removing the child from the environment or manipulating it in some other fashion.

At times the treatment of a parent may be concurrent with the direct treatment of the child. Usually the two are treated by different therapists, to avoid such complications as the competitive struggle for the attention of a single therapist. There is another, rather paradoxical, reason for having such a tandem arrangement. If the parent has a separate therapist, there is a greater possibility that the therapy of the parent will not be too exclusively related to the needs of the child. Even though the original recommendation for treatment of the parent was motivated by the needs of the child, it will usually be found that the parent in treatment is more likely to make progress if he or she feels that his or her interests are not being neglected and that he or she has a right to happiness and to therapy on his or her own. To have a therapy of one's own, like a "room of one's own," can satisfy deep needs and can provide a basis for improvement which then can be reflected in a more productive relationship with the child.

These comments on the parent as a patient suggest the relevance of a more general comment, that, even when the parent is not officially a patient, a therapeutic attitude toward the parent (and other relatives) is worth having. When the parent obviously is behaving in a disturbing fashion toward a child, it is easy for the child's therapist to develop hostile attitudes toward the parent in their incidental contacts. Such hostility often provokes unmanageable guilt or counterhostility in the parent, which may then be expressed toward the child. Consequently, the therapist's attitude toward the parent should, in general, be one of regarding the parent as being, in a sense, an incidental patient also and thus of having toward the parent a noncondemning, accepting attitude along with an attitude of firmness and an expectation of sincere attempts at more mature behavior. Strongly critical attitudes to relatives of patients or strongly sympathetic and forgiving attitudes are valuable only in special instances, when they happen to meet the dynamic needs of the relatives themselves. Such attitudes are to be used, not as an expression of the therapist's emotional reactions, but as a technique of helpfulness to the relatives and the patient, and only when the therapist has some conviction that they are dynamically correct.

*b*) *Direct psychotherapy.*—"Direct psychotherapy" is the category of procedures which influence the patient directly and which may be classified as (1) suppressive, (2) supportive, (3) relationship, and (4) expressive psychotherapy.

(1) *Suppressive psychotherapy.*—Suppressive psychotherapy employs such techniques as authoritative firmness and commands, the ignoring of symptoms and complaints, placebos used with dogmatic assurance, suggestions under hypnosis to repress symptoms, comparable waking suggestion, exhortation, and persuasion. Essentially, in this approach, the therapist acts as a dictator, as an adjunct to the forces of repression, as an omniscient and omnipotent father who expects to be obeyed.

Such an approach is aimed in part at the suppression or re-repression of unconscious material which is threatening to erupt, and at a strengthening of the usual defenses. In part, it is intended to counteract the secondary benefits of neurotic illness, such as the striving for attention and sympathy and the use of symptoms to control the environment.

It shades over into the next variety, supportive psychotherapy, and in some instances actually is a productive variety of supportive psychotherapy, if it is used in a deliberate attempt to meet a patient's need for a strong, firm, guiding, controlling hand.

In general, however, present-day psychiatry has little respect for the suppressive techniques, recognizing that they are often used without reference to the actual psychodynamic problem and that, even if they have some effect at times, they leave the problem unsolved and the patient seriously vulnerable to subsequent stresses and strains.

(2) *Supportive psychotherapy.* — Supportive psychotherapy uses such components as a warm, friendly, strong-leadership type of support and reassurance; help in the development of hobbies and outlets (e.g., in occupation and recreation); symptomatic medication; adequate rest and diversion; the removal of external strain; hospitalization; the provision of a period of necessary dependence; and guidance and advice in practical issues. Group psychotherapy also may have a valuable supportive effect.

Essentially, supportive therapy uses those techniques which will make the patient feel more secure, reassured, accepted, protected, encouraged, safe, less anxious, and less alone. In good part, even a supportive psychotherapy must be individualized and be dependent on the understanding of the specific individual. For example, in one patient symptomatic medication will have excellent supportive value; in another it may mobilize sharp anxiety about the development of a drug addiction. Its goal is a rather limited one, that of offering support during a period of illness or turmoil and at times of restoring or strengthening the defenses and integrative capacities which are temporarily impaired during the illness. It provides a period of acceptance and dependence when the patient is acutely in need of help in meeting his frustrations, his guilt, and his anxiety or the external pressures which are too great for him to handle.

Often supportive psychotherapy shades over into relationship therapy or is combined with it. And supportive psychotherapy may use a limited amount of expressive psychotherapy, such as the verbalization of unexpressed emotions. The verbal expression of emotion has the value of some relief of emotional tension. And, in a therapeutic situation, the expression of emotion and its subsequent discussion may lead to a greater objectivity in evaluating a current problem. In this fashion the patient may achieve some relief of anxiety and symptoms and get help, through superficial insight, in reaching some sort of solution of a current problem or reactive upset.

The therapist must keep in mind the fact that supportive help may foster regressive tendencies and too great a dependency. He must keep in mind the obligation to avoid the development of undue dependence and the need for a persistent weaning to a resumption of independence.

In practice, supportive psychotherapy is of value in psychiatric conditions such as these: relatively mature individuals in reactive upsets largely based on extraordinarily severe environmental pressures (e.g., some traumatic neuroses, some reactive depressions); individuals who, in general, have made a rather good adjustment and are in what seems to be only a temporary period of pressure, of turmoil, of temptation, or of indecision; individuals who have been fairly responsible and giving in their life-adjustment but who now are required to give beyond their psychologic means (e.g., a wife whose husband is behaving in a more infantile fashion than usual) and who need to be given to, so that they will have more to give; individuals who are extremely resistant to expressive psychotherapy and those who the therapist concludes are fundamentally too sick to respond to expressive psychotherapy; and, finally, patients who have no drive toward a fundamental change in their adjustment and are essentially interested in a restoration of a more comfortable previous adjustment.

In some instances a period of supportive psychotherapy may lead to the joint decision that expressive psychotherapy is the procedure of choice. And the reverse in part may be true; during an expressive psychotherapy the therapist occasionally must be flexible enough to provide a period of supportive therapy.

It must be added that in the present transitional period of a plethora of patients and a paucity of psychiatrists, supportive psychotherapy at times is used not as the procedure of choice but of practical necessity.

(3) *Relationship therapy*.—Before embarking on a description of relationship therapy, a transitional comment should be made, contrasting the types of psychotherapy with regard to one essential difference, viz., the goals of therapy. It can be said that, in contrast to the supportive type of psychotherapy (described in the preceding section), a relationship psychotherapy (described in this section) and an expressive psychotherapy (to be described in the following section) have more extensive goals. The latter two types aim not only at a restoration of the *status quo ante*, at the re-establishment of a former equilibrium, but also at a change in personality patterns and at a decrease in vulnerability to external pressures.

Then, to contrast these two, it can be said that a relationship therapy has more limited goals and techniques than does expressive psychotherapy. The differences will become apparent in the description of the two in this and the subsequent section.

The present section—an attempt at a delineation of relationship therapy—provides difficulties in presentation and clarification. The concept of a relationship therapy is fundamentally a simple one, and yet it is so much a matter of atmosphere and feeling and personal interplay that a clear phrasing of its essence in brief form is difficult to achieve.

Perhaps a relationship therapy can best be described as a fairly prolonged period of contact of patient and therapist in which the therapist can maintain, without much conscious effort, a good therapeutic attitude of the sort described in previous pages of this chapter. In response to such a therapeutic attitude, the patient behaves in various ways, and there develops an interplay of feeling, of communication, and of new experience. In such a growing relationship certain therapeutic experiences occur, which may be listed in part as follows: (*a*) the experience of being accepted as of value, or potentially so, and of not being condemned or rejected because of defensive distortions; (*b*) the growth of an identification with some of the more successful techniques and adjustments of the therapist as they may fit the individual needs of the patient; and (*c*) spontaneous corrective emotional experiences, based on the fact that the therapist does not respond in the manner expected by the patient. These points will be elaborated in subsequent paragraphs.

The essence of the technique of a relationship therapy can be phrased in this way: It consists of a series of interviews in which current and past life-problems and situations and conscious conflicts and wishes and fears are discussed but in which the therapist is less interested in the dynamics of the problems than in the fostering of a good therapeutic relationship. The cornerstone of the relationship is that during the interviews the therapist has toward the patient the sort of attitude that is characteristic of a good father or mother or of a good older brother or sister.

In such an attitude and such a relationship the element of support must play a vital role, of course; a good parent or a good older sibling does offer support. In fact, a relationship therapy may, at times, use some of the specific techniques of a supportive therapy. And, in a sense, relationship therapy can be considered a protracted variety of supportive therapy, in that the therapist may see the patient over a period of months or years (usually once a week or so) in an atmosphere of friendliness and support. And such a sustaining relationship has some value on that basis alone; it offers a limited satisfaction of some of the deep needs for acceptance and dependence which develop in many patients in an attempt to counterbalance their neurotic frustrations, their guilt, and their anxiety.

But in this technique of relationship therapy the therapist avoids being too supportive, because he hopes not only to offer sustaining help but also, through his therapeutic attitude of being nonjudgmental, noncondemning, nonsubmissive, nonanxious, noncontrolling, firm, consistent, and realistic, to have a modifying effect on the patient's personality. He knows that the constant playing of the note of supportiveness is often not enough. He knows, further, that a too emphatic or a too prolonged sounding of that note may infantilize the patient. And the therapist wants the patient to obtain more from the therapy than the security and reassurance that comes from feeling supported and sustained.

Consequently, the therapist would like his attitude to include all the attitudes that can characterize the helpful parent or older sibling. A good father is not too supporting; the therapist must not be. A good father sets limits to unacceptable behavior; so must the therapist. A good father can point out mistakes; so can the therapist. A good father is not frightened by threats; nor is the therapist. A good father can be firm without hostility; so can the therapist. A good father expects a growth in self-reliance; and so should the therapist. A good father gives respect and acceptance; so does the therapist. A good father is not always good and can make mistakes; the same goes for the therapist. A good father need not try to be the perfectly good father or completely well adjusted with his children; nor need the therapist with his patients.

A further contrast of supportive therapy and relationship therapy is this: The therapist's basic role in a relationship therapy is not that of a supporting crutch but rather that of a firm, helpful friend, who wants to help and be sustaining but expects the patient to be as self-reliant and independent as he can be. The therapist would prefer to help the patient see facts and issues and alternatives, so that he can make his own decisions, rather than to try to make the patient's decisions for him. The therapist expects to disagree as well as to agree, even though the patient hopes for complete agreement and supportive approval.

Another comment to indicate that a relationship must go beyond a purely supportive attitude: The therapist hopes that his attitude of having, on the one hand, a sincere tolerance toward certain aspects of the patient's life toward which the patient had been too self-critical and self-condemning and of having, on the other hand, a clear recognition of the need for a firm, realistic setting of limits about the acting-out of unacceptable behavior will be of value in helping the patient to become mature. He hopes that such a bilateral attitude will help the patient toward a more reliable and successful variety of inner control and social adjustment and hence to a greater independence.

Such a relationship, then, may lead to specific experiences and responses and modifications in the patient. Of these, two may be singled out for special comment: (*a*) the development of healthy identifications and (*b*) some corrective emotional experiences.

The therapist hopes that some of his own more mature attitudes, which become evident in the relationship, will be incorporated by the patient as part of his own attitudes, if they seem appropriate, just as a son may incorporate some of the attitudes of a good father. In other words, the therapist hopes that the patient will, through a process of identification, adopt some of the therapist's more successful defenses and adjustments. Such identifications may tend to counterbalance some of the patient's less healthy identifications with the unfavorable influences of his childhood and lead to a greater strength, to a diminution of anxiety and defenses, and, more generally, to an increase in integrative capacity.

Further, the therapist hopes that some corrective emotional experiences will occur spontaneously, viz., that the patient will somehow be influenced by the fact that the therapist's attitudes and responses are different from the ones which his personality sickness has led him to expect from others. Such a contrast between expectation and actuality (e.g., between the expectation of being able to provoke the therapist to rejection and the actuality that it does not happen) can lead to distinct modification in patterns of interpersonal relations. (It is to be noted that in a relationship therapy there is merely the general expectation that a persistently good therapeutic attitude is likely to lead to some corrective emotional experiences. In an expressive psychothera-py, however, more specific corrective experiences are likely to occur, because specific patterns are being worked through and because there may be some planning for the occurrence of spe-cific corrective experiences which the therapist regards as cen-tral for the treatment.)

To rephrase the processes just described, it may be said that, fundamentally, a relationship therapy provides the therapist with an opportunity to behave in a fashion different from the behavior of the patient's parents and, in a sense, to neutralize or to reverse the mistakes of the parents. If the patient had overly authoritarian parents, the therapist's friendly, nonauthoritarian attitude means that the patient has an opportunity to adjust to, to be led by, and to identify with a new type of parent-figure. And, in a similar fashion, patients who had overly indulgent, overly seductive, overly passive, or inconsistent parents can now have a new start-ing point, of being, in a sense, brought up again by a parent who is not making such mistakes or who may be responding in a way quite different from the patterns of the parents.

In many cases the mere fact that the therapist is responding fairly maturely provides enough of a contrast with the mistaken attitudes of the parents. In other instances, however, it may be wise for the therapist to emphasize the contrast, i.e., of being quite permissive if the parents were destructively restrictive or of being emphatically firm if the parents were destructively indul-gent. Obviously, in many instances the patient cannot quickly adjust to, or be influenced by, such a contrasting attitude. Hence a relationship therapy is to be regarded as a slow process, which may take months or years.

Such a phrasing of the pattern of a relationship therapy may give the false impression that the therapist is placing the total responsibility for the patient's problems in the laps of the parents. Actually, serious problems may arise in childhood even when the parental attitudes are fundamentally sound. For example, a child, with little or no provocation from the parents, may develop hos-tile, destructive impulses toward the parents and then expect hostile, destructive retaliation from them. In such a setting he may develop severe anxiety, be provocative toward them, or be defensively resistant. And, at that point, believing his parents to be hostile people, he may identify with his "hostile parents" and consequently have a pattern which persists. And, of course, in such a situation, even mature parents may be bewildered and anxious and be provoked to hostility, which then can be a focus for conflict and identification in the child.

A relationship therapy can fit such a pattern as the one just described, as well as the patterns in which the primary responsibility is the parents'. In the pattern in which the child's destructive feelings initiated the interaction, a relationship therapy can be effective in this way: When the patient becomes hostile to the therapist and expects hostility in return, as an adult he is now better able to see the actual fact that he is not receiving a retaliatory hostility. (As a child, he was less able to distinguish fact from fancy.) He now can see that his hostility is not met with hostility; the effect is that of having him realize that his own hostile impulses are not so dangerous as they seemed, that parents or parent-figures are not so unfriendly as he thought, and that he no longer need identify with an image imbued with hostility. In addition, if the parents had, out of bewilderment, actually responded with hostility, the fact that the therapist does not, again offers a chance for a corrective experience.

At this point the comment should be made that one of the basic propositions of this chapter is that relationship therapy is a pervasive substrate of many of the forms of expressive psychotherapy discussed below. Further, one unsolved problem of psychotherapy, to be answered by further research, has to do with the possibility that some therapeutic results ordinarily credited to expressive therapy are in actuality to be credited to the concomitant therapeutic relationship.

A relationship therapy of itself is suitable for many varieties of psychogenic illness. It is especially to be chosen when the patient is too resistive to attempts at an expressive psychotherapy or is considered too ill for this type of treatment; and it is indicated when the skill and training of the therapist are not adequate for such psychotherapy or, on a more positive basis, when a gradual maturing process based on the elaboration of new foci for identification is regarded as the most promising line of modification.

Relationship therapy can form the backbone of the work of the psychiatrist whose training was not psychodynamically oriented; it is the vehicle for the success of many psychiatric social workers; and it can provide the best line of approach for the growing group of internists and other physicians whose psychosomatic interests call for the development of techniques of psychotherapy. Such a statement, of course, does not eliminate the possibility of the interweaving of a certain amount of expressive psychotherapy into relationship therapy, in the work of those whose training and skill are adequate.

(4) *Expressive psychotherapy.*—This is a broad and unsatisfactory term to include a variety of special techniques and procedures. Perhaps the essential characteristic of all of them is that they attempt to go beyond the goals of a supportive and of a relationship therapy. The goals of the various forms of expressive psychotherapy not only include the goals of the above-mentioned techniques, viz., a restoration of a disturbed equilibrium, the formation of new foci for identification, and the occurrence of spontaneous corrective emotional experiences; they also include the goals of a greater awareness of the determinants of the illness, an emotional reorientation and a more mature perspective with regard to these determinants, an increase in ego capacity and strength, and specific and central corrective experiences.

A variety of procedures may be called "expressive" or "exploratory" or "uncovering," and again there is a great deal of overlapping of techniques and terminology. The most superficial variety of expressive psychotherapy is a frank discussion of personal problems, of impulses, life-situations, and conflicts which are quite conscious to the patient but which he ordinarily would not discuss with others. This would include a sort of confession and ventilation of "worries," family problems, doubts, impulses, conscious anxieties, guilt feelings, etc., and a joint study of current conflicts and remembered past life-situations as they seem to relate to neurotic reactions or psychosomatic disorders. Such a series of discussions of conscious problems would include, of course, a good therapeutic attitude on the part of the psychiatrist, with the constructive effects hoped for in a relationship therapy. In addition, however, in this type of expressive psychotherapy, there is the added goal of some increase in understanding and insight. The therapist in such a program would not give interpretations of unconscious material but would limit himself to a clarification of conscious problems, to a linking of events and feelings with reactions and symptoms—a linkage which the patient had not noticed previously on his own. Even such superficial insight may lead to an increase in perspective and objectivity, to a lessening of anxiety, and to some undercutting of future automatic responses.

In addition, such a discussion of conscious issues may give the therapist a chance to correct the patient's misinformation on personal problems—a correction which may lead to some diminution of anxiety. Further, the verbalization of vague or unclear worries may have some therapeutic effect, since the process of verbalization itself may make the problem more specific and less vague. Vague dangers often seem greater than clear ones. Consequently, the process of verbalization may lead to a better perspective and objectivity.

This combination of superficial expressive psychotherapy with relationship therapy may then be deepened at times by the inclusion of a varying amount of dealing with unconscious material, via free association, understanding of the transference, some dream material, etc. Such psychotherapy goes by a number of labels, such as "brief psychotherapy," "therapeutic interviewing," or "psychoanalytically oriented psychotherapy." Intensively supervised training, with adequate emphasis on transference and countertransference problems, is a *sine qua non* for this type of therapy. (It is unnecessary to specify the details of this variety of psychotherapy, since it can be visualized quite simply as the deepening of relationship therapy and "conscious" expressive therapy described above, by the use of some of the facets of psychoanalysis, to be described in the following paragraphs.)

If, now, in other cases, the psychotherapy deals extensively and intensively with unconscious problems (with, however, as much attention to conscious problems and reality situations as the material calls for); if the therapeutic sessions are frequent enough to give extensive information about the complexities of the patient's patterns; if the emphasis is predominantly on dealing with transference and resistance and on the working-through of defenses to uncover and express preconscious and unconscious pathogenic material; if the patient can productively be given insight into the ways in which his patterns unconsciously have led to distorted attitudes to the therapist; and if both dynamic and genetic material play an important role in therapy, the technique is called a "psychoanalysis."

Since this is a textbook of dynamic psychiatry rather than of psychoanalysis per se, the technical aspects of psychoanalysis will not be considered in detail.

A psychoanalysis is built on the basis of a relationship therapy, with the above-mentioned effects of a persistent therapeutic attitude (nonjudgmental, etc.) and the possibility of new foci for identification and of corrective experiences. It deals also with the clarification of conscious anxieties and conflicts. Its additional and specific characteristics are the following: Its emphasis is on dealing with unconscious conflicts, with the goal of uncovering and verbalizing various unconscious drives and emotions and of alleviating unconscious anxieties. It places great emphasis on an understanding of unconscious problems as expressed in transference distortions. One of its major goals is the achievement by the patient of an increased insight into his unconscious trends, with a possibility of better integration, now that the impulse is to be dealt with by the adult ego rather than by the relatively weak ego of childhood. This process can be rephrased as the bringing into consciousness of unacceptable impulses so that they may be dealt with by conscious and adult acceptance or renunciation or modification rather than by repression, with its symptom-forming consequences. Another of the major goals of psychoanalysis is the corrective emotional experience of having previously unconscious and automatic attitudes, now directed toward the therapist, brought into consciousness and of seeing that they are reacted to by the therapist in a way far different from the patient's expectations.

As part of its emphasis on the exploration and expression of unconscious material, a psychoanalysis makes extensive use of dreams and the associations to them, of the various indications of hidden transference and defensive reactions, and of close observation of the sequence of ideas in free association, i.e., the type of expression of thoughts and feelings which occurs when one puts aside the usual attempt to censor one's talk or to present one's ideas or memories in a logical fashion.

In a sense a psychoanalysis deals with material on a "deeper level." This can be specified as meaning (*a*) that there is an extensive attempt to understand the unconscious dynamics, in addition to the conscious dynamics; (*b*) that interpretation of unconscious material plays a more important role than clarification of conscious material does; and (*c*) that the significance of the past in the formation of current problems is emphasized, as well as the significance of the current unconscious patterns and problems themselves.

Another variety of expressive psychotherapy is play therapy in children. In this, the child's play, when he is alone with the therapist, acts as a technical substitute for dreams and free association. The play may start with the spontaneous choice of one of a variety of toys and play situations, or the play situation may be planned by the therapist to facilitate the expression of anxiety-provoking impulses, e.g., the use of a family of dolls, on which the child may displace his interpersonal patterns. The goal of such therapy is either the development of a capacity for a greater expression of throttled emotions, in a safe and supervised therapeutic situation, or the use of the material so revealed for the development of insight and understanding or for the corrective living experience in the transference. Depending on the depth of the therapy, such work may be called "psychoanalytically oriented play therapy" or "child analysis."

Hypnotherapy is another variety of expressive psychotherapy, in which hypnosis is used in part to facilitate the expression of unconscious material, which then may be handled therapeutically.

Narcosynthesis is a comparable technique of facilitating the expression of suppressed or repressed material through the technique of the intravenous injection of sodium pentothal or sodium amytal to the point of thorough relaxation but not sleep. This technique seems to be effective chiefly when there have been recent severe traumatic experiences, which stirred impulses and anxiety to a degree that could not be handled without repression and symptom formation.

Certain varieties of group therapy (the open discussion, in a small group, of common or universal problems or of individual problems) not only have supportive value, as mentioned above, but also permit the expression of hidden anxieties and conflicts, and some insight and corrective experiences in relation to the leader and to the others of the group.

It is not possible to state in any brief fashion the indications and contraindications for the varieties of expressive psychotherapy. Essentially, they are more suitable for neurotic problems than for psychotic, since a relatively intact ego is essential for the integration of "expressed" material. Modifications of the techniques described, however, make them usable with some psychotic patients during their hospital stay. In general, the expressive psychotherapies are suitable for patients who are willing to cooperate in such a procedure, who in the diagnostic evaluation of the psychiatrist are capable of constructive modification through the expressive techniques, and who cannot be given adequate help through simpler procedures.

As a postscript to the above description of the varieties of psychotherapy, the following may be added: Except for certain previously repressed material which is uncovered in rather intensive expressive psychotherapy, the material brought by patients to psychotherapeutic sessions is approximately the same in all varieties of psychotherapy. The essential difference is what happens after the patient brings the material. Expressed with great oversimplification, the following contrast can be made. In any variety of psychotherapy the patient may tell the therapist of an anxiety dream or a nightmare of a small animal with big sorrowful eyes about to be devoured by an enormous spider. In a *suppressive* therapy the therapist would insist that the patient stop being concerned about dreams and stop being anxious over inconsequential nothings and would order him to forget his dreams and jump out of bed in the morning. In a *supportive* therapy the therapist might comment that dreams are disturbing at times to everyone, that this is a common enough type of dream, and that perhaps some mild sedative for sleep might temporarily be of value. In some cases he may try to get the patient to talk freely of his fears. In a *relationship* therapy the therapist would put to himself the question of whether in the dream he is the devouring spider or the endangered small animal or whether the patient is either. He is alerted to the probability that in the treatment the patient may be afraid or may soon be afraid either of being hurt or of hurting. He may make no direct comment to the patient about the dream other than a supportive comment, and then later help to steer the patient into some discussion of his conscious fears. Largely he uses the dream to put the question to himself as to whether he has done anything to frighten the patient or whether he has permitted the patient to frighten him, and so helps himself to continue in a good therapeutic attitude. In an *expressive* therapy that does not go deeply into unconscious material the therapist may use the dream material in the fashion just mentioned as part of relationship therapy but, in addition, may lead the discussion to some expression of the patient's fears, his thoughts about them, etc., and, noting the material touched on, be led to some clarification or interpretation of the patient's fear of women, etc. In an expressive therapy of a deeper variety, the therapist would have the patient associate freely to the elements of the dream and then or later give an interpretation of the unconscious problems revealed by the combination of the dream, the associations, and the patient's attitudes. In such a therapy, if the material justified it, the interpretation given (the latent meaning of the dream) may well be that the patient was deeply afraid of being devoured by women figures (and now by the therapist) because of his own desire to open his eyes wide to see what he felt he should not see. (Implicit in this is the attitude that the therapist knows of his impulses and will not punish him.) In other instances, the interpretation may be that the patient regards himself as the omnipotent devouring spider and expects the therapist to cower in fear. (And implicit in this is the fact that the therapist does not regard the patient as omnipotent or frightening, and that the therapist is not cowering in fear.)

## 2. THE TRAINING AND SKILL OF THE THERAPIST IN THE USE OF SPECIFIC TECHNIQUES

It is clear that special training must be called for in many of the techniques mentioned above. Only a neurosurgeon should remove a brain tumor. Only a psychiatrist trained in electro-convulsive therapy (as well as in general and dynamic psychiatry) should give that variety of shock therapy. Only an accredited psychoanalyst should do psychoanalysis.

Because of the overlapping of the fields of knowledge and of training, some varieties of therapy may be done by specialists in several fields. A psychiatric social worker, adequately trained (working either in a psychiatric clinic or in an agency which has close supervision by psychiatrists), may make use of some aspects of the techniques of supportive therapy, relationship therapy, and expressive therapy essentially limited to conscious material. Her work will largely be oriented to the patient's environmental and family problems, and her special experience in social pathology and family constellations can be specific assets in therapy. A clinical psychologist, if his training is adequate, may do the same varieties of psychotherapy while working as part of a psychiatric clinic team, although his primary responsibility is in the field of teaching, research, and the use of special diagnostic tests. The internist or general practitioner who has had no special training in psychotherapy should limit himself to supportive techniques, whereas, if he has had special training, his skills may include the use of relationship therapy and superficial expressive psychotherapy based on conscious material. The psychiatrist whose training was largely nondynamic should limit himself to supportive therapy, relationship therapy, expressive therapy dealing with conscious material, general care of psychotic patients, and shock therapy. The psychiatrist whose training included intensively supervised dynamic psychotherapy may, in addition, make "brief psychotherapy" the focus of his practice. The psychiatrist whose training included full training in psychoanalysis may use the method of psychoanalysis.

### 3. PRACTICAL ASPECTS OF TREATMENT

To recapitulate: The therapist must take into consideration the diagnostic formulations (clinical, dynamic, and genetic) and the transference and countertransference phenomena apparent during the exploratory period. He must consider the various types of acceptable therapy and their applicability in terms of the specific problem at hand. He must pay attention to the problem of the goals of treatment in the individual patient and fit the potentialities of the various treatment procedures to the needs and potentialities of the patient. Further, he must consider his own training and skill or those of the therapists to whom he might refer the patient.

In addition, his decisions about therapy must take into full consideration many practical issues. The age of the patient, his level of intelligence, the presence of serious physical defects, his cultural and educational background, his geographical location in respect to treatment—all are of importance in determining the feasibility of the therapy which may seem indicated.

The elements in the family constellation which foster improvement and those which block progress must be evaluated. The destructive aspects of the environment in which the patient must stay during treatment or to which he must return after treatment are often of crucial importance, particularly in childhood.

The resources of the community may have to be assessed as well. If private hospitalization is indicated, the availability of a vacancy in a good hospital, at a rate which the patient or the family can afford to pay, must be determined. If the patient should have ambulatory private care, the availability of an adequately trained therapist cannot be taken for granted. If the patient is unable to pay for private care, the existence of a good clinic in the community is crucial. (And if the patient's therapy would be benefited by his paying a small fee, the clinic should provide such a fee system as one of its therapeutic activities.)

The purpose of these final paragraphs, however, is not to give a full survey of practical considerations—rather it is to call attention to the danger that the therapist may become so fascinated by the discoveries of modern psychiatry and by the dynamic problems of the individual patient that he will minimize the need to consider the current realities. But when the therapist recognizes the urgent necessity of having his planning be realistic and appropriate, the practical issues in any individual situation become obvious and pertinent.

## BIBLIOGRAPHY

1. AICHHORN, A. *Wayward Youth* (New York: Viking Press, 1945).
2. ALEXANDER, F. *Fundamentals of Psychoanalysis* (New York: W. W. Norton & Co., 1948), pp. 272–302.
3. ALEXANDER, F., and FRENCH, T. M. *Psychoanalytic Therapy* (New York: Ronald Press, 1946).
4. ALEXANDER, F., and HEALY, W. *Roots of Crime* (New York: Alfred A. Knopf, 1935).
5. BENNETT, A. E. "The Role of Psychotherapy in Electroshock Therapy," *Am. J. Psychiat.*, 105:392, 1948.
6. BINGER, C. *The Doctor's Job* (New York: W. W. Norton & Co., 1945).
7. BRENMAN, M., and GILL, M. M. *Hypnotherapy* (New York: International Universities Press, 1947).
8. COLEMAN, J. V. "Patient-Physician Relationship in Psychotherapy," *Am. J. Psychiat.*, 104:638, 1948.
9. DIETHELM, O. *Treatment in Psychiatry* (New York: Macmillan Co., 1951).
10. FEDERN, P. "Psychoanalysis of Psychoses," *Psychiat. Quart.*, 17:1, 246, 470, 1943.
11. FENICHEL, O. *Problems of Psychoanalytic Technique* (Albany, N.Y.: Psychoanalytic Quarterly, Inc., 1941).
12. FENICHEL, O. *The Psychoanalytic Theory of Neurosis* (New York: W. W. Norton & Co., 1945), pp. 547–89.
13. FINESINGER, J. E. "Psychiatric Interviewing. I. Some Principles and Procedures in Insight Therapy," *Am. J. Psychiat.*, 105:187, 1948.
14. FREUD, A. *Introduction to the Technic of Child Analysis* (London: George Allen & Unwin, 1931).
15. FREUD, S. *A General Introduction to Psychoanalysis* (New York: Boni & Liveright, 1935); or *Introductory Lectures on Psychoanalysis* (London: George Allen & Unwin, 1917).
16. FREUD, S. *New Introductory Lectures on Psycho-analysis* (New York: W. W. Norton & Co., 1933).
17. FREUD, S. Papers on Technique, in *Collected Papers*, Vol. 2 (London: Hogarth Press, 1924).
18. FROMM-REICHMANN, F. *Principles of Intensive Psychotherapy* (Chicago: University of Chicago Press, 1950).

19. GARRETT, A. *Interviewing: Its Principles and Methods* (New York: Family Welfare Association of America, 1942).

20. GRINKER, R. R., and SPIEGEL, J. P. *Men under Stress* (Philadelphia: Blakiston Co., 1945).

21. HENDRICK, I. *Facts and Theories of Psychoanalysis* (New York: Alfred A. Knopf, 1939).

22. HINSIE, L. E. *Concepts and Problems of Psychotherapy* (New York: Columbia University Press, 1937).

23. JESSNER, L., and RYAN, V. G. *Shock Treatment in Psychiatry* (New York: Grune & Stratton, 1941).

24. KALINOWSKI, L. B., and HOCH, P. H. *Shock Treatments and Other Somatic Procedures in Psychiatry* (New York: Grune & Stratton, 1946).

25. KLEIN, M. *The Psycho-analysis of Children* (London: Hogarth Press, 1932).

26. KNIGHT, R. P. "A Critique of the Present Status of the Psychotherapist," *Bull. New York Acad. Med.*, 25:100, 1949.

27. KNIGHT, R. P. "The Psychoanalytic Treatment in a Sanitarium of Chronic Addiction to Alcohol," *J.A.M.A.*, 111:1443, 1938.

28. KUBIE, L. S. *Practical Aspects of Psychoanalysis* (New York: W. W. Norton & Co., 1936).

29. KUBIE, L. S. "The Nature of Psychotherapy," *Bull. New York Acad. Med.*, 19:183, 1943.

30. LEVINE, M. "An Orientation Chart in the Teaching of Psychosomatic Medicine," *Psychosom. Med.*, 10:111, 1948.

31. LEVINE, M. *Psychotherapy in Medical Practice* (New York: Macmillan Co., 1942).

32. LEVY, D. M. "Attitude Therapy," *Am. J. Orthopsychiat.*, 7:103, 1937.

33. LEVY, D. M. "Trends in Therapy: Release Therapy," *Am. J. Orthopsychiat.*, 9:713, 1939.

34. LORAND, S. *Technique of Psychoanalytic Therapy* (New York: International Universities Press, 1946).

35. MENNINGER, K. *The Human Mind* (3d ed.; New York: Alfred A. Knopf, 1945), pp. 363–416.

36. NUNBERG, H. *Practice and Theory of Psychoanalysis* (New York: Nervous and Mental Disease Publishing Co., 1948), pp. 75, 105, 174.

37. POWDERMAKER, F. "The Techniques of the Initial Interview," *Am. J. Psychiat.*, 104:642, 1948.

38. *Proceedings of the Brief Psychotherapy Council* (Chicago: Institute for Psychoanalysis, 1942, 1944, 1946).

39. ROSEN, J. N. "The Treatment of Schizophrenic Psychoses by Direct Analytic Therapy," *Psychiat. Quart.*, 21:3, 1947.

40. SARGENT, W., and SLATER, E. *An Introduction to Physical Methods of Treatment in Psychiatry* (Baltimore: Williams & Wilkins Co., 1948).

41. SCHILDER, P. *Psychotherapy* (New York: W. W. Norton & Co., 1951).

42. SLAVSON, S. R. *The Practice of Group Therapy* (New York: International Universities Press, 1948).

43. Spock, B., and Huschka, M. *Psychological Aspects of Pediatric Practice* (New York: New York State Committee on Mental Hygiene, 1938).
44. Szurek, S. A. "Remarks on Training for Psychotherapy," *Am. J. Orthopsychiat.*, 19:36, 1949.
45. Witmer, H. L. (ed.). *Teaching Psychotherapeutic Medicine* (New York: Commonwealth Fund, 1947).
46. Whitehorn, J. C. "Psychotherapy," in *Modern Medical Therapy in General Practice*, 1 (Baltimore: Williams & Wilkins Co., 1940), 3.
47. Whitehorn, J. C. "Guide to Interviewing and Clinical Personality Study," *Arch. Neurol. & Psychiat.*, 52:197, 1944.

# PART III

# INFLUENCE OF PSYCHOANALYSIS
# ON ALLIED FIELDS

# XII

## THE PSYCHOSOMATIC APPROACH IN MEDICINE

FRANZ ALEXANDER, M.D., AND THOMAS S. SZASZ, M.D.

### WHAT IS PSYCHOSOMATIC MEDICINE?

THE psychosomatic approach in medical research and therapy consists in the co-ordinated application of somatic (i.e., anatomical, physiological, pharmacological, and surgical) methods and concepts, on the one hand, and psychological methods and concepts, on the other. Interest in the mutual influence of physiological and psychological processes is by no means new, as evidenced by such German expressions as were popular in the last century—*Psychophysiologie* (Wundt) or *Psychophysik* (Fechner). What is new in the modern psychosomatic approach is that both the physiological and the psychological processes are studied with the same scientific standards. This progress, like all fundamental scientific progress, became possible by improved methods. It is only since the advent of the psychoanalytic technique that psychological processes can be studied with precision. As a result, generalities, such as, for example, that the emotional state of a person may have a profound influence upon the course of any disease, can now be replaced by the precise study of these psychological influences.

Psychological processes are the functions of the central co-ordinator of the organism, i.e., of the highest integrative centers of the central nervous system. Essentially they are similar to other processes in the organism. The most important difference is that they are perceived subjectively. Accordingly, these processes can be studied by psychological techniques. Psychological methods, however, differ in many respects from all other methods used in medicine, such as physics, chemistry, anatomy, and physiology. Hence the co-ordination of these two types of approach meets with inherent difficulties, which are being overcome only gradually.

When psychoanalytic interest first turned to the problems of organic medicine, some pioneers, notably Georg Groddeck (51, 52, 53), attempted to understand somatic processes entirely *as if* they were the same as psychic processes and symptoms. He applied psychoanalytic concepts to physiologic processes, without due recognition of the fact that the latter require different conceptual tools for adequate description and understanding. The results thus arrived at were often bizarre, such as "interpreting" the fever of an infectious illness as "meaning" sexual excitement, or the increased blood flow to an organ, for whatever reason, as "meaning" a displaced erection.

Another example of such conceptual confusion may be seen in the approach of certain so-called "organicists." We are referring to the persistent attempts, both past and present, to find some histological or biochemical alteration in the central nervous system which would "explain" the neuroses or schizophrenia. Such findings, even if present, would no more explain the specific psychological pictures found in various psychiatric syndromes than the discovery of the syphilitic basis of paresis could explain the various psychic symptoms which occur in patients with this disorder.

The two examples cited are, of course, counterparts of each other. They illustrate the inappropriateness of simply transposing the concepts of psychology into physiology or vice versa. The creation of an *integrated conceptual system* which would combine the basic principles of these two diverse scientific approaches thus appears to be one of the most important goals of present-day research in psychosomatic medicine.

The current psychosomatic approach in medicine can be considered as a logical outcome of the basic orientation of Freud. From the beginning, Freud's approach to psychology was consistently biological. He considered psychological processes as functions of the living organism, which, like all other bodily functions, are in the service of survival and propagation. This, in his time, was in stark contrast to the traditional approach of psychology, which had its origin in philosophy. Since Descartes, emphasis has been placed upon the fact that all our knowledge about the surrounding world is based on such psychological processes as observing, knowing, and understanding (*cogito, ergo sum*). Hence the belief that psychological phenomena cannot be explained from external facts and that all other sciences are secondary to psychology. This epistemological emphasis gave psychology an extra-territorial status which was, in a sense, above and beyond all other sciences, and introspection was considered the only legitimate approach to psychic life.

Freud's biological orientation is best exemplified by his concept of the mental apparatus, the main function of which he considered to be the preservation of the equilibrium (stability) of the organism by satisfying its instinctual (biological) needs and protecting it from excessive external stimuli (45). This task it achieves by the perception of internal or instinctual needs, by the perception of existing conditions in the external environment upon which the satisfaction of instinctual needs depends, and, finally, by the confrontation of the data of internal and external perception with each other ("integrative function"). The ultimate function of the mental apparatus, however, is an executive one: the control of co-ordinated voluntary behavior, which is based on the integration of the data of internal and external perception by reasoning. According to Freud, all neurotic symptoms can be considered as failures of these functions; they are substitutes in fantasy for adequate, integrated acts. Whenever the relief of instinctual tensions by suitable co-ordinated behavior fails, these tensions seek other outlets. Neurotic symptoms are adaptations occurring in the face of such failures of adequate discharge of instinctual tensions; they are often inadequate, autoplastic substitutes for adequate, alloplastic action (44). Neurotic symptoms vary greatly in their effectiveness in relieving (draining) instinctual tensions; often they can relieve tensions only partially, and they may create secondary conflicts, leading to new tensions.

Often these chronic emotional tensions elicit chronic responses (dysfunctions) in the vegetative system, which have been called "functional" disorders, such as "nervous indigestion," diarrhea, cardiac neurosis, etc. The understanding of such conditions requires the co-ordinated use of psychological and physiological methods (9, 31, 88).

## EARLY PSYCHOANALYTIC CONTRIBUTIONS

It is of interest to note that the first studies of Breuer and Freud (21) concerned themselves with hysterical conversion symptoms, i.e., with disorders in which certain isolated bodily changes occur in the field of the skeletomuscular and sensory systems (paralyses, contractures, and sensory disturbances). Such symptoms are motivated by unconscious thought-processes which cannot find outlet in motor behavior because of repression. Accordingly, they have a specific "meaning," which can be interpreted like any psychoneurotic symptom.

Otherwise, psychoanalytic research during the first two decades of this century was not primarily concerned with psychosomatic problems. This was the era during which the main interest of psychoanalysis was the exploration of unconscious processes. In addition to conversion hysteria, the chief syndromes studied were anxiety hysteria, obsessive-compulsive neurosis, depressions, and certain sexual and behavior disorders. In so far as the physiological processes or disorders were studied and interpreted, the pattern of thought was along the mechanism of hysterical conversions.

Among the early psychoanalysts, both Abraham and Ferenczi were interested in certain problems which today we would designate as psychosomatic, and both made important contributions to these problems. Abraham applied his concepts concerning the oral and anal stages of libido development to the explanation of certain disorders of the gastrointestinal tract. He described with great precision those emotional attitudes which in normal child development accompany the ingestion of food and the elimination of feces (1, 2, 3, 4).

He further pursued Freud's view that the infant's first attitude toward the contents of his bowels is a "coprophilic" one, i.e., the infant considers his feces at first a part of his own body and a valuable possession. In the course of toilet training he acquires the idea that he has to give up this possession in order to please his parents (mother), and subsequently he develops an attitude of disgust as a reaction formation against his earlier, repressed attitude toward bowel functions. Thus the excremental act becomes associated with hostile sadistic (soiling) impulses. Neurotic patients under emotional stress often regress to these emotional reactions. Such regressions may be important in many gastrointestinal disturbances in later life.

Ferenczi, too, was interested in many of the nonverbal (nonpsychological) means by which emotions may be expressed within the organism (36, 37, 39). Many of his thoughts concerning the psychological implications of fundamental physiological processes, such as growth and propagation, have influenced later psychosomatic research. In particular, his discrimination between the erotic and the utilitarian functions of different physiological processes has been further pursued by the theoretical formulations of Alexander and French.

Ferenczi also made extensive use of the concept of regression, the importance of which he demonstrated in all types of biological phenomena. In his concept of "patho-neurosis," he emphasized the fact that all injuries to the body may favor an autoerotic preoccupation with the affected organ (36). Although this term has not gained acceptance, Ferenczi's concepts concerning the narcissistic regression which occurs as a result of physical trauma or organic disease—including problems of war neurosis—have had a deep influence on subsequent psychoanalytic thinking (38). In a psychoanalytic study of patients with general paresis, made in collaboration with Hollos, Ferenczi for the first time used the concept of adaptation of the personality to its organic defects (57).

As has been emphasized before, most of the early psychosomatic contributions, particularly those of Jelliffe (59–63) and Groddeck (53), attempted to interpret physiological dysfunctions outside the neuromuscular and sensory systems with the same conceptual tools as had been used successfully in respect to hysterical conversion symptoms. In his early writings Felix Deutsch (27, 28, 29) also followed the same trend and tried to interpret many physiological disorders as hysterical conversions which express a definite unconscious psychic content.

One of the few early authors who did not fall into the foregoing methodological error is Paul Schilder. His book *The Image and Appearance of the Human Body* (78) contains a wealth of clinical observation and hypotheses. Schilder's concept of body image is closely connected with the psychoanalytic concept of the ego as a system of perception and perhaps also as an "entity." It has an important bearing on the problem of what constitutes a hysterical conversion.

## THE PSYCHOSOMATIC ERA IN MEDICINE

In the last twenty years a new phase of psychosomatic research developed which was largely initiated by the conceptual clarification of the difference between hysterical conversion symptoms and vegetative responses to psychological stimuli (Alexander, 8). It was recognized that the similarity between a hysterical conversion symptom, such as the paralysis of a limb, on the one hand, and the vegetative responses to emotions, such as increased gastric secretion or increased blood pressure, on the other hand, consists merely in the fact that both conditions are "psychogenic," that is to say, they are caused by a chronically unrelieved emotional tension. The mechanisms involved, however, are fundamentally different, both physiologically and psychodynamically (8, 9). The hysterical conversion symptom is an attempt to relieve an emotional tension in a symbolic way; it is a symbolic (displaced) expression of a definite emotional content. This mechanism is restricted to the voluntary neuromuscular or perceptive systems whose functions are to express and relieve emotions. In contrast to this, a vegetative neurosis consists of a psychogenic dysfunction of a vegetative organ which is not under the control of the voluntary neuromuscular system and which therefore does not express any (primary) psychological meaning. The vegetative symptom is not a substitute expression of the emotion but its (normal) physiological concomitant. The pathologic nature of the condition consists primarily in the fact that, under continued emotional stimuli caused by unresolved conflicts, the vegetative responses become chronic. In time they may lead to irreversible tissue changes, resulting in clear-cut organic syndromes. This view introduced a new etiological concept into medicine: that organic illness may result, at least partially, from chronic neurotic conflicts.

This distinction between *two fundamentally different types of symptom formation* (conversion and vegetative neurosis) has become generally accepted, although it is frequently stated in somewhat different terms. It may be noted also that, according to Fenichel (35), the basic difference between what we today call "organ-neurotic"[1] symptoms on the one hand, and psychoneurotic symptoms, on the other, was recognized by Freud a long time ago. In a paper on psychogenic visual disturbances (43), Freud suggested the distinction between two types of psychogenic symptoms, differentiating the functions of an organ as it serves sexuality or utility. This distinction corresponds to Freud's views at that time (1910) concerning the duality of instincts (i.e., sexual and ego instincts). This idea was later taken up and elaborated by Ferenczi (36, 39).

1. The terms "organ neurosis" and "vegetative neurosis" are used synonymously.

The foregoing difference between two types of symptom formation was stated in still another way by Edward Glover, as follows:

Following this approach it is possible to draw two fundamental distinctions between the psychoneuroses and all psychosomatic disorders, first, that the *process of symptom-formation in the psychoneuroses follows a standardized psychic pattern*, and second, that *the psychoneuroses have psychic content and meaning. Psychosomatic disorders*, on the other hand, although influenced by psychic reactions at some point or another in their progress, *have in themselves no psychic content, and consequently do not represent stereotyped patterns of conflict*. Should they develop psychic meaning, it may be assumed that a psychoneurotic process has been superimposed on a psychosomatic foundation [48, pp. 170–71].

Thus both Alexander and Glover emphasize that organ-neurotic symptoms do not express any *primary* psychic meaning; in addition to this, Alexander connects hysterical symptoms with the voluntary neuromuscular and sensory perceptive systems, whereas Glover defines an additional difference in terms of the presence or absence of standardized or stereotyped patterns of conflict. Both these factors deserve further comment.

Glover's second distinction between psychoneuroses and psychosomatic disorders refers to the existence of a standardized pattern of conflict in the former and its absence in the latter. This point is of interest, since it has a bearing on the problem of specificity of somatic symptoms. In contrast to the specific pattern in which, for example, phobias or obsessions develop, the development of somatic symptoms in Glover's opinion is not governed by similar specific *psychological* patterns; he relates the nature of the choice of these symptoms to a number of determinants, such as constitutional factors, the depth of regression, the nature of the distribution of libido, etc.

Concerning the restriction of hysterical conversion symptoms to certain structures—defined on an anatomical and physiological basis—Szasz called attention to the fact that this rule applies only to motor (or discharge) symptoms. Thus, for example, in the case of hysterical pain the symptom does not depend upon any special type of peripheral innervation, such as the cerebrospinal conduction system. The mechanism in such a case does not rest on primarily physiological foundations but rather on the patient's own *body image*. That is to say, such a symptom may occur or, more precisely, may be referred to any part of the body which has a psychic representation. We may further note in this connection that when we think of "psychosomatic responses" we have in mind, as a rule, only motor or discharge phenomena. This follows inevitably from the fact that perception is, in the last analysis, a function of the ego or of the total psychological integration of the person at any particular time. Discussion of this interesting and important problem of perception in general and pain in particular, however, would lead us too far afield, and we cannot, therefore, pursue it any further at this time other than to state that here lies what appears to us a relatively unexplored area of psychosomatic research.

Gradually more and more systematic studies of emotional factors of different organic diseases were undertaken in different research centers. The fundamental theoretical concept underlying the psychosomatic studies conducted at the Chicago Institute for Psychoanalysis (10) was that emotional states do not express themselves in external behavior only but that the internal physiological processes also respond to every emotional state in an adaptive manner. This concept leaned heavily on Cannon's experimental studies of the physiological changes which regularly follow certain emotional states, such as anger and fear (22). These investigations, however, went further than studying the internal physiological responses to such basic emotional states as rage and fear. On the basis of their clinical studies, Alexander and his co-workers came to the conclusion that specific emotional states elicit specific physiological responses. They postulated, for example, that oral-incorporating cravings have a specific effect upon gastric secretion and motility; that rage, depending on its different psychological representations, may influence either the neuromuscular, the gastrointestinal, or the vascular system. In these studies the psychological processes observed were not brought into connection with the entire disease picture but rather with a specific physiological process, such as gastric secretion, vascular contraction, or muscular tension.

At the same time, Dunbar (30, 31, 32) and her collaborators paid more attention to the overt personality features which are commonly found in patients with certain organic disturbances. Stimulating though these studies were, they did not reveal any specific causal connection between psychological and organic processes. It is probable that what Dunbar observed were frequent and typical defense reactions against some basic conflicts which were present in certain organic diseases. In other words,

Dunbar observed rather distant end-results of the various psychological mechanisms which are more directly connected with disturbed organic functions.

At the present stage of development one of the central problems in psychosomatic medicine is that of the specific nature of the emotional stimuli involved in different organic disorders.

## THE PROBLEM OF SPECIFICITY

There are three main schools of thought concerning this problem. According to the first view, mentioned above, the psychological factors which influence or disturb the functions of the vegetative organs are as specific as those which have been established in cases of conversion hysteria. They have an ideational content, a symbolic meaning, which can be interpreted in psychological terms: the affected visceral organ expresses the unconscious content, just as a hysterical conversion symptom is a symbolic expression of repressed psychological content. In psychoanalysis this view is the oldest one and at present is largely abandoned.

The second school of thought expresses a view which tends in the opposite direction. According to it, the nature of the active emotional factors may not determine the nature of the vegetative disturbance. Many different psychological stimuli may call forth the same vegetative responses. The nature of the vegetative disturbance depends largely on constitutional factors or on a previously acquired vulnerability of the affected organ. This view takes over only one component of the Freudian concept of hysterical conversion, namely, that of "bodily compliance." Under the influence of emotions, organic disturbances may develop according to the existing vulnerable spots within the organism. The person with a susceptible gastrointestinal system will react to emotional conflicts with stomach or bowel disorders. The person whose Achilles' heel is in the circulatory system will respond to emotional disturbances with cardiac or vascular symptoms. The vulnerability of the involved organ may be due to heredity, previous organic disease, or some other factors.

The third view which has been the working hypothesis of the investigative work at the Chicago Institute for Psychoanalysis takes an intermediary position between these two approaches. It does not discount the concept of the vulnerability of the affected organs, but it adds another factor, based primarily on

Cannon's original formulations (22, 23). According to this view, to every emotional state there corresponds a characteristic physiological response which in itself is not pathologic but is an integral part of the emotional state. Stimulation of the sympatho-adrenal system, resulting in increased carbohydrate metabolism, faster heart action, and elevation of blood pressure, together with a relative inhibition of digestive functions, are all constituent parts of the state of rage. The physiological concomitants of anxiety are similar to, although probably not identical with, those of rage. Both states are common in emergency situations. Relaxation and emotional withdrawal from external affairs go with a physiological state which is the opposite of that found in emergency situations. The physiological concomitants of a relaxed state are characterized by increased anabolic and storing processes. The gastrointestinal functions are stimulated, while the functions of the skeletal muscles and of the circulatory and respiratory systems are inhibited. These changes—both in emergency and in the relaxed state—are adaptive reactions of the vegetative organs to the total situation in which the organism finds itself. They fulfil a physiological function. This theory gives full recognition to the local vulnerability of the affected organs but at the same time postulates a certain specific correlation between the emotional state and its physiological concomitants or sequelae: the nature of the emotional state determines the type of physiological response. The coexistence of both factors (the somatic local vulnerability of the affected organ and the specific emotional constellation) is responsible for the organic disturbance.

As has been mentioned before, Dunbar's point of view differs from the foregoing, inasmuch as it postulates certain overt personality features characteristic of different diseases. These features appear in overt behavior and can be described by personality profile studies, as proposed by Dunbar.

Alexander (9) emphasized that the specific correlation is not between overt personality features and vegetative response but between the latter and certain, mostly unconscious, emotional constellations which may be present in very different types of personalities and which may appear and disappear during the life of the same person. Accordingly, the specific relationship between disease and psychological factors is much less static than is postulated by Dunbar's concept.

## PSYCHOSOMATIC MECHANISMS

In the present stage of psychosomatic medicine, there is a certain number of theoretical conceptions of a general nature which are utilized rather widely by workers currently active in this field. These conceptions rest on many well-established observations concerning psychophysiologic interrelations; they show the influence particularly of the views of Darwin, Cannon, and Freud.

### VOLUNTARY BEHAVIOR

Psychologically, voluntary behavior can be described in terms of motives and goals. The physiological functions which are suited to achieve certain goals can thus be understood in terms of their utility, much as in the case of certain functions of a machine. These physiological functions are mediated by the voluntary nervous system, their end-organs being the striated musculature. From a nosological viewpoint, disturbances in these functions may give rise to hysterical conversion symptoms. (In a wider sense, there are many other types of failures in co-ordinated voluntary behavior, comprising essentially all disturbances in interpersonal relations. The mechanisms here described are not presented and cannot be used as a basis for a rigid classification of psychiatric syndromes.)

### EXPRESSIVE INNERVATIONS

Expressive innervations are specific physiological processes, such as weeping, laughing, blushing, sighing, etc., which take place under the influence of specific emotional tensions (Darwin, 26). The physiological systems involved in these patterns of behavior include both the voluntary (cerebrospinal) and the autonomic nervous systems; moreover, in expressive innervations skeletal muscles may become activated through extra-pyramidal pathways, in contrast to the pyramidal conduction system which activates voluntary movements. Psychologically, expressive innervations cannot be understood in terms of utilitarian goals; they are discharge phenomena, and their only goal or "utility" is to secure relief from emotional tension. Thus weeping, for example, helps to discharge the painful feelings associated with grief. Disturbances of these functions are usually classified with hysterical conversion symptoms (e.g., hysterical laughter or weeping). However, it would be more nearly correct to regard such disturbances as bridging the gap between hysterical conversions and vegetative neuroses, since they combine features of both. In blushing or hysterical weeping, for example, the symptom may indeed be regarded as a hysterical conversion, since it expresses a specific unconscious psychological meaning in a bodily change; however, since the physiological pathways activated in this process include certain functions of the autonomic nervous system, a characteristic feature of a vegetative neurosis is also present.

### PSYCHOSEXUAL PHENOMENA

Psychosexual phenomena are essentially similar to expressive innervations. Indeed, it is, par excellence, by means of sexual activity that the organism can rid itself of emotional tensions. Only in certain mature manifestations of sexuality is the aim of race preservation served also. The pregenital forms of sexuality discharge instinctual tensions which cannot be described in terms of utility, from the point of view either of self-preservation or of race preservation. The physiological mechanisms in sexual phenomena consist in complicated and not yet fully understood combinations of voluntary innervations, together with autonomic and hormonal changes (e.g., copulation, erection, ejaculation, orgasm, periodic changes in sexual receptivity, etc.) (15, 40). Because of this complex participation of cerebrospinal, autonomic, and endocrine responses, the disturbances of sexual functions cannot be rigidly classified as hysterical conversions or vegetative neuroses; different sexual disturbances may include features of both mechanisms, in varying proportions (e.g., frigidity and amenorrhea). The psychological aspects of these phenomena have been well explored by psychoanalytic studies of the last fifty years. Their physiology is still largely unknown.

### VEGETATIVE RESPONSES

Vegetative responses consist of visceral reactions to emotional stimuli. Most of the current psychosomatic studies are concerned with these mechanisms.

1. *Adaptive responses, the "vegetative retreat," and "regressive innervations."*—As was postulated by Cannon (23), the main function of the sympathetic division of the autonomic nervous system is the regulation of internal vegetative functions in relation to external activities, particularly in emergency situations.

Thus adaptive responses in emergency situations consist of the stimulation of those functions which are needed for fight or flight; this is accomplished by the activation of the sympatho-adrenal system.

In the relaxed state, on the other hand, there is normally a withdrawal of interest from the environment, and the vegetative responses corresponding to this state are under the dominant influence of the parasympathetic branch of the autonomic nervous system; this results in stimulation of the digestive and storing (anabolic) functions and in a relative diminution in catabolic functions. While these responses are appropriate in the relaxed state, some patients react to effort, anxiety, and certain conflict situations with emotional withdrawal, and the corresponding vegetative responses ensue. In such cases these responses are paradoxical and can be interpreted as regressive solutions of the necessity to meet the emergency situation with adequate externally directed responses. This type of autoplastic response was designated by Alexander (9) as the "vegetative retreat."

Following upon this general schema, Szasz (87) found it possible to interpret certain autonomic dysfunctions more specifically as regressions to earlier, infantile modes of autonomic functioning. He also emphasized that, instead of speaking of a preponderance of one or the other branch of the autonomic nervous system or of an "autonomic imbalance" in psychosomatic disorders, what characterizes many of these syndromes is a localized *parasympathetic (cholinergic) hyperfunction* (e.g., peptic ulcer, diarrhea, asthma, neurodermatitis, etc.); *these autonomic dysfunctions represent regressions in specific physiological activities.* For example, the vagal hyperactivity of the patient with peptic ulcer was shown to be similar to the vagal preponderance which exists during the first two years of life, at a time when the sympathetic supply to the gastrointestinal tract is not yet fully developed (87). Similarly, some cases of diarrhea could be shown to be related to a reactivation of the gastrocolic reflex mechanism which is most active during infancy (85). On the basis of such examples, together with certain theoretical considerations, it was suggested that such patterns of autonomic response (localized parasympathetic hyperfunctions) be designated as "regressive innervations"; in contrast to this type of response, certain chronic sympathetic excitations of organs or organ-systems were designated as "concomitant innervations."

2. *Life-situations, emotions, and physiology.* — Harold G. Wolff, Stewart Wolf, and their associates studied a large number of physiological reactions under experimentally induced emotional states. Their study of the subject with gastric fistula, "Tom," now belongs among the medical classics (91). Their method in this case consisted of making careful observations of gastric activity, together with certain physiological measurements, under varying life-situations and in response to experimentally induced emotional conditions. They made similar studies on the eye (74), on the mucous membranes of the colon (50), bronchi (81, 82), nose (58), and on patients with essential hypertension (90) and diabetes mellitus (55, 56). Wolff interprets many of these reactions as serving the purpose of warding off or keeping out noxious stimuli. Illustrative of such an interpretation is the following:

> Conspicuous among defensive protective reactions are those involving the nose and airways. It has been observed that in reaction to assaults and threats, certain individuals occlude their air passages and limit the ventilatory exchange by vasodilatation, turgescence, hypersecretion and contraction of smooth and skeletal muscle. The changes, especially in the upper respiratory airways, give rise to a variety of symptoms, notably pain and obstruction, the latter often leading to secondary infection, and the prolongation of morbid processes. Also the individual exhibits a behavior pattern and attitude of a non-participation in interpersonal relations [94, p. 1075].

Wolff's interpretation (92, 94) is essentially an extension of Cannon's basic philosophy concerning the mechanisms of "fight or flight" to a great many physiological reactions not considered or accounted for by Cannon. Yet Wolff's hypothesis contributes little toward the solution of the problem of specificity of symptoms, as it holds no clue to the question of why one particular organ-system should be affected in a particular case rather than in another. Moreover, although Wolff sometimes refers to the infantile prototypes of such reactions, he does not utilize the psychoanalytic concept of "regression." It is therefore implied that the reactions mentioned are considered *defensive in a temporally current sense* (that is, they are considered *currently useful*). It is readily seen that the psychoanalytic interpretation of such symptoms is similar, but with the difference that such symptoms are viewed as *regressions to earlier developmental patterns of reaction (defense), which are reactivated as a result of some current conflict*. The chief value of the work of Wolf and Wolff lies in their numerous and accurate observations concerning a wide va-

riety of psychosomatic reactions. They do not differentiate, however, between conscious and unconscious psychological processes
and make no reference to the psychoanalytically well-established
phenomenon of regression, a conception without which the "defensive" nature of many physiological dysfunctions cannot be
explained.

3. *Endocrinological responses in chronic stress.*—Physiological
adaptations to stress occur in every part of the body. In addition
to psychological adaptations, the most extensively studied and
best-understood physiological changes which occur in response
to stress are those mediated by the voluntary and autonomic
nervous systems. That the endocrine system participates in the
body's defenses in such situations has been known for some time,
but it was only recently that a comprehensive theory concerning
these endocrine reactions has been put forward. Hans Selye (79,
80) co-ordinated a vast number of observations under the name
of the "general adaptation syndrome"; this term designates a
complex chain of events, initiated by a variety of stressful situations ("stressors") and mediated by *hormonal* mechanisms. According to this theory, the first hormonal response to stress is the
"alarm reaction." In the case of prolonged stress, chronic hormonal defensive reactions ensue ("the stage of resistance"); and it
is these chronic and excessive hormonal changes, mediated primarily by the anterior pituitary and adrenal cortex, which lead to
various pathologic changes in end-organs, designated as "diseases
of adaptation" (e.g., arthritis, periarteritis nodosa, etc.). Understanding of the precise influence of psychological factors upon
the endocrine system is still largely unexplored territory.

4. *Dissociation of physiologically co-ordinated functions.*—
Sydney G. Margolin (68) and his associates recently reported
that, in a patient under psychoanalytic observation, under certain
circumstances various gastric functions may become dissociated;
for example, there may occur changes in gastric motility and the
secretion of hydrochloric acid and pepsin which do not run parallel to each other but vary in an independent and apparently
random manner. Hitherto, most psychosomatic studies were concerned with hyperfunction or hypofunction. These observations
point to dissociation of an organ's functions as another possible
disease-producing mechanism. Szasz (83, 84) has raised a similar
question in connection with the normally associated functions of
the salivary and gastric glands. He noted that hypersalivation

occurs frequently in pregnant women, whereas the incidence of duodenal ulcers in such cases is extremely low. The question was raised whether the secretory activities of the salivary and gastric glands might become dissociated under such circumstances. The significance of these observations remains to be evaluated and depends on further studies of the phenomenon of dissociation of the functions of single organs or organ-systems.

## Psychological Factors in Vegetative and Psychosexual Disorders

During the last twenty years a great many psychosomatic studies concerned themselves with the detection of the role of specific emotional factors in different organic diseases. The essential features of the conceptual framework of these studies were described briefly in the previous section ("Psychosomatic Mechanisms"). It may be added now that each of the syndromes to be described will fall into one of two categories, depending on whether psychological factors lead to the physiological disturbance or vice versa. Examples of the first type of psychophysiologic interrelationship are found in cases of duodenal ulcer or asthma, and of the second type (i.e., physiological factors leading to psychological changes) in cases of diabetes mellitus and in the psychological changes accompanying the menstrual cycle in women.

In this chapter we cannot deal with the detailed result of the numerous psychosomatic studies reported in the literature. Only the most salient features of the best-established observations (largely based on psychoanalytic studies) will be summarized.

These studies consist primarily of the description of typical psychodynamic constellations which are found consistently in different organic diseases. Although these findings are largely empirical, in the conditions most extensively investigated the psychophysiological correlations are consistent with well-established physiological data. Thus, for example, the stimulation of gastric secretion by sustained and unrelieved receptive urges makes sense, so to speak, physiologically, since feeding activates gastric secretion and, at the same time, probably represents the earliest gratification of receptive urges. Similarly, the presence of chronic unrelieved aggressive impulses in hypertension is consistent with certain aspects of the physiology of rage; that is, elevation of the blood pressure is an integral part, on the physiological level, of the affect of rage.

On the other hand, the exact etiological significance, in specific individual syndromes, of many of the psychodynamic conflicts which will be described here is still far from being established. It is thus possible that some of the psychodynamic configurations which are now correlated with physiological changes may themselves represent derivatives of more basic conflicts. Further careful psychoanalytic studies of patients suffering from these diseases may thus necessitate modifications in current hypotheses.

Finally, it should be noted that the role of *quantitative* (psychic-economic) factors in the development of the various syndromes is not taken into account by formulations stressing psychodynamic factors only. This is a shortcoming of practically all current psychosomatic studies and is probably due, at least in part, to the methodological difficulties encountered in dealing with quantitative factors. There is, of course, no way of "measuring" the intensity of the various impulses which participate in a conflict. However, careful psychoanalytic observation makes it possible for the analyst to estimate the *relative* strength of various instinctual forces and of the defenses against them. Economic considerations appear indispensable for a complete understanding of physiological dysfunctions. The role of quantitative factors may also help in elucidating the connection between some so-called "psychosomatic" diseases and psychosis (13, 47). Cases have been reported in which the remission of psychotic symptoms is followed by the development of psychosomatic symptoms and vice versa. This relationship has been observed between ulcerative colitis and paranoid schizophrenia and between asthma and paranoid schizophrenia.

## GASTROINTESTINAL DISTURBANCES

There are few vegetative functions which play such an important role in the emotional life as does the ingestion of food. From early life on, eating is associated with the feeling of security, of receiving love and care, and also with greed, possessiveness, and envy. The neurotic conflicts centering around these basic emotions may variously contribute to disturbances of the appetite (bulimia and anorexia) and of swallowing (nervous vomiting and cardiospasm) and also to dysfunctions of the digestive system (duodenal ulcer, constipation, diarrhea). What seems to be best established is that the accentuation and inhibition of the wish to receive love and protection, being deeply associated with feeding, may activate or inhibit almost any phase in the incorporation and digestion of food. Those functions which are under the control of autonomic innervations are activated or inhibited by emotional stimuli on the principle of the conditioned reflex. This is best demonstrated by the influence of the receptive cravings upon gastric secretion, which involves the following sequence of events: the wish to receive, to be taken care of, is associated on the psychological level with the wish to be fed and, physiologically, with increased gastric secretion (5, 11).

As was emphasized above, the recognition of these psychological components of illness does not constitute the full etiological theory of gastrointestinal disturbances. Similar emotional conflicts involving dependent receptive urges are found in individuals who do not suffer from any disorder of gastrointestinal functions. Still unknown coexisting local physiological or anatomical factors must be assumed to explain pathological developments as a result of this type of emotional conflict situation. In addition, quantitative (psychic-economic) factors may also play a role in determining the precise results of such conflict situations.

The excremental functions are also connected with distinct emotional attitudes from early life onward. These have been well described by the early psychoanalytic authors, particularly by Freud, Abraham, and Jones. Possessiveness, the sense of duty and obligation, the desire to give, the hostile impulses in the form of soiling, and early infantile sexual theories about pregnancy and birth (child = feces) have all been well established in fifty years of psychoanalytic studies. All these emotional attitudes influence the functions of the gastrointestinal tract and may contribute to their dysfunctions (different forms of diarrhea and constipation).

While the influence of this type of emotional attitude upon the excremental act itself, which is under voluntary control, does not raise particularly difficult theoretical questions, their influence upon peristalsis is more obscure. Recently, Szasz (85, 86) suggested the possibility that disturbances of peristalsis of the colon and rectum may result from variations in oral tendencies, through the mediation of the gastrocolic reflex. This theory rests upon what is considered as the basic rhythm of gastrointestinal activity, viz., the sequence of events in the nursing infant—hunger, feeding, defecation, and sleep. Activation of the upper portions of the gastrointestinal tract, by parasympathetic stimulation, is generally accompanied by inhibition of the colon and rectum, whereas a decrease in vagal tonus is accompanied by increased activation of the lower bowel. According to this theory, activation of oral cravings is thought to be paralleled by an increase in vagal activity, and this leads to a relative inhibition of colonic and rectal function and thus to constipation. It is postulated that satisfaction of the oral-intaking needs (either in reality or symbolically) or, more commonly, their inhibition by guilt on account of the sadistic nature of the impulses is paralleled by a decreased vagal activity; thus, through the chain of events indicated, there is increased stimulation of the sacral parasympathetics supplying the colon and rectum, and diarrhea ensues. The foregoing mechanisms may account for the effects of oral tendencies on lower gastrointestinal functions. While the role of such "oral mechanisms" appears to be considerable in many cases of constipation and diarrhea, it is likely that so-called "anal mechanisms" may also affect the functions of the colon and rectum. In other words, anal-erotic impulses may activate reflex mechanisms originating from the ano-rectal region (95).

### BRONCHIAL ASTHMA

According to French, Alexander, *et al.* (41), the inhibition of the urge to cry seems to be the nuclear emotional factor in these cases. The function of crying in the infant is to call for maternal help and attention. Later the same effect is achieved by more complex physiological functions (speech), which, like crying, involve the expiratory phase of respiration. The inhibition to confess has been established by these studies as a superimposed factor upon the inhibition to cry. The fear of being separated from mother or the maternal figure brings about the urge to regain maternal love through confession of forbidden thoughts and impulses. If this urge is inhibited, the patient who has an allergic sensitivity may respond with a typical disturbance of the respiratory function known as "asthma."

As in the field of gastrointestinal disorders, here, too, the psychological factors appear usually in combination with specific somatic factors (allergic sensitivity). The coexistence of both factors explains why in many cases the symptoms may disappear by bringing about certain changes in either one of these two types of factors—the psychological or the allergic. In most cases, only the combination of both types of factors produces the illness.

### RHEUMATOID ARTHRITIS

In this condition, as in essential hypertension, the central dynamic factor is thought to be the inhibition of hostile impulses. In these cases, however, a frequent finding is also an early propensity toward the muscular expressions of aggressive impulses. At the same time, there is a consistent history in early childhood of parental restriction of locomotory freedom. Often as a rebellion against this, there is, in arthritic women, a history of tomboyishness in pre-puberty, with great stress on physical exercise, indicating the presence of intensive muscle eroticism (Johnson, Shapiro, and Alexander, 64). In these studies correlations were attempted only between psychological factors and their possible relationship to chronic muscular tension. How chronic muscular tension may participate in the pathogenesis of the disease entity known as "rheumatoid arthritis" is not clear and requires further study (49).

### ESSENTIAL HYPERTENSION

Among the great variety of cardiovascular disturbances, the most extensive studies have been made on essential hypertension. A continuous struggle against hostile impulses is the central issue described by most authors who have studied this condition (Binger *et al.*, 20; Alexander, 6, 7; Saul, 76). The inhibition of aggressive self-assertive impulses is frequently due to a conflict expressed by the overcompensation of an underlying repressed excessive dependence: for example, the fear of losing the affection of others through hostile behavior. Characteristic findings are temper tantrums in early childhood and the frequently sudden change, mostly during puberty, from openly aggressive behavior to excessive control.

### SYNCOPE

As emphasized by Engel (33), the term "syncope," or fainting, denotes only a symptom which may be due to a variety of causes. He also suggested that the underlying pathological processes which lead to syncope may be most conveniently classified according to three basic mechanisms: "1. Altered cerebral metabolism due to circulatory disturbances; 2. Altered cerebral metabolism due to metabolic factors; 3. Psychological mechanisms not involving any known disturbance in cerebral metabolism or circulation" (33, p. 5).

The two most common types of fainting in young adults are vasodepressor and hysterical. The physiological mechanism underlying vasodepressor syncope is that of a sudden fall in blood pressure; although the fainting reaction may be initiated in any position, extreme hypotension and unconsciousness are much more likely to occur in the erect than in the recumbent position, because of the hydrostatic effect of gravity. Psychologically, fainting of this type tends to occur in situations of fear and danger, particularly when the overt expression of fear must be suppressed. Both the physiological and the psychodynamic aspects of this syndrome were studied and described with great care by Engel and Romano (33, 34, 75). Vasodepressor syncope is thus a typical example of a vegetative neurosis. In hysterical fainting, on the other hand, there are no physiological disturbances of the cardiovascular system, and the symptom represents the substitutive or symbolic expression of a repressed instinctual impulse.

### MIGRAINE

The physiological mechanisms involved in migraine have been studied by many workers, and there is general agreement concerning the role of vasomotor disturbances of the cranial arteries (93). There is disagreement, however, as to whether vasoconstriction is the primary disturbance and vasodilatation is a compensatory reaction or whether vasodilatation has an independent origin. There is also extensive literature concerning the emotional factors which may induce or contribute to these local changes in cranial blood flow. Most authors have noted the significance of repressed destructive impulses (Fromm-Reichmann, 46; Wolberg, 89; Wolff, 93). As has been stated above, the same emotional factors appear as the outstanding psychological feature in essential hypertension and in arthritis. Whether specific psychological (dynamic and economic) factors are responsible for the fact that one patient develops hypertension, another arthritis, and a third migraine headaches is still an open question. The hypothesis that the nature of the hostile impulses is important in determining the resulting physiological disturbance still needs further validation. According to Alexander (9), fully consummated aggressive behavior has three phases: (1) The conceptual phase: the preparation of the attack in fantasy, its planning and mental visualization. (2) The vegetative preparation of the body for concentrated activity. This consists in changes in metabolism and circulation. (3) The neuromuscular phase: the consummation of the aggressive act itself through co-ordinated muscular activity. The nature of the physical symptoms may depend upon the phase which is accentuated or in which the complete psychosomatic process of hostile attack becomes arrested or inhibited. If the process is arrested after the first phase, migraine headache may develop. If it progresses to the vegetative stage, hypertension may result. And if the hostile behavior is inhibited only in its last phase, namely, the actual hostile attack, arthritic symptoms will be favored. The somatic compliance resulting from vulnerability of the involved system must also be considered as a determining factor.

### HYPERTHYROIDISM

The significance of emotional factors in thyrotoxicosis has long been known through numerous clinical observations. On the basis of the studies of a number of investigators (Lidz and Whitehorn, 66, 67; Conrad, 24; Mittelmann, 73; Ham *et al.*, 54), the following features appear characteristic of this syndrome. In some cases hyperthyroidism develops suddenly following exposure to a traumatic situation; this syndrome was accordingly designated as "shock-Basedow." Usually, however, the disease develops less precipitately, and one often finds a lifelong urge toward accelerated maturation; this is thought to be a more or less specific defense against anxiety on the part of these patients (Ham *et al.*, 55). It was accordingly suggested that this continuous urge for self-sufficiency, so dominant in these patients from early childhood onward, may constitute a chronic stimulus for thyroid function, finally leading to hyperthyroidism. The fact that the primary physiological function of the thyroid gland is closely related to growth and metabolic rate is consistent with this hypothesis. The physiological details of the mechanism—of how such continual stress may stimulate thyroid hyperfunction —remain to be explained.

### DIABETES MELLITUS

Interesting psychoanalytic studies of patients with diabetes have been reported by Daniels (25) and Meyer *et al.* (70). It is difficult to ascertain the etiological significance of the psychological observations described in these cases. One of the chief difficulties in elucidating the psychosomatic aspects of this syndrome is the fact that the physiological mechanisms responsible for the development of diabetes are not fully understood. Present studies (Benedek, Mirsky *et al.*, 18) indicate that in this disease the typical psychological phenomenon—which appears as an insatiable oral need, similar to that seen in bulimia—may be an adaptation on the part of the organism to a probably hereditary metabolic insufficiency. Much of the psychological material observed in these cases can thus be interpreted as various defenses of the ego against the perception and demands of this excessive oral need.

### FATIGUE STATES

Certain recurrent or chronic fatigue states connected with disturbances of the carbohydrate-regulating mechanisms offer in many respects an opposite picture from that found in arthritis, hypertension, and migraine. This picture consists in emotional withdrawal from activity and rebellion against the necessity for continued effort, particularly against routine work undertaken without zest. According to McCulloch, Carlson, Alexander, and Portis (69, 12), continued zest and interest, much like rage, have a stimulating effect upon carbohydrate metabolism. If the organism has to perform effort-requiring accomplishments over a prolonged period of time without interest in the performance, it appears that the promptness of the carbohydrate regulation necessary for effort suffers. This may explain why extreme fatigue attacks frequently develop in persons who have to engage in such effort-requiring activities under external or internal compulsion without having interest in their task. Attacks of fatigue are particularly likely to occur when the patient has given up hope of achieving some cherished aim.

### SKIN DISEASES

Although the influence of emotional factors on diseases of the skin has been known, in one way or another, ever since biblical times (Job), precise data concerning psychophysiological interrelations in this organ-system are still relatively meager. The most extensively studied conditions are neurodermatitis, eczema, and urticaria. On the basis of psychoanalytic observations in patients with neurodermatitis, Miller (71, 72) emphasized the importance of sado-masochistic and exhibitionistic trends. Scratching, which is of paramount importance in most skin disorders, once they have developed—and may even be of some etiological importance in neurodermatitis—often expresses specific psychological conflicts; the role of both hostile and erotic (masturbatory) impulses in this activity is well established (14). In urticaria a specific correlation of the symptom with inhibited weeping has been described by Saul and Bernstein (77). Kepecs *et al.* (65) have recently described some experimental studies concerning the relationship between weeping and exudation into the skin. They found that weeping is accompanied by increased fluid secretion into the skin (using an experimentally produced blister), whereas inhibition of weeping results, first, in a drop in exudation rate, followed by a rise if the inhibition is sustained.

Itching and scratching, leading to skin changes as a result of chronic traumata to the skin, are closely related to erotization of different parts of the body (such as the anus); in such cases, scratching often provides a conscious erotic pleasure and is clearly a masturbatory equivalent.

### DISTURBANCES OF SEXUAL FUNCTIONS

The existence of an intimate interrelation between emotions and sexual functions is a matter of common knowledge. Indeed, what we now consider a relatively new approach to medicine, namely, the psychosomatic approach, had already characterized the earliest psychoanalytic studies concerned with the problem of sexuality. In his essay *Three Contributions to the Theory of Sex* (42), Freud described certain behavioral manifestations of infants and children which he considered the developmental precursors of adult sexual activities. Indeed, a precise description of the "psychosexual development" of human beings was one of the first discoveries of psychoanalysis.[2] The course of the psychosexual development of the individual forms the core of the development of the entire personality (17).

For a proper understanding of disturbances of the sexual functions, precise knowledge of the normal functions of these organ-systems—as in the case of all other organ-systems—is essential. We shall not undertake a detailed presentation of this information here but will merely indicate briefly the interrelations between

2. It is of interest to note that the term "psychosexual" attempted to bridge the gap between the psychological and the somatic aspects of behavior, to which later the much-criticized term "psychosomatic" was applied.

certain endocrine functions and sexual behavior. In the male the full development of mature sexual function is dependent on the normal development of testicular function, which takes place during puberty under the influence of pituitary stimulation. The secondary sex characteristics of the male develop in response to androgenic stimulation. Similarly, in the female the development of mature sexual function depends on the activation of the ovaries by the pituitary; but, whereas in the male the testes produce but a single type of hormone, in the female there is a cyclical production of two different types of hormones—estrogens and progesterone, the hormones which control menstruation.[3]

Some disturbance of sexual function occurs in every neurosis and psychosis. A classification of such dysfunctions is, however, extremely difficult. The various terms in common usage designating sexual disturbances do not refer to syndromes or disease entities but are rather *descriptions of symptoms*.

The term "impotence" actually refers to a number of symptoms which are all characterized by some disturbance in performing the act of intercourse with orgasm. It may include such varied manifestations as lack of interest in the sexual act, inability to have or maintain an erection, premature or retarded ejaculation, or intercourse and ejaculation without orgasm, etc. From the psychological point of view, the most important conflict in all these symptoms is usually related to *castration anxiety*, that is to say, to unconscious fears connected with injury to the penis; on an even deeper unconscious level this may be equated in some cases with fears of complete annihilation and death. In addition to this basic factor—which may be regarded as a common denominator among all symptoms of sexual dysfunction—a number of other psychological factors may be of varying importance. Foremost among these is the nature of the *pregenital organization of the libido* in the particular person; in other words, the relative importance of oral, anal, urethral, skin, and other bodily areas in the childhood sexual history of the individual. In connection with this we may also mention the importance of *infantile sexual theories*, which often have the profoundest influence on the later development and manifestations of the sexual drive.

Parallel with the foregoing psychological phenomena, there occur physiological changes in the genitals which lead to the

3. For a more detailed consideration of this subject, as well as of the various psychosexual dysfunctions, see Benedek (16).

actual somatic manifestations of the disorder. The precise physiological changes responsible for many of these symptoms are still poorly understood, as, indeed, are the exact hormonal and neurophysiological control of erection and ejaculation (40). There is an intimate connection between anal, urethral, and genital functions (39).

The psychosexual dysfunctions of women may be divided into two large groups: (1) disturbances connected with the act of intercourse and (2) disturbances connected with the process of menstruation and childbearing. *Frigidity* is probably the commonest dysfunction. The psychological motivations of this symptom are analogous to those of impotence in men; they usually relate to fears of being damaged by the penis and of fears of pregnancy and childbirth. The term "frigidity," like "impotence," does not refer to any single condition but denotes a rather wide variety of phenomena, ranging from severe phobic abhorrence of intercourse and vaginismus to cases where the sexual act may be pleasurable in varying degrees but is without orgasm.

Disturbances of menstruation and childbearing are numerous and complex. The interplay between the various hormonal stimulations and emotions, as seen during the menstrual cycle, has been discussed elsewhere (17). Severe disturbances of menstruation, including complete amenorrhea, may be the physiological manifestation of severe conflicts over sexuality with profound inhibition of sexual functions.

Conflicts related to childbearing may find expression in such diverse symptoms as pseudocyesis, sterility (which may consist of an inability to conceive as well as an inability to carry a pregnancy to term), or hyperemesis gravidarum and may lead to postpartum psychosis.

One of the most significant psychosomatic studies belonging to this field is that of Benedek and Rubenstein (19). These authors attempted to correlate the psychological attitudes in women with changes in the estrogen and progesterone level occurring during the ovarian cycle. They found that increased estrogen production goes with an increased turning of libidinal interest toward heterosexual contacts. To the increased progesterone production following ovulation, on the other hand, there corresponds a turning of the libidinal charge toward the self (narcissistic regression).

## PROBLEMS OF THERAPY

It was emphasized that psychosomatic medicine, as a method of investigation, consists essentially in the combination of the investigative techniques of medicine and psychoanalysis. It follows that there is no such thing as a specific technique of psychosomatic therapy. The psychosomatic approach must rather be considered as a universal principle of medicine (one could say a medical "Weltanschauung") which should be applied to every patient, for every patient, in addition to being the carrier of a diseased organ, is also an individual human being whose emotional reactions are involved in the specific disease process. The nature of the psychophysiological interaction may vary from case to case; in some, psychological (interpersonal) stress may be etiologically related to the ensuing disease, while in others the person's emotional reactions are of an essentially reactive nature to a primarily somatic (e.g., genetic, traumatic) disease process.

Knowledge of personality development and psychodynamics is increasingly considered one of the basic sciences of medicine, to be taught to every physician. Psychopathology, at the same time, is seeking its place as a counterpart of somatic pathology. And, accordingly, psychiatric diagnosis and management are becoming indispensable in an integrated therapeutic approach to all chronic diseases. Although every physician must be able to make at least a rough psychological diagnosis, decisions concerning psychotherapy—as in the case of other specialized treatments—must rest with the psychiatric specialist. It is important to emphasize that whenever the psychological approach consists in more than providing emotional support, that is to say, whenever it attempts to penetrate behind the ego's defenses and uncover etiological factors, it is likely to activate emotional tension and cause an exacerbation of somatic symptoms. Indeed, we are only now beginning to understand the functional value of somatic illness for the total personality. Also in patients with organic disease psychological treatment may have to be supplemented by, or intelligently co-ordinated with, somatic measures, whenever the latter type of treatment is indicated. Finally, it should be noted that attempts to treat patients with certain organic diseases through psychoanalysis are of relatively recent origin and that the analysis of such patients often presents special problems, not unlike the problems encountered in the analysis of psychotic patients.

## BIBLIOGRAPHY

1. ABRAHAM, KARL. "The First Pregenital Stage of the Libido," in *Selected Papers* (London: Hogarth Press, 1927), chap. xii.
2. ABRAHAM, KARL. "The Narcissistic Evaluation of Excretory Processes in Dreams and Neurosis," in *Selected Papers* (London: Hogarth Press, 1927), chap. xvii.
3. ABRAHAM, KARL. "Contributions to the Theory of the Anal Character," in *Selected Papers* (London: Hogarth Press, 1927), chap. xxiii.
4. ABRAHAM, KARL. "The Influence of Oral Erotism on Character-Formation," in *Selected Papers* (London: Hogarth Press, 1927), chap. xxiv.
5. ALEXANDER, FRANZ. *The Medical Value of Psychoanalysis* (New York: W. W. Norton & Co., 1936).
6. ALEXANDER, FRANZ. "Psychoanalytic Study of a Case of Essential Hypertension," *Psychosom. Med.*, 1:139, 1939.
7. ALEXANDER, FRANZ. "Emotional Factors in Essential Hypertension," *Psychosom. Med.*, 1:173, 1939.
8. ALEXANDER, FRANZ. "Fundamental Concepts of Psychosomatic Research: Psychogenesis, Conversion, Specificity," *Psychosom. Med.*, 5:205, 1943.
9. ALEXANDER, FRANZ. *Psychosomatic Medicine: Its Principles and Applications* (New York: W. W. Norton & Co., 1950).
10. ALEXANDER, FRANZ; FRENCH, T. M.; *et al.* *Studies in Psychosomatic Medicine: An Approach to the Cause and Treatment of Vegetative Disturbances* (New York: Ronald Press, 1948).
11. ALEXANDER, FRANZ, *et al.* "The Influence of Psychologic Factors upon Gastrointestinal Disturbances: A Symposium," *Psychoanalyt. Quart.*, 3:501, 1934.
12. ALEXANDER, FRANZ, and PORTIS, S. A. "A Psychosomatic Study of Hypoglycaemic Fatigue," *Psychosom. Med.*, 6:191, 1944.
13. APPEL, JESSE, and ROSEN, S. R. "Psychotic Factors in Psychosomatic Illness," *Psychosom. Med.*, 12:236, 1950.
14. BARTEMEIER, L. H. "A Psychoanalytic Study of a Case of Chronic Exudative Dermatitis," *Psychoanalyt. Quart.*, 7:216, 1938.
15. BEACH, F. A. *Hormones and Behavior: A Survey of Interrelationships between Endocrine Secretions and Patterns of Overt Response* (New York: Paul B. Hoeber, 1948).
16. BENEDEK, THERESE. "The Functions of the Sexual Apparatus and Their Disturbances," in FRANZ ALEXANDER, *Psychosomatic Medicine* (New York: W. W. Norton & Co., 1950), chap. xv.
17. BENEDEK, THERESE. "Development of the Personality," *this volume*, chap. iv.
18. BENEDEK, THERESE; MIRSKY, I. A.; *et al.* Unpublished observations.
19. BENEDEK, THERESE, and RUBENSTEIN, B. B. *The Sexual Cycle in Women: The Relation between Ovarian Function and Psychodynamic Processes* ("Psychosomatic Medicine Monographs," Vol. 3, Nos. 1 and 2 [1942]).

20. BINGER, C. A. L.; ACKERMAN, N. W.; COHN, A. E.; SCHROEDER, H. A.; and STEELE, J. H. *Personality in Arterial Hypertension* (New York: American Society for Research in Psychosomatic Problems, 1945).

21. BREUER, JOSEPH, and FREUD, SIGMUND. *Studies in Hysteria* (New York: Nervous and Mental Disease Publishing Co., 1936).

22. CANNON, W. B. *Bodily Changes in Pain, Hunger, Fear, and Rage: An Account of Recent Researches into the Function of Emotional Excitement* (New York: D. Appleton & Co., 1929).

23. CANNON, W. B. *The Wisdom of the Body* (New York: W. W. Norton & Co., 1939).

24. CONRAD, AGNES. "The Psychiatric Study of Hyperthyroid Patients," *J. Nerv. & Ment. Dis.*, 79:505, 1934.

25. DANIELS, G. E. "Analysis of a Case of Neurosis with Diabetes Mellitus," *Psychoanalyt. Quart.*, 5:513, 1936.

26. DARWIN, C. R. *The Expression of the Emotions in Man and Animals* (London: J. Murray, 1872).

27. DEUTSCH, FELIX. "Psychoanalyse und Organkrankheiten," *Internat. Ztschr. f. Psychoanal.*, 8:290, 1922.

28. DEUTSCH, FELIX. "Zur Bildung des Konversionssymptoms," *Internat. Ztschr. f. Psychoanal.*, 10:380, 1924.

29. DEUTSCH, FELIX. "Der gesunde und der kranke Körper in psychoanalytischer Betrachtung," *Internat. Ztschr. f. Psychoanal.*, 12:493, 1926.

30. DUNBAR, FLANDERS. *Psychosomatic Diagnosis* (New York: Paul B. Hoeber, 1943).

31. DUNBAR, FLANDERS. "Psychosomatic Medicine," in SANDOR LORAND (ed.), PSYCHOANALYSIS TODAY (New York: International Universities Press, 1944), pp. 23–41.

32. DUNBAR, FLANDERS. *Mind and Body: Psychosomatic Medicine* (New York: Random House, 1947).

33. ENGEL, G. L. *Fainting: Physiological and Psychological Considerations* (Springfield, Ill.: Charles C. Thomas, 1950).

34. ENGEL, G. L., and ROMANO, JOHN. "Studies of Syncope. IV. Biologic Interpretation of Vasodepressor Syncope," *Psychosom. Med.*, 9:288, 1947.

35. FENICHEL, OTTO. *The Psychoanalytic Theory of Neurosis* (New York: W. W. Norton & Co., 1945).

36. FERENCZI, SANDOR. "Disease- or Patho-neuroses," in *Further Contributions to the Theory and Technique of Psycho-analysis* (London: Hogarth Press, 1926), Paper No. 5.

37. FERENCZI, SANDOR. "The Phenomena of Hysterical Materialization," in *Further Contributions to the Theory and Technique of Psychoanalysis* (London: Hogarth Press, 1926), Paper No. 6.

38. FERENCZI, SANDOR. "Two Types of War Neuroses," in *Further Contributions to the Theory and Technique of Psycho-analysis* (London: Hogarth Press, 1926), Paper No. 11.

39. FERENCZI, SANDOR. *Thalassa: A Theory of Genitality* (New York: Psychoanalytic Quarterly, Inc., 1938).

40. FORD, C. S., and BEACH, F. A. *Patterns of Sexual Behavior* (New York: Harper & Bros., 1951).

41. FRENCH, T. M.; ALEXANDER, FRANZ; *et al. Psychogenic Factors in Bronchial Asthma*, Parts I and II (Psychosomatic Medicine Monographs, Vol. 1, No. 4; Vol. 2, Nos. 1 and 2 [1941]).

42. FREUD, SIGMUND. *Three Contributions to the Theory of Sex* (4th ed.; New York: Nervous and Mental Disease Publishing Co., 1930).

43. FREUD, SIGMUND. "Psychogenic Visual Disturbance According to Psychoanalytical Conceptions," in *Collected Papers* (London: Hogarth Press, 1925), Vol. 2, Paper No. 9.

44. FREUD, SIGMUND. *Inhibitions, Symptoms and Anxiety* (London: Hogarth Press, 1936).

45. FREUD, SIGMUND. *An Outline of Psychoanalysis* (New York: W. W. Norton & Co., 1949).

46. FROMM-REICHMANN, FRIEDA. "Contribution to the Psychogenesis of Migraine," *Psychoanalyt. Rev.*, 24:26, 1937.

47. FUNKENSTEIN, D. H. "Psychophysiologic Relationship of Asthma and Urticaria to Mental Illness," *Psychosom. Med.*, 12:377, 1950.

48. GLOVER, EDWARD. *Psycho-analysis: A Handbook for Medical Practitioners and Students of Comparative Psychology* (2d ed.; New York: Staples Press, 1949).

49. GOTTSCHALK, L. A.; SEROTA, H. M.; and SHAPIRO, L. B. "Psychologic Conflict and Neuromuscular Tension. I. Preliminary Report on a Method, as Applied to Rheumatoid Arthritis," *Psychosom. Med.*, 12:315, 1950.

50. GRACE, W. J.; WOLF, STEWART; and WOLFF, H. G. *The Human Colon* (New York: Paul B. Hoeber, 1951).

51. GRODDECK, GEORG. "Ueber die Psychoanalyse des Organischen im Menschen," *Internat. Ztschr. f. Psychoanal.*, 7:252, 1921.

52. GRODDECK, GEORG. "Traumarbeit und Arbeit des organischen Symptoms," *Internat. Ztschr. f. Psychoanal.*, 12:504, 1926.

53. GRODDECK, GEORG. *The Book of the It: Psychoanalytic Letters to a Friend* (New York: Nervous and Mental Disease Publishing Co., 1928).

54. HAM, G. C.; ALEXANDER, FRANZ; and CARMICHAEL, H. T. "A Psychosomatic Theory of Thyrotoxicosis," *Psychosom. Med.*, 13:18, 1951.

55. HINKLE, L. E., and WOLF, STEWART. "Experimental Study of Life Situations, Emotions, and the Occurrence of Acidosis in a Juvenile Diabetic," *Am. J. M. Sc.*, 217:130, 1949.

56. HINKLE, L. E.; WOLF, STEWART; *et al.* "Studies in Diabetes Mellitus: Changes in Glucose, Ketone, and Water Metabolism during Stress," in *Life Stress and Bodily Disease* (Baltimore: Williams & Wilkins Co., 1950), chap. xxii.

57. HOLLOS, STEFAN, and FERENCZI, SANDOR. *Psychoanalysis and the Psychic Disorder of General Paresis* (New York: Nervous and Mental Disease Publishing Co., 1925).

58. HOLMES, T. H.; GOODELL, HELEN; WOLF, STEWART; and WOLFF, H. G. *The Nose: An Experimental Study of Reactions within the*

*Nose in Human Subjects during Varying Life Experiences* (Springfield, Ill.: Charles C. Thomas, 1950).

59. JELLIFFE, S. E. "Dupuytren's Contracture and the Unconscious: A Preliminary Statement of a Problem," *Internat. Clin.*, 3:41st ser., 184, 1931.

60. JELLIFFE, S. E. "Psychoanalysis and Internal Medicine," in SANDOR LORAND (ed.), *Psychoanalysis Today* (New York: International Universities Press, 1944), pp. 12–22.

61. JELLIFFE, S. E. "Psychopathology and Organic Disease," *Arch. Neurol. & Psychiat.*, 8:639, 1922.

62. JELLIFFE, S. E. "Somatic Pathology and Psychopathology at the Encephalitis Crossroad: A Fragment," *J. Nerv. & Ment. Dis.*, 61:561, 1925.

63. JELLIFFE, S. E., and EVANS, E. "Psoriasis as an Hysterical Conversion Symbolization," *New York State J. Med.*, 104:1077, 1916.

64. JOHNSON, A. M.; SHAPIRO, L. B.; and ALEXANDER, FRANZ. "A Preliminary Report on a Psychosomatic Study of Rheumatoid Arthritis," *Psychosom. Med.*, 9:295, 1947.

65. KEPECS, J. G.; ROBIN, MILTON; and BRUNNER, M. J. "Relationship between Certain Emotional States and Exudation into the Skin," *Psychosom. Med.*, 13:10, 1951.

66. LIDZ, THEODORE. "Emotional Factors in the Etiology of Hyperthyroidism: The Report of a Preliminary Survey," *Psychosom. Med.*, 11:2, 1949.

67. LIDZ, THEODORE, and WHITEHORN, J. C. "Life Situations, Emotions, and Graves' Disease," *Psychosom. Med.*, 12:184, 1950.

68. MARGOLIN, S. G.; ORRINGER, DAVID; KAUFMAN, M. R.; *et al.* "Variations of Gastric Functions during Conscious and Unconscious Conflict States," in *Life Stress and Bodily Disease* (Baltimore: Williams & Wilkins Co., 1950), chap. xliv.

69. McCULLOCH, W. S.; CARLSON, H. B.; and ALEXANDER, FRANZ. "Zest and Carbohydrate Metabolism," in *Life Stress and Bodily Disease* (Baltimore: Williams & Wilkins Co., 1950), chap. xxiv.

70. MEYER, ALBRECHT; BOLLMEIER, L. N.; and ALEXANDER, FRANZ. "Correlation between Emotions and Carbohydrate Metabolism in Two Cases of Diabetes Mellitus," *Psychosom. Med.*, 7:335, 1945.

71. MILLER, M. L. "Psychodynamic Mechanisms in a Case of Neurodermatitis," *Psychosom. Med.*, 10:309, 1948.

72. MILLER, M. L. "A Psychological Study of a Case of Eczema and a Case of Neurodermatitis," *Psychosom. Med.*, 4:82, 1942.

73. MITTELMANN, BELA. "Psychogenic Factors and Psychotherapy in Hyperthyreosis and Rapid Heart Imbalance," *J. Nerv. & Ment. Dis.*, 77:465, 1933.

74. RIPLEY, H. S., and WOLFF, H. G. "Life Situations, Emotions, and Glaucoma," *Psychosom. Med.*, 12:215, 1950.

75. ROMANO, JOHN, and ENGEL, G. L. "Studies of Syncope. III. The Differentiation between Vasodepressor Syncope and Hysterical Fainting," *Psychosom. Med.*, 7:3, 1945.

76. SAUL, L. J. "Hostility in Cases of Essential Hypertension," *Psychosom. Med.*, 1:153, 1939.

77. SAUL, L. J., and BERNSTEIN, CLARENCE, JR. "The Emotional Settings of Some Attacks of Urticaria," *Psychosom. Med.*, 3:349, 1941.

78. SCHILDER, PAUL. *The Image and Appearance of the Human Body: Studies in the Constructive Energies of the Psyche* (London: K. Paul, Trench, Trubner & Co., 1935).

79. SELYE, HANS. "The General Adaptation Syndrome and the Diseases of Adaptation," *J. Clin. Endocrinol.*, 6:117, 1946.

80. SELYE, HANS. *The Physiology and Pathology of Exposure to Stress: A Treatise Based on the Concepts of the General-Adaptation-Syndrome and the Diseases of Adaptation* (Montreal: Acta, Inc., 1950).

81. STEVENSON, IAN. "Variations in the Secretion of Bronchial Mucus during Periods of Life Stress," in *Life Stress and Bodily Disease* (Baltimore: Williams & Wilkins Co., 1950), chap. xxxviii.

82. STEVENSON, IAN, and WOLFF, H. G. "Life Situations, Emotions, and Bronchial Mucus," *Psychosom. Med.*, 11:223, 1949.

83. SZASZ, T. S. "Psychosomatic Aspects of Salivary Activity. I. Hypersalivation in Patients with Peptic Ulcer," in *Life Stress and Bodily Disease* (Baltimore: Williams & Wilkins Co., 1950), chap. xliii.

84. SZASZ, T. S. "Psychosomatic Aspects of Salivary Activity. II. Psychoanalytic Observations concerning Hypersalivation," *Psychosom. Med.*, 12:320, 1950.

85. SZASZ, T. S. "Physiologic and Psychodynamic Mechanisms in Constipation and Diarrhea," *Psychosom. Med.*, 13:112, 1951.

86. SZASZ, T. S. "Oral Mechanisms in Constipation and Diarrhea," *Internat. J. Psycho-Analysis*, 32:196, 1951.

87. SZASZ, T. S. "Psychoanalysis and the Autonomic Nervous System," to be published in *Psychoanalyt. Rev.*

88. WEISS, EDWARD, and ENGLISH, O. S. *Psychosomatic Medicine* (2d ed.; Philadelphia: W. B. Saunders Co., 1949).

89. WOLBERG, L. R. "Psychosomatic Correlations in Migraine: Report of a Case," *Psychiat. Quart.*, 19:60, 1945.

90. WOLF, STEWART; PFEIFFER, J. B.; RIPLEY, H. S.; WINTER, O. S.; and WOLFF, H. G. "Hypertension as a Reaction Pattern to Stress: Summary of Experimental Data on Variations in Blood Pressure and Renal Blood Flow," *Ann. Int. Med.*, 29:1056, 1948.

91. WOLF, STEWART, and WOLFF, H. G. *Human Gastric Function: An Experimental Study of a Man and His Stomach* (2d ed.; New York: Oxford University Press, 1947).

92. WOLFF, H. G. "Protective Reaction Patterns and Disease," *Ann. Int. Med.*, 27:944, 1947.

93. WOLFF, H. G. *Headache and Other Head Pain* (New York: Oxford University Press, 1948).

94. WOLFF, H. G. "Life Stress and Bodily Disease—a Formulation," in *Life Stress and Bodily Disease* (Baltimore: Williams & Wilkins Co., 1950), chap. lxix.

95. YOUMANS, W. B. *Nervous and Neurohumoral Regulation of Intestinal Motility* (New York: Inter-Science Publishers, 1949), chap. xvi.

# XIII

## SOME RELATIONSHIPS BETWEEN SOCIAL ANTHROPOLOGY AND PSYCHIATRY

### Margaret Mead, Ph.D.

URING the last twenty-five years anthropologists and psychiatrists, particularly psychoanalytically oriented psychiatrists, have worked together and have found it increasingly easy to understand each other. Each group has found it valuable and rewarding to take problems which the other has uncovered and attempt to carry them further. This working relationship has several roots. Field anthropology and psychiatry are sciences which depend as much on the skill and insight of the practitioner as upon the theoretical framework within which the practitioner operates. Both rely on the observation of living persons, talking, walking, and acting, and upon the investigator's being able to use disciplined insights into his own behavior as part of the observations which he makes. So the well-analyzed psychiatrist is able both to observe and to use the way in which a patient activates his own special preoccupations, and the anthropologist with field experience is prepared to follow the intricate trail of his own difficulties of adjusting to, and understanding the behavior of, an alien people, to arrive at a pattern very different from his own. He must learn to recognize inversions of emotional expression, to know when laughter may be a sign of grief or the deepest quiet the sign of anger, which in his own society would have been accompanied by loud outbursts of rage; he must learn to experience empathically shame in his upper arms or fear as a chilliness of the buttocks or raised body hair on the big toe, to realize what it means to keep knowledge in the stomach under food or to place the seat of decision in the back of the neck.

And, like the psychiatrist, the anthropologist suffers the strains, pays the penalties, and reaps the rewards of intensive attention to a world not his own, a world in which the slightest muscle twitch and a suspended syllable of his subjects must be seen in terms of a pattern, of a system of behavior, which, however bizarre, is nevertheless recognized as lawful and understandable. Both are trained in the recognition of pattern—the psychiatrists in the patterns of particular individuals who have woven the threads of their experience into a special idiosyncratic fabric; the anthropologist in the patterns shared by groups of individuals who have selected, not over a single lifetime, but over many lifetimes, from the institutions and ways of behavior available to them those particular social forms which, fitted together, make a whole within which it is possible for a group of people to maintain and reproduce themselves (13). So, as the psychiatrist listens and comes to understand the way in which a patient has selected and rejected from among the admonitions and models of behavior presented to him by parents and siblings, teachers and schoolmates, from the beliefs and practices, prayers and superstitions, ways of eating, drinking, gambling, saving, and spending, to express his own needs, so the anthropologist sees each existing culture as a more or less coherent and functioning synthesis of political and social forms, ways of organizing work, and exchange, ownership, and inheritance, marriage and education. Where the psychiatrist takes as a relevant datum, "This patient's mother was a devout Roman Catholic, but after the age of eight he steadfastly refused to attend church," the anthropologist takes as data, "Part of the imported ceremony consisted of magic designed to cause other men's wives to run away to the giver of the ceremony, but the Arapesh refused to accept this magic, saying it would only cause trouble"; or "Among surrounding tribes, the Peyote cult, with its emphasis upon visions obtained under the influence of drugs, spread like wildfire, but the Zuni Indians steadily refused it." In the patient who resists his religious environment, the psychiatrist can trace the individual patterning which makes the refusal meaningful and which is, in turn reinforced by the refusal, just as each time the Arapesh, preferring smooth relationships, refuse a form of troublesome magic, they both exercise a highly patterned attitude and reinforce that attitude once again (68, Part I). In the recognition of such patterns, psychiatrist and anthropologist learn to rely on the internal consistency of the behavior of their subjects: in the patient, in the way in which similar or complementary types of behavior appear in treatment of parent, employer, analyst, friend, and in the interpretation of losses or gains in the outer world; in the members of a society, in the way in which the layout of a house, the conception of the body, the organization of a meeting, and the construction of a dramatic performance show the same systematic and intricate relationships. Neither psychiatrist nor anthropologist is concerned with simple quantitative relationships between single variables or with how often a patient dreams a significant dream or a people enact a particularly revealing ceremony, but rather in the structure of the dream, the plot of the ceremony. The frequency with which a certain type of dream is dreamed or offering made to the gods, to be meaningful to psychiatrist or anthropologist, has to be reinterpreted as part of a whole pattern of behavior, in which its frequency is only one attribute, its intricacy and intensity represent other dimensions—dimensions which neither discipline yet has precise tools for measuring.

But, while both disciplines begin with the same data—the observed behavior of living individuals, in which the observer is the delicate recording instrument (and no mediation of written documents or questionnaires can take the place of the living behavior)—and both are interested in problems of patterns and the delineation of systematic interrelationships, once the initial observation is made, the two disciplines order them differently. Consider, for instance, a new patient, who, instead of shaking hands, pats the psychiatrist gently on both shoulders. This patting behavior, atypical in a society in which shaking hands is customary, will be noted and referred in time to a large number of other behaviors of that particular individual, to his capacity for forming ties with men, to his ease of body contacts, to his ready and unconventional bodily expressiveness which has not stayed within socially prescribed limits, etc. In time, when this observation is integrated with other observations of the same individual, the psychiatrist will come to understand him, his particular way of relating himself to the world, his particular handling of the sensations of his own body. But the anthropologist, who enters a strange tribe, where the head man comes forward and pats him carefully and gently, will proceed differently. He, too, will note the pat, note its difference from greetings among surrounding tribes; he will note his own response to the pat and whether he feels reassured or frightened by it (but will refer his response, in turn, to his own previous experience in his own and other cultures); but the identity of the men who pat him will be significant in structural terms of age, rank, role, etc. If all the group pat him except one man, he will note this fact, so that later it can be referred to the status of the man—perhaps he is a visitor or a sorcerer or a widower—and if status fails to explain his apparently aberrant behavior, his nonpatting may be either a sign that there are several possible ways of greeting a stranger, that there is high tolerance of individual variations in behavior of this type, or that the nonpatter is pathological and is or is not recognized as such. But the anthropologist's next step is to observe many other behaviors of many other individuals; and for his type of conclusions it is not necessary that his observations of greetings and farewells, challenges and boasts, funeral orations and addresses to the gods, be performed by the same person. All the members of the group he is studying contribute detail after detail to his understanding of the shared behavior of the entire group—behavior which they share because they have been reared by a group of people who live in the same society together and participate in a common way of life. As the psychiatrist aims at building up a picture of a single personality and then proceeds from that to an understanding of various types of personality or, specifically, of various types of maladjustment, in which he groups together individuals showing predominantly hysterical manifestations or those of a compulsive type, the anthropologist aims at building up a picture of a culture and proceeds from that to an understanding of how different types of cultures function and change (33, 62).

Historically, as the two disciplines have a common bond in the strength of their method of observation and their capacity to include the observer (47) systematically within the observation, so they have faced certain common pitfalls. Both disciplines, as currently practiced, work without the relevant historical data. The anthropologist faces a people without any written records, who in each generation reshape their memory of past events or the interpretation of the natural landscape or the origin of a particular invention according to their heart's desire. So the Cheyenne, of whom we know from other evidence that they became a tipi-dwelling people only a few generations ago, tell a tale of the origin of their tipi dwelling at the beginning of the world; the Samoans, who we know must have arrived on their small archipelago in canoes not too many centuries ago, place the origin of all Samoans in the ancient village of Fitiuta and, although converted to Christianity and not disputing the general doctrine of the Garden of Eden, reply gently to objectors, "*Tasi le mea* ["There is just one thing to say in objection to your point"], the

*Samoans* originated in Fitiuta." Sometimes we have external evidence that the particular origin claim, line of migration, or steps in an invention are not true; but more often we have no way of checking the pasts of the people whom we study and have, instead, to take their view of the past as relevant data on the present alone, part of their way of placing themselves in the world. The psychiatrist faces the same problem when the patient whose father died twenty years ago describes his father as a cruel torturer. In particular cases, investigators may be sent out to assemble data on the father's character; and external evidence may be collected that the father was, indeed, the torturer which his son's present image of him suggests or that he was, on the contrary, very gentle and indulgent. More usually, the psychiatrist, armored by long experience against participating in the patient's affect, takes the data on the patient's father as data on the patient alone, depending on the patient's behavior to him, the patient's interpretation of whether he is or is not torturing or indulging him, to supply the outline of his possibly false or possibly true interpretation of the past. But sometimes, although decreasingly, anthropologists and psychiatrists alike fall into the snare of attempting to reconstruct the far-distant past from the particular residue which remains in the memories of those who live and speak today. This imputation of real existence to unseen events, whether in the past or in the present, leads not only to such constructs as Freud's *Totem and Taboo* (28), in which it is difficult to distinguish between great symbolic insight and imputed history, or the more recent attempt of Zilboorg (86) to defend the importance of women by substituting a theory of primal rape of the mother for primal murder of the father. Methodologically, both disciplines are faced with a dual problem of extracting full meaning from the data given them by the patient on the couch or by the last member of a subdued people who remembers a head-hunting raid. In such reports, especially of past behavior which has been rejected under contact with European standards and values, the cannibal feast or the taking of the tokens of virginity of the bride may take on a very different affective quality from that which it had when it was the fully accepted and well-articulated practice of a living, still complacent culture. In our own society, in which social mobility is so prevalent, the body habits of parents of a different social or ethnic group may be reinterpreted by the adult and given a meaning which they lacked at the time. Both disciplines arouse the criticisms of those sciences which have concentrated so hard on questioning the hitherto believed that they feel repelled by the necessary willingness of anthropologists and psychiatrists to believe in the hitherto unknown and unbelievable, and so are particularly sensitive to every error, every failure of these students of living behavior to recognize the limitations of their data.

Interest in history provides another snare for the unwary, because of the necessary concentration of the psychiatrist upon a single human being, who had a beginning in the union of sperm and egg and a single consecutive life-history, culminating in the hour of observation in the psychiatrist's office. Concentrated upon understanding the organization of this single identifiable personality, the psychiatrist gets from his anamnesis material, from the patient's view of his parents and playmates, data which appear to have sequence and to present a cause-and-effect pattern. "I was born just ten months after my sister. My mother had to wean my sister because she was pregnant, and she refused to nurse me. I was put on a bottle but nothing agreed with me. I vomited all the time." And today this patient responds to unpleasant situations or rejection by nausea. Subsequent studies of small children, followed through periods of many months when it was possible to show the interrelationships between maternal care and child response, have substantiated many of the theories based upon such anamnestic records to the extent that the phrasing came to be, "A rejecting mother *may* produce in her child a rejection of the substitute food which is offered." The anthropological phrasing would be: "Within this society, breast feeding and weaning are articulately regarded as signs of affection or rejection." In societies on which there is historical documentation the anthropologist may know and be able to take into account changes in such attitudes and in the total social configuration. This concentration of the psychiatrist on the particular series of learning which the patient shows, which must be understood if the patient is to improve and in which it is a completely valid method to exclude the great mass of social and economic events within which the learning occurred, is likely to become in the hands of social scientists a way of interpreting all social life as one in which a given set of maternal or parental practices are themselves determinative rather than mediative in relation to the growing child (2, 73). But the anthropologist's focus is upon ongoing societies, none self-contained, forever interacting, inter-marrying, exiling their members, receiving immigrants, borrow-ing institutions, altering and reinterpreting the inventions avail-able to them, within which generation after generation of chil-dren learn to be members of those societies. Patterns of cultures survive through generations of changing personnel; language spoken by one race will be spoken by a different race in the future; religions originating in one continent are transformed many times, reshaped and enriched, as they pass from people to people. Speculations about the particular origins of such basic human attitudes as those toward incest do not serve our purposes so well as does careful observation on the existing attitudes through a known period of history or over a geographical area, except as data on those who are speculating. For the most fruit-ful interchange between psychiatrist and anthropologist—the one working with adult patients, the other with an ongoing culture as embodied in adults—the questions "What is the pattern? How does he—or it, the society—function?" are the most appropriate ones, recognizing that in each case the only past which can be fully studied is that which is represented in the present. By studies of the present we may build up the material for a thor-ough study of social change.

This relationship between the psychiatrist's data on *how* a given patient is handling himself in the world and the anthropolo-gist's data on *how* a given group of people is handling their lives in the world is the first step in interaction between the two disci-plines. Here each uses his particular skill without reliance on the theoretical tools of the other, and each throws light upon the meaning of the other's material. The psychiatrist is protected against regarding the particular nexus between his patient's indi-vidual pattern and the particular Western Euro-American, Ju-deo-Christian cultural pattern of which his patient is a part as human nature and is given material for placing our own historical ways of doing things beside those of many other social alterna-tives. The anthropologist is given an understanding of the psy-chodynamics of human behavior, which makes it possible for him to see the ceremonies and rituals, the family forms and kinship patterns, the burial rites and harvest festivals which he records, as the patterned expressions of the psychologically intelligible human beings who embody them.

A few of the ways in which such findings of anthropologists

may be used will be discussed before going on to the much closer area of co-operation between psychiatry and anthropology which has come with the study of children, from child analysis, on the one hand, and the detailed study of primitive children, on the other. In this, instead of comparing synchronic patterns, in which understanding can come not from how they developed but merely from what is their present form, anthropologist and child psychiatrist follow identified living children over time, through a process of rapid growth; and a whole new field of understanding of the process of personality in culture is opened up. But the very fascination and increased freedom which come to members of both disciplines when they move in a field which they have joined together to make many times wider have tended to make each lose sight of the fundamental insights of the other, based on labors which are, of necessity, not shared in these co-operative undertakings—the eight or more hours a day of listening by the analyst, the concentrated months of living every minute in a strange, faraway culture by the anthropologist. The familiarity with the ways of the human psyche which the analyst thus gains, the practiced knowledge of the intricate nature of cultural process which the anthropologist gains, may not be fully allowed for.

## KNOWLEDGE OF OTHER SOCIAL FORMS

One of the basic contributions which cultural anthropology can make to psychiatry is in describing the many varieties of the family structure (61), within which the growing child develops his pattern of interpersonal relations, his conception of his own sex and of his relations to both sexes. There are societies like the Trobriand Islanders (50, 51), in which the father's physical paternity is passionately disavowed—along with the disavowal that any substance can permanently enter the body, even food, which merely passes through; like the Todas (78), in which one of the fraternity of husbands of the same woman may be credited with fathering a child born many years after his death, if no other brother has performed the appropriate acknowledgment ceremony. We find societies, like Dobu (26), in which the dwelling house is treated virtually as a connubial couch into which no stranger may enter and from which the adolescent son is forced out to wander about, looking for some young girl who will surreptitiously take him in, until dawn makes it necessary for him to flee before a prospective mother-in-law, who, alert for possible victims, may wake and seat herself in the doorway, blocking his path. It is in Dobu, too, that the whole balance of power between husband and wife swings back and forth as the couple resides in alternate seasons, now in the wife's village, now in the husband's, always among a group hostile to the spouse who does not belong. In contrast, we find the Samoan household (58), consisting of some ten to twenty persons, in which the husband-wife pairs almost disappear in the hierarchical, co-operative structure, with a titled householder at the head, in which each child performs duties appropriate to its age and sex and growing boys and girls are separated by a taboo imposed by the little boy, when he, who has been lugged about and cared for by his sister-nurse, "feels ashamed." In such a structure, understandably enough, the violent hates and jealousies of the Dobuan village are missing. Or we find the pattern of Zuni (13), where the houses were owned by a lineage of women, in which the sons and brothers preserved a ceremonial place; men married and went to live in the houses of their wives and mothers-in-law and always remained to some degree strangers, who might, almost any day, find their clothes lying in a bundle on the roof—a signal that they were no longer wanted in the houses where their children belonged. We can find almost every possible variation in household arrangements—from the lonely, isolated family life of the Ojibwa (46), where single families may live alone for months, to the crowded tenement life of Borneo (41), where forty or fifty families live under one roof and marriages have to be postponed for years until a new tenement with rooms for new marriages is again built; from the completely patriarchal husband presiding over a whole group of wives, as in many parts of Africa (43), to the less frequent pattern of one wife for a group of brothers, and the variant institution of Tibet (74) in which a group of brothers inherit their father's second wife when he becomes old. We can find mothers-in-law who must always be addressed as "Third person, plural number," and never seen, as in Manus; mothers-in-law who may be married simultaneously with their daughters to the same man, as in Arapesh; or the Navajo situation in which a man may wed a widow with a daughter and later discards the mother, marries the daughter, and observes a strictly taboo relationship toward the former wife (77). Brothers and sisters may be tied together by the closest of sentimental bonds, as in Manus (64, 66), or separated by a taboo which is never relaxed until old age, as in Samoa (58; 67, pp. 117–18; 70).

It is unnecessary to multiply examples indefinitely; a moment's imaginative thought will supply the variety of experience available to the child born and reared within such different family structures, with all the possibilities of diffusion, compartmentalization, or concentration of affects. In the isolated biological family the parent of opposite sex becomes the only model for adult behavior toward persons of opposite sex; in large extended families a variety of adults of the same sex may offer contrasting patterns or a blurred and generalized version of what it is to be a woman or a man. Or each individual adult may play sharply differentiated roles in regard to the children, so that a man is stern to his own son but plays the role of a "male mother" to his sister's son, a woman may be indulgent and warm to her own daughter but play the role of a "female father" to her brother's daughter (21, 43, 75). While the small biological family tends to rear individuals who will, in turn, concentrate their available attitudes of dependency, affection, passion, possessiveness, etc., on their wives, it is possible, as in Manus (66), to specialize these attitudes to different relatives, so that a man feels sentimental affection for his sister, jocular gay sexual easiness for his female cross-cousin (whom he may not marry but whom he may fondle in public), and possessive disrespect for his wife.

As the known lives of individuals in our own society are seen to be given form by the oedipal situation, it becomes abundantly clear that such differences in family structure will give exceedingly different forms to the ways in which small children learn to deal with their springing sexual attachments to the adults of both sexes with whom they are reared. Identification with one's father's father, which makes it possible to joke with him (29) or in some societies even to call one's father's mother "wife" and treat her with pornographic boldness, is a different solution of the relationship to a stern father from that offered by a society in which one's father honors his father until his death. When Freud's descriptions of the oedipus complex were first subjected to anthropological scrutiny, the criticism concentrated upon such differences in form, the need for a wider, more abstract phrasing to describe situations in which power was divided between father and mother's brother or in which a child was cared for by half-a-dozen female members of a household in which the head was often not his father. These early theoretical extensions had a certain rigidity, because of the assumption that the content from the child's side was fixed by the nature of his growth processes, as one might conceive of a plant, growing upward according to a fixed principle, thrusting through barriers or turning aside when the barriers were too great or dividing when they were multiple. Such a formulation assumed some sort of biological residue of an assumed biological normality, in which a rivalry situation between child and parent of own sex was somehow given, even though some cultures were able to dodge and overlay this essential position with peculiar, somehow secondary, arrangements. This interim theoretical position thus kept traces of the thinking based on the family form on which the first detailed psychoanalytic observations were made. The phrasing today would be that the oedipal situation, in the widest meaning, is a way of describing what any given society does with the fact that children *and* adults are involved in the growing child's sexual attitudes, especially toward the parent of opposite sex. The possibilities of heavily cathected experience are inherent in the nature of human growth and human parenthood, unequally stressed in different forms of family structure and household arrangements. Crises of relationship between parents and children may occur in early childhood, in adolescence, at marriage, with own parenthood, at the retirement or death of the parent; and on each occasion the adult's behavior can be seen not merely as a living-out of own childhood experience but as adult reaction to the behavior of children. Thus the current crisis in American middle-class men when their daughters marry or have a first child may be referred to the cult of youth fostered throughout adolescence and maturity in the American middle-class male at least as much as to any specific pattern of pregenital behavior.

Or we may consider the way in which cultures handle types of ambivalence toward the dead (63). Setting aside the more complex problems of the nature of ambivalence itself, the extent to which its development in the individual is a response to the experiences the infant undergoes as compared with the inherent contradictoriness of primary thought-processes, there is still room to explore the ways in which different societies have handled the mixed attitudes that the living entertain toward the dead. Cultures differ enormously in the prescription of acceptable attitudes, in enjoining an emphasis upon grief and bereaved love with no hint of overt hostility, so that guilt over repressed hostile wishes is intensified; or in tabooing grief and stressing only fear and hostility, in which case the feelings of attachment and affection are the ones which must be repressed; or in working out some acceptable patterned combination of both attitudes.

Among the Chukchee and the Koryak of aboriginal Siberia the whole emphasis is laid upon the complete removal of the dead, the equipment of the spirit so that it will never return, the bewildering and baffling of the spirit so that it cannot find its way back to the abode of its relatives. In discussing the Siberian practices, Bogoras' (14) and Jochelson's (42) own words are reproduced so as not to mar their accounts by the introduction of less vivid paraphrases. After death, among the Chukchee, "one man must stay all the time with the body, because should it be left alone it might revive and do harm. . . . Among other taboos connected with the funeral must be mentioned the interdictions against beating the drum for three nights during the time of the ceremony. The beating of the drum might call the deceased back to the house. . . . At every hitch in this task [that of dressing the corpse in its burial clothes] the followers admonish the dead one, saying 'Leave off! Make haste! You have to go away, do not be so obstinate.' " After reaching the grave and going through a number of ceremonies "the 'fortifier' [officiant] cuts the throat of the corpse and leaves the body." This last stroke is to prevent the spirit of the deceased from following the people of the cortege and is considered quite indispensable. On the way home the order of march is reversed, and many ceremonies and incantations are performed—the fortifier throwing behind him several small stones, which become a "mountain"; a bunch of grass, which becomes a "forest"; and a cup, which becomes a "sea"—magical defenses against the return of the dead. On the return home "all the members of the procession, holding one another by the hand, form a large ring, which is encircled by that part of the thong that was taken home from the funeral . . . each one cuts off the part nearest himself."

A notable feature of the mourning ceremonies of the Koryak, whose culture has many traits in common with the Chukchee, is the taboo against the manifestation of grief until after burial. The elaborate grave clothes cannot be finished until after death, and this sometimes entails two or three days' sewing. "While the dead person is in the house, he is considered as a member of the family and the people try to make it appear as though nothing had happened. It is supposed that he is participating in the meals of the family and in card playing."

While Chukchee and Koryak observances contrast with our own traditional insistence on emphasizing the grief of the mourners and speaking only good of the dead, the Bagobo (12) of the Philippines have institutionalized both attitudes. They share a very widespread belief in multiple souls but have given it a special twist by distinguishing a right-hand soul, which is beneficent, and a left-hand soul, which is malevolent. The *takawanan* ("good soul") is associated, in native thinking, with those factors of existence which stand for life, health, activity, and joy, while the *tebang* ("bad soul") is associated with factors that tend toward death, sickness, sluggishness, pain:

> The left-hand soul becomes a *buso* ["demon"]. Like other *buso*, he digs up dead bodies, tears the flesh from the skeletons and devours the flesh; like other *buso*, he stands under the house of the dying, or hovers over it to drink the watery blood of the corpse.... An intelligent adult differentiates perfectly the tripartite nature which tradition has assigned to man,—there is a physical body that the *buso* will dig up and eat after it has been put under the soil; there is a good *takawanan* that goes to the One Country to continue its existence in a less substantial and more highly idealized manner than on earth, although moved by like interests and like emotions to those that motivate him here, and, finally, there is an evil *tebang* that turns into a horrible man-eating *burkan*, perpetually roaming over the earth like a prey animal, and preserving not a single tie or a single interest to bind him to the friends and activities of his mortal life.

A more ingenious device for permitting the free play of ambivalent attitudes toward a single individual or toward one's self could hardly be imagined. All that is evil, all that is detestable, in one's living thought, in one's dream experiences, all the socially nonacceptable, thoroughly disreputable attitudes, can be fastened upon this left-hand soul, who is even open to the accusation of having actually left the owner's body to carry out its evil purposes. Similarly, after death, all the relief, the hostility to the dead, the fear of an invasion of the reorganized lives of the survivors by the troublesome memory and presence of the dead—all these can be projected upon the *tebang*, which is even robbed of all sense of personality or memory of its former associates. That the conflict is not quite resolved is shown by the fear that the good soul may try to take others with it on its long journey. But the grief over the loss of a loved one, the wish to cherish one who is dead and to care for him, are taken care of in the disposal of the right-hand soul, which journeys to the One Country and is so loath to leave its dear ones behind that it must bathe in the dark waters of a river of forgetfulness before it is contented to remain in a country where "the rice ... is of immaculate whiteness, and each grain as big as a kernel of corn; the camotes are the size of a great round pot, and every stick of sugar cane is as large as the trunk of a cocoanut-palm."

A full appraisal of the effect of such institutionalized mourning practices on those who live within the culture of which they are a part is possible only if the student divorces their present content and function from their origin. If the student approached the precautionary measures of the Koryak in terms of their probable origin, he would use psychiatric data on guilt and obsessive precautions to interpret these procedures as indications of extreme guilt in those Koryak who practice the precautions. But, if it is realized that such institutions may have developed many thousands of miles or thousands of years away, in a quite different setting, and have gone through many transformations, it is then possible to concentrate upon the way in which the present usages facilitate the behavior of individuals who live within them. A child who fears its mother so much that he spontaneously invents horrible fantasies of devouring witches is in very different plight from a child whose tradition presents him with images of witches in comparison to which his own negative affects toward his mother seem pallid. Individuals reared within the pattern of mourning current in Western culture twenty-five years ago are forced to suppress any expression of negative attitudes toward the dear departed, and, in cases where strong hostility and death wishes have been felt, what may be merely a conscious conflict in many individuals may show itself as severe disturbance in others.

But the way in which the particular ceremonials or myths or religious usages of any society are related to the types of infantile and childhood experience within that particular society is a matter which has to be very fully understood before the role which any ceremonial like those described above can be accurately assessed. If each human society were a self-contained unit, repeating over hundreds of years the same cycle of life and death, we might fairly expect to find, on the basis of what we know both of individual psychodynamics and of the nature of human culture, that the myths and the rituals, the kinship terms, and the ways in which the language was spoken and the vocabulary used —if not its actual grammar—would be perfectly fitted together with the recurrent experiences of deprivation and indulgence, with the way in which childhood and adolescence, maturity, parenthood, and death were handled. It might be expected that the individual's way of feeling about intercourse would have a one-to-one relationship to early learning at the mother's breast whether there were witches in folklore side by side with mothers who behaved in a most unwitchlike way, or witchlike mothers without direct reflection in the folklore, or mothers and folk witches whose behavior was identical. Each of these and many other possible and more complicated relationships between folk-lore and everyday practice would be systematic. Data on adult practice would be perfect data on the forms of childhood experi-ence, while full data on childhood experience would make it pos-sible to extrapolate to the formal relationships and emphases of some other aspect of the culture. But, even here, unless we could assume, as we have no basis for doing, that the *whole* culture had been evolved on the spot—language, marriage, tool-using, meth-ods of burying the dead or determining an inheritance, dance form, or folk tale—the childhood experience would never explain the whole content of the culture, would never explain such as-pects as the grammar of the language, the invention of cremation, the existence of marriage itself, or the belief in a supernatural. All such aspects of culture must be explained historically and be assumed to have passed through many peoples, changing their forms, it is true, in each people's hands, as the acting and inter-pretation of Hamlet varies from one century of English history to another or is given a different twist by Madariaga in 1948 (49). The particular twist, the reinterpretation of some usage which a people share with many neighbors, can be seen as inti-mately related to their particular childhood experience, just as a patient's preference for one Shakespearean character above an-other may be taken as a datum, without the assumption that he himself would ever have been able to conceive of Hamlet or Macbeth. The *particular* form which a ceremony takes, in con-tradistinction to other versions, may be interpreted as throwing light on the basic formative experiences of childhood. But the whole of the ceremony, in its most individualized and most wide-spread forms, must be considered in order to understand how the culture functions, what choices are offered those born within it, what leeway is offered to the impulses which we must assume are potential in all human beings but which are differently realized in different periods of history and in different human societies. Thus it comes about that a ritual which shows deep marks of fear or appeasement of devouring gods may actually function quite differently, in one society by allaying anxiety, in another by accentuating it.

The closest we can come to scientific study of origins of ritual or myth, as opposed to speculative reconstructions, is in the study of change, in which we can follow the transformations of widespread, psychologically relevant themes, as different peoples reshape them. If we investigate what happens to a widespread fairy tale like "Jack and the Beanstalk" when transplanted from Europe to the United States, we find some very interesting transformations (16). Giants are very old folklore figures, of such relevance to the universal experiences of childhood that it is a quite tenable assumption that stories of giants might be reinvented again and again. However, in the case of such a European folk tale as "Jack and the Beanstalk," the story must be seen as having a long and unrecoverable history. In the tale recorded from the southern mountains in the United States (18), instead of the accident in which Jack is duped into accepting a handful of beans for his cow, which, when thrown away, turn into the beanstalk, we have a scene in which the mother gives a bean she finds on the floor to Jack and tells him to plant it. Instead of stealing the giant's money bag, goose that laid the golden egg, and harp, Jack steals a rifle, a knife, and coverlet off the giant's bed; passive fantasy symbols have become much more active. In the European version Jack's father appears in various ways: sometimes he is killed or imprisoned by the giant; sometimes he is rescued by Jack, and the family is restored. In the American story the father is entirely absent (31, 56, 84). In a more recent American version (30) the giant's wife, who is a relatively harmless and ineffective figure in the European tales, has been transformed into a dangerous and menacing figure. We could then ask not only what happens in the lives of American children out of which such changes in the story grow but also what comfort American children take from the story so transformed. The answer to the first question, about the distinctive forms of the tale in America, would be data on the particular cultural psychodynamics of Americans as compared with Europeans. The answer to the second would be data on elements in the culture available to American children, who, like all children everywhere, are smaller than their parents but are unlike all children, in that some children have no myths of giants available to console them.

Perhaps one of the most imposing collections of data which anthropology can present is that on the prevalence of overt sexual inversion. Primitive peoples represent the whole gamut: we find societies which institutionalize transvestitism for both males and females in which transvestites of each sex live as married couples with members of their own sex (19); societies in which transvestitism of only one sex is officially recognized (sometimes accompanied by the most severe penalties for the other sex) (61, pp. 416–17); societies in which one facet of a complementary homosexual relationship is cultivated but the other completely disallowed (8, 67); societies in which there is no cultural recognition of any sort of the possibility of identification with the other sex that is more than a light occupational whim, a slightly greater toughness of muscle in a girl, or a slightly softer skin in an occasional boy (58). We find societies like the Navajo, in which a male transvestite was admired because he could do all that either a man or a woman could do, occupationally, and other American Indian societies in which male bravery was so highly valued that children were subjected to continuous scrutiny and ruthless ordeals, under the pressure of which and with the known possibility of transvestitism a certain number of males in each generation chose to "change" rather than to be brave, to accompany the war party as tellers of tales rather than as warriors (37).

Devereux has provided a detailed description of the elaborate behavior of transvestites among the Mohave (19). Male transvestites insisted upon the terms appropriate to the genitalia of women being applied to their genitalia, equating the penis with the clitoris, the testes with the labia majora, and the anus with the vagina. The female transvestites were equally insistent on the reversed nomenclature. These transvestites lived as spouses with members of their own sex and were referred to by the pronoun appropriate to their assumed role. The male transvestite imitated menstruation by drawing blood from a scratch, submitted to the entire puberty ritual for females, and required from his male partner the observances demanded from the husband of a girl who menstruates for the first time. These males also went through symbolic "pregnancies," observed the pregnancy taboos, and, whereas Mohave women deny their pregnancies in public, these homosexuals boasted of them. In the absence of their husbands they stuck rags and bark under their skirts, and finally drank a decoction of mesquite beans said to cause severe constipation; the eventual pains were treated as labor pains, and, finally, the transvestite went to the bush, squatted like a parturient woman, and later pretended it had been a stillbirth, going through mourning ceremonies for the imaginary child. All these observances were known and recognized in the society, and teasing the transvestites by pointing out their pretenses was a frequent, although sometimes dangerous, form of humor.

We may place beside these Mohave observances the behavior of two New Guinea tribes. In New Guinea we have observations on two tribes, barely fifty miles apart, in one of which, the Arapesh (71), passive receptivity and gentle parental behavior are emphasized for the males, with assertive behavior first disallowed and later inculcated as a necessary but disagreeable social duty. During a long period of indulgent nursing, the infant is encouraged to adopt a passively receptive attitude toward a willingly giving mother and a father who treats him as gently as the mother; later the small boy cares for younger siblings, becomes the custodian of his own growth, and grows his wife. Relationships among adolescent boys are warm and affectionate, but there I found no recognition of explicit homosexual practice or of transvestitism.

Near by, on the Sepik River, live the Iatmul (8, 67),[1] who share with the Arapesh the widespread institution of a men's cult into which males are initiated at puberty. Kinship system and forms of social organization are sufficiently alike to identify these two peoples as belonging to the same culture area. This anthropological concept of the "culture area" is essential in making the distinction between differences in particular versions of widespread practices and responsibilities for their origin. Within a culture area we can assume historical connections. As Iatmul and Arapesh are both known to be cultures in this New Guinea culture area of which the men's initiatory cult is a constant feature, we can treat their contrasts in behavior as variations on a common theme which are significant data on their cultural character struc-

1. Also unpublished field work of Bateson and Mead (1938).

ture. Among the Iatmul the baby is taught to demand food before it is fed, is held at arm's length by the mother, and is treated as a bit of incarnate assertiveness as strong as the mother, who must angrily compel it to her will. All children are classified with the women, as opposed to the initiated males, and the boy sees his father either at home playing a rather aimless role or at a distance performing spectacular dramatic ceremonies for the benefit of an audience of women and children. Little boys give evidence of strong female identification, carry babies about by choice, play at housekeeping, and in posture they often cannot be distinguished from girls. Within the adult culture there is elaborate ceremonial transvestitism on particular occasions: when the exploits of their sister's sons are celebrated, mother's brothers dress in shabby old female garments and pantomime passive female activities, such as receiving bright orange fruits in the anus or rubbing the anus on the nephew's shin; and father's sisters dress up in festive male attire, scraping male lime spatulas in gourd lime containers. The initiatory ceremonial is filled with the most explicit type of ceremonialism, in which the miserable novices are treated as the abused wives of the bullying initiators. In the one village of Tambunum where I worked in 1938, eleven words for sodomy were in continuous use as abusive terms between everyone, regardless of sex. And yet homosexuality is prevented within the group, not because the psychological groundwork in extreme passive female identification and overcompensatory braggart male assertiveness is not well laid down but through the simple device of tabooing male passivity of any sort. Little boys, hearing continually of sodomy, often attempt to practice it, but slightly older boys respond by thrusting sticks into the hands of each and forcing them to fight each other. Unprotected buttocks remain a temptation through life; men in the men's house frequently move from one place to another in the group with their small wooden stools held protectingly over their anuses. A riot can be precipitated between the moieties in a men's house because a mischievous boy has thrust the wooden fire tongs into the exposed anus of a stooping feeble old man. As reliance is placed entirely on tabooing all passive male homosexuality at the same time that the active side is cheerfully elaborated, the stranger or the work boy from another tribe becomes an immediate prey. Iatmul boys away at work have a reputation for exercising to the fullest on people like the Arapesh the capacities which their own culture has first stimulated and then disallowed by the simple expedient of actively interdicting the necessary complementary behavior.

It is noteworthy that in tribes where there is no recognition of transvestitism or of any sort of inversion an occasional individual will still show deviance in preference for the behavior or occupation of the opposite sex. But whether many individuals will find expression for a potentiality or not seems to depend, finally, on the cultural expectations.

So far we have discussed the way in which differences in various types of formal arrangements in family structure, marriage patterns, concepts of the soul, and mourning for the dead could throw light upon an understanding of human psychodynamics, check tendencies to read our own special local social forms into theories, and broaden our view of the many potentialities which each human being has for constructing viable ways of life. But data on different forms of marriage and kinship alone do not provide us with any direct material on psychodynamics. We may speculate as to whether a child's responses to his parents will not take very different forms in a society like Zuni, where the mother and mother's mother are the property owners and the father is a visitor; we may construct hypotheses about the way in which a socially recognized theory of dual souls—one good, one bad— might serve to give a different form to the required suppression of ambivalent attitudes toward the dead among the Bagobo; but these remain mere theoretical extrapolations from present observations upon the way in which our own family structure and mourning practices are reflected in the analysis of individual patients, in the dreams and products of the insane.

### Studies of Character Formation

Obviously, the next step for an understanding of the extent to which differences in culture make possible differences in character structure is detailed studies of the process of character formation. In the conventional anthropological frame of reference there is no need to make a series of observations on a single individual, but rather one should make masses of observations on individuals of identified status within which regularities of culture can be distinguished. When anthropologists study personality in a culture involving the hypotheses of dynamic psychology, it is still necessary to establish sequences of cultural experience which can be related to our systematic knowledge of the growth process; to study, for instance, the way in which the infant is fed, carried, cleansed, put to sleep; how the child learns to sit, crawl, walk, talk, swim, control its sphincters and relate its genital behavior to social demands; and what the cultural definitions of experience are which enable it to interpret the unidentified impulses and tensions in its own body and to steer its way among the objects of the external world. In order to translate the findings on psychodynamics from one culture to another,[2] we need to invoke the most basic knowledge we have about growth sequences (69) and about learning (9). Knowledge of growth sequences makes it possible to see the way in which children learn the culture into which they are born against a systematic background in which readiness for an activity or dominance of one phase of an activity in the child can be fitted together interpretively with the behavior of the rearing adults and surrounding older children. It is possible to follow the customary practices and the observed responses of groups of individuals in a cross-sectional study of a society, so that, at the end of a year's observation, the anthropologist can bring away a statement of the way in which the infant, the young child, the older child, and the adolescent learn and, in turn, stimulate regular responses from the adults, thus becoming a contributing human segment of the cultural circle.

When such observations are made, we find that there are consistent sequences (70), that the Arapesh (67, 68, 71) treat birth as a woman's mystery from which men are excluded, where the midwife is the woman who has most recently given birth (a characteristic preference for emotional closeness to experience rather than for any disciplined competence); that the life or death of the newborn is phrased in terms of the ability of the parents to feed it properly as "saving it" or not "saving it"; that the infant is put to the breast at once and throughout infancy is fed lovingly, the mother first carrying it in a net bag against her bare back curled up in a fetal position, later in a sling beneath her breast, even suckling it as she climbs a steep mountain side

2. Kardiner (44, 45) has been particularly interested in working from psychodynamic conceptions to an interpretation of culture based on materials collected by anthropologists, while Erikson (23, 24), Roheim (80), and Gorer (34) combine actual work with informants, in the anthropological tradition, with the use of psychodynamic concepts.

with fifty pounds of yams suspended from her forehead carrying bag. Running parallel with the warmth and giving quality of Arapesh life, there is an element of clumsiness, a lack of precision of adjustment, from the midwife, who may never have been present at any delivery except her own, through the bathing of the baby in cold water, not with a view to hardening it, but simply through lack of the idea of warming the water; through frequent periods when the baby may have no food because the mother has gone on a journey and failed to get back in time or failed in some plan to have another woman feed the child; through failure to teach the child any sort of precise manual habits. Children sit at the top of the house ladder and cry to be taken down, when other New Guinea children would climb up and down easily; cut themselves with knives, which they are given simply because they cry for them; and go into temper tantrums which no one knows how to stop if refused food, when there is none. Thus in a thousand details of the way the body is handled, the sequences in which events are learned to occur, the culture is communicated to the child, and his character becomes an embodiment of it.

We may contrast this method of intercommunication, in which the mother gives warmly but clumsily and the child learns to accept without discriminating accurately the details of the giving and the taking and later in life becomes a prey to sorcery fears and fears of seduction, depletion, etc., proceeding from the relatively unmotivated, temporarily hostile moods of his neighbors, given form by outside sorcerers, with the sequence of learning among the Manus of the Admiralty Islands (25, 64, 65, 66). Here no woman who has not had a child may be present at birth, the mother is isolated with her young infant during a month when her husband cannot come near her, the feeding is seen as giving milk rather than as giving the breast, the mother resisting while the father insists that she give the child *food*. The infant is held very little but is laid instead on a mat on the floor and is not carried about until it can itself hold onto its mother's neck, leaving her hands free to punt a canoe. It is taught as soon as it can crawl not to touch other people's possessions and learns a high degree of bodily control, precision of movement, and ability to distinguish sequences of events objectively, "tying a canoe badly, rope slips, canoe floats away," rather than of the type "falling, knee hurts, hungry, where is mother." The adult preoccupation with the use of the body in the external world and with the handling of things is translated to the child, first, by treating the suckling situation as one in which milk passes from mother to child, later by great emphasis on learning sphincter control and prudery in regard to all excretory functions. The Manus child grows up as an efficient, tool-using, well-co-ordinated active youngster, fitted to observe the outer world, almost completely devoid of fantasy life of any sort. He will grow up into a man who classifies sexual activity with excretion as shameful, who has respect for those who are actively engaged in affairs of exchange and manipulation of objects, exacting of himself and others, building himself a high standard of living under great handicaps (for the Manus own nothing but their marketable skills of fishing, canoe-building, sailing, and trading), and dying young.

Manus and Arapesh cultures are alike, in that neither has significant elaborations of fantasy, in art, in religious ritual, in philosophizing. They present contrasting pictures, in that the Manus emphasizes relationship to objects (67) to such an extent that the body itself becomes an object, the breast a feeding tube, the phallus, capped with a white shell, something to shake at a rival in an economic transaction, the soul of a dead parent a guardian who can help one go fishing, to be discarded into anonymity as soon as it fails to be useful. The body as a well-co-ordinated machine-like affair concerned with taking in and giving out other objects is the model—a model for planned, incessant, effective activity.

To return to the Arapesh, where the passive feeding situation with a giving parent and a taking child remains the model throughout life, the striking emphasis is not on the externalization of attention and the disallowance of sensuousness, as among the Manus, but rather on the continuance of a mild, passive approach to the environment in which hunting is phrased as "walking about looking for (the appearance of) a quarry" and the ideal form of hunting is waiting in the village until a dream advises one that some animal has fallen into a trap set miles away in the bush. Both cultures are one-sided in their emphasis: in neither is the growing child presented with the symbolic forms which mediate in beautiful and intricate ways between the child's early experience of the world and the participation in that world which the organizational forms of his society, the exigencies of making a living, demand.

But there are many cultures which do provide such an elaborate set of artistic and religious forms, where the adults who rear
the children move, themselves remembering but in transformed
ways, their own preverbal experiences, in ritual and design, in
musical pattern and dance form, make the same paths available to their children. The Balinese child (6, 7, 10), suspended
in a sling on its mother's hip, passively, almost flaccidly, re-
laxing in such a way that it adjusts to her movement without
experiencing bumps or jolts, wakes and sleeps in her arms, during the long temple ceremonies, at the play where brothers will
chase and terrorize each other in mime, whereas in everyday
life no such behavior is permitted; where the witch is openly
attacked by her young male victims, who nevertheless fall helpless before her magic; where men and women in trance turn
razor-sharp daggers against their own breasts, in an ecstasy of
concentrated inwardness but are not harmed or even fatigued.
In her treatment of her baby, the mother will tease, stimulate, and
withdraw, the child will go through a sequence of stimulation,
deposition by younger children, and, in turn, will see the younger depossessed. Sequences in which climax is broken coincide in
his own life-cycle with the dramatic rituals at which he is a spec-
tator. The highly patterned, elaborated, released artistic skill of
many generations has gone into fashioning a medium, within
which individuals, who, when tested by our tests, are indistin-
guishable from schizophrenics in our culture, are able to live,
marry, bear children, and maintain a society, in which there is
food enough for all and hardly any recognition of fatigue, in
which the old learn as easily as the young, in which men learn
new skills, not by observing the outer form of the activity—as the
Manus would—but by following the inner movement of the one
who is already skilled, surrendering to the tempo of his body (11,
52, 53, 54, 57, 59).

From series of observations of this sort we begin to build a picture of the consistencies which can exist among the cultural
forms with which an individual is presented, the way in which
the individuals who embody those forms will communicate
them, the way in which the infant with his human potentialities
responds and, by responding, permits the adult to take the next
step in himself living out the full cycle as it has been formalized
within a society. To form such a picture as this, we need accurate, detailed observation of each age, from infants in arms to the

oldest gaffer and crone, observations of a people as they work, at their ceremonies, during life-crises. Retrospective accounts of childhood experiences, accounts given by adults of what they think was done to them or what they think they did to children, while suggestive and, when placed beside our general knowledge of character formation, often permitting us to form useful hypotheses, are no substitute here for observation, minute, day-by-day, of each step in the process. In homogeneous, slowly changing societies, all the observations can be made simultaneously; we do not need to follow single individuals through their lives in order to understand the general course which personality development takes; and it is possible to relate specific materials, such as projective tests, dreams, artistic constructions, of individuals at any age to the total cycle of which they are a part.

## USE OF INDIVIDUAL PRODUCTIONS

A principal problem of communication between anthropologists and psychiatrists becomes the selection of forms of material from other cultures which are readily translatable in terms of the psychiatrists' clinical experiences. Three lines of communication have been developed. Detailed observations on child training are readily interpretable by child analysts, who themselves deal with children in the course of a process of change. For full translation, the observations should be on particular children, so that a variety of behaviors of a single individual can be presented within the whole cultural context. Then it is possible to see how a given child, developing within a socially prescribed pattern of feeding, carrying, weaning, etc., has developed its particular idiomatic version of experience. Because the clinician's ear and eye are trained to study and understand those individuals in whom the process of learning allowed for by the society has to some degree miscarried, accounts of the behavior of the traumatized child in another society (58, 64, 71), the orphan, the physically handicapped, the hyperreactive, form perhaps the best communication, provided that the clinician can keep in mind that here, as in his own cases, it is the individual *in whom* the process has miscarried who is being studied. Jules and Zunia Henry's (38, 39) records of play behavior among Pilaga children combine this advantage of presenting the record of the traumatized child against a background of the behavior of those children who are developing within their culture, according to expectation.

The individual's account of his own life is a useful form of recording. As illustrations I will quote briefly here from three verbatim records from a Winnebago Indian, collected by Paul Radin (76) in 1910, a Lepcha of Sikkim (Kurma), collected by Geoffrey Gorer (34) in 1936, and an Arapesh of New Guinea, Unabelin (68, Part V), collected by myself in 1931—all males. From the Winnebago Indian:

Father and mother had four children and after I was born. An uncle of my mother named White Cloud spoke to her before I was born and told her, "You are about to give birth to a child who will not be an ordinary individual." These were the words he addressed to her. It was then that my mother gave birth to me. As soon as I was born, indeed as I was being washed—as my neck was being washed—I laughed out loudly.

I have been told that I was a good tempered child.

During childhood my father told me to fast and I obeyed him. Throughout the winter, every morning, I would get up very early, crush charcoal, and then blacken my face with it. As soon as the sun rose would I go outside, and there gazing steadily at the sun, make my prayer to the spirits, crying.

Thus I acted up to the time that I have memory of things. . . .

## From a Lepcha of Sikkim:

My next memory is being frightened of my baby brother crying. Mother told me not to go near him as he was a devil, *Sang-rong moong*. Some time before my elder sister was fetched from where she was stopping; I slept with Mother till she was delivered and afterwards with my sister.

Some time later I and my brother and sister and Mother were all sitting on the verandah when Passo's wife arrived carrying a big bamboo full of water; she leant it against the fence and said to Mother, "I'd like to have that boy to look after; please give him to me." Mother replied, "I don't know if he wants to, but if he does you can fetch him and take him home with you." Then Passo's wife said to me "I am going to take you home with me and I will love you. I have got meat at home and boiled rice pudding [*tok-tok*]; if you come home I will give it to you." I said I did not want to go, so then she said "Let us go anyhow, you can eat it and after that you can come back." Then she took me to her house and gave me *tok-tok*. In the evening I wanted to go home but Passo's wife said to me "There is a devil Sang-rong moong in your house who will eat you if you go." I was not frightened of that and tried to get away but they fastened the door shut and would not let me go.

## From an Arapesh of New Guinea:

[Here I asked a question: Tell me about the admonitions which your father gave you.]

When my father bore us, he tabooed meat, he did not drink cold water.

He did not drink coconut juice. He did not drink sugar cane juice. My mother also abstained from all these things. . . .

My father did not sleep with other women. He waited. He waited. When his child was tall, when his child could walk, when his child no longer wished to drink at the breast, then he could sleep with women. He waited. Later he had intercourse with his wives.

But this new generation, my generation, they are no good. When their children are still small they have intercourse with wives. They are worthless. My father did not eat food in other hamlets. He did not eat food given him by other people. He was afraid it would harm his children. He followed all these taboos when my eldest brother was born. He [my brother] flourished. He grew tall. Later they sorcerized this brother of mine. He fell from a tree and was killed. Of this, I told you before. Now my father slept with my mother. She was pregnant with my sister. He tabooed well. He waited. When my sister had grown big, my mother was pregnant with Polip. She bore Polip. They waited. They waited. Then my mother bore me. They waited. When I was big she bore Yagulai. When he was big she bore my little sister. Now my mother was old. She was finished with child bearing. My father was too old. All of my fathers were old men too.

Rorschach records, Thematic Apperception Tests, and drawings made in response to definite suggestions have also been used as ways in which behavior in other cultures could be caught in a form which would make it amenable to interpretation by psychiatrists in our society and, conversely, make their insights more useful to anthropology. These materials may be used in different ways. A group of Rorschachs may be presented on a single culture, and the psychiatrist attempt to work out the regularities of the cultural character structure, using the individual protocol merely as data upon the general form, as Oberholzer did with the Alorese material (20), as projective tests were analyzed in the Indian study (83), etc., in which proportions of form and movement, of whole or detailed responses, are used to define different modal tendencies within another culture; or content sequences may be analyzed to show characteristic handling of highly toned situations, as Abel has done for French and Chinese (3, 4).

Where projective tests are so used, all that we have is another statement of characteristic forms of behavior which can also be derived from art, ritual, folk themes, etc. Such material, however, has the advantage that the psychiatrist, who is likely today to be working more with protocols on tests than with art or ritual, can see the cultural differences.

The difference in culture patterns can be demonstrated by a few examples.

Children's replies to a special set of Thematic Apperception Test pictures (40):

### HOPI PROTOCOLS

The woman is talking. She is the mother. She tells them to help her. They will.

He is an old man. He sit down. He is sick. He will die.

He is their uncle. He tell them they did wrong to fight. They not fight anymore.

They are looking at the turtle. And the mother is nursing the baby.

They are Hopis and the mother tells her boy to go out to the field. They are weeds. He will hoe them.

Here are Hopis and they are waiting to get married. They will be happy.

The boy is crying because the mother scolded him. He not want to do what she say. He will.

These people are learning to dance good. People will see them. They will dance right.

He is crying. He did not want to do what he was told. He will spank.

### NAVAJO PROTOCOLS

This woman is grinding. You use this to take the flour off the stone. These two men are telling stories. The boy is sitting up here and thinking. One of these men say to the woman. "What are you grinding?" These are the plants.

This is the father and this is the white man, and the horse. Looks like they are talking together about the ring. The Indian says it is a pretty ring. What man has the ring.

This is grandmother and there are the flowers. He is smelling them.

They are singing and this one is going to shake hands with the other.

These two are going to dance. This man wants these two to dance.

This man is trying to whip the horse. Because they want to go faster.

The girl is standing there. She is thinking about something.

It is an old man. Maybe he is watching those flowers. Maybe he is all alone and that is what he is thinking about. He thinks they are pretty.

When whole protocols are available for individuals on whom other material is also recorded, which unfortunately has not been the publication practice during these years when the use of projective tests has been developed, then it is possible for the psychiatrist actually to compare the general context, the anamnestic material, and the performance on a Rorschach. Such materials provide limbering-up exercises for the clinician, most of whose time is devoted to individuals within one cultural pattern, as, for example, when Harrower and Miale originally wished to interpret the adjustment of my Arapesh informant Unabelin as due to a position of social leadership, because this seemed to them the best explanation of how he could have maintained a good adjustment in spite of strong internal tension (68, Part V). When I asked whether they could conceive of some alternative solution, they suggested a culture which was highly permissive to individual fantasy but made little institutionalized use of it. This second suggestion is an exact description of Arapesh culture. Each such joint attempt should expand the psychiatrist's understanding of the projective tool, as well as increase the anthropologist's ability to use psychodynamic concepts.

Dreams provide another context in which it is possible to move easily from one cultural context to another, as there is no material to date which suggests that the general psychological pattern of dreaming is not cross-cultural. Earlier discussions of dream symbolism wasted a great deal of energy elaborating the point that water, or fire, might mean different things in the dreams of members of different cultures, simply failing to raise the argument to a high enough level of abstraction. If the dream in any society is approached with an understanding of dream process, of mechanisms such as condensation, and if the psychiatrist is fully aware of the extent to which the particular symbolism of his patients' dreams are culturally patterned and of the way in which each patient's idiomatic interpretation of life, type of imagery, pattern of repression, etc., will be manifested in dreams, then dreams become very useful cross-cultural material. If the dream can be separated from the clinical context, it provides an ideal stage on which to study the innermost extent of cultural patterning of preverbal bodily experience, just as the tools and scientific thought of a people provide us with data on the extent to which culture produces a medium for dealing with the observed nature of the external world. More psychologically immediate, perhaps, than the differences between the arts and rituals of different cultures are the differences in what they make of dreaming. Where dreams are articulated into the social life, as the basis of religious vocation, artistic design, or social event, they become as recognizably culturally patterned as the rhythmic design of a song or the plot of a myth, and, instead of being merely the crudest, although quite recognizable, outline of a pattern of culturally regular repression and disallowance of bodily impulses, the expressions themselves are transformed and elaborated.

The most significant study of primitive dreams, still unpublished, was made by Kilton Stewart (82), who collected dreams in three primitive societies: the Negrito of Luzon, the Yami of Botle Tabago, and the Senoi of Malaya. These three cultures had very different attitudes toward dreams. The Yami disapproved of them entirely as a source of religious inspiration. The Negrito shaman had a special type of dream in which the dream character directly helps the sick. The Senoi train their dreamers so that destructive characters and events are converted into constructive forms. The dreams of children and adolescents in the three societies were remarkably similar. So: "I dreamed that I saw a big snake and I ran very fast" (Negrito); "I dreamed that I went to the top of a mountain. Suddenly I fell and was injured" (Yami); "I dreamed that I went out for a walk. A tiger saw me. I ran away and climbed a tree. Then I woke up" (Senoi).

In contrast, we find among adults the following:

"I dreamed that I saw an *anito* [dream character] walking in the forest. As soon as I bent to get a potato, the *anito* made a fearful sound and came upon me. I jumped up and ran home" (Yami).

But the Yami make no use of dreams except as a basis for ritual behavior. An example of such a dream is:

I dreamed that I fought with an *anito* and defeated him. Four days later I got a sick back and prayed and offered it horns of deer. Soon after this, this sickness was well cured.

I dreamed that I was going to take a bath in the river. On the way I saw a big giant who was going to eat me [Negrito].

This was the unelaborated dream of an ordinary adult, but a Negrito shaman dreamed the following:

One night I dreamed that I went to catch fish in the river. After fishing, I returned home. On my way home, I met a horse which ran after me. As soon as I reached home, I became sick. When I was already very ill, an old woman appeared and gave me medicine. After this, she advised me not to eat more than one-half chopa of rice and if one ate more than this, one would die. From that time, I got well and the old woman disappeared at once; and I think the old woman who gave me medicine was Jesus Christ and the horse was a fairy. However, the horse did not harm me, but I stopped fishing in that place.

Then compare this ordinary adult Senoi dream:

I dreamed that I went out of my house to visit a snare that I had set for mouse-deer. On the way, a tiger appeared. As for me, I ran and climbed up a near-by tree. Then I woke.

with a Senoi shaman's dream in which a destructive instrument is transformed creatively:

During the clearing of our last rice plantation, late one evening I was giving the last few strokes of the axe to the trunk of a huge Tualang tree. As it fell, it hurled me down on the ground. When it had fallen, I went home to sleep and in my dream, the spirit of the Tualang sang to me, a song which I still sing to this day:

> "You hurled me down-stream to the left,
> You I hurled up-stream to the right,
> If indeed you would like my help,
> I would like to help you."

This record gives us, in a medium immediately translatable into materials upon which psychoanalytical insights have fed, intimate detailed data on the way the conceptual model of experience provided by the body can be given form and meaning in cultures which make use of it. In such cases dream thought need not become a disturbing rival form, opposed to "rational thought." It is possible to see that the only alternatives are not either high adjustment to the external world, paid for by a break with this early preverbal way of thought, which is completely relegated to an unconscious, kept precariously out of ordinary waking functioning, or a break-through of a kind of thinking so culturally unpatterned that it obscures adjustment to the external world, such as is found in schizophrenia. In those societies in which there is articulate social use of these primary processes of thought, it is not only the extraordinarily gifted individuals who are able to preserve their creativity—as in our society—but each member of the society is provided with a medium through which the inarticulate ways of thought of the infant and the culturally disciplined mature observation of internal and external world can be articulated into a pattern which provides meaning to both. We know too little of the cultural conditions for creativity, but there are suggestions that types of reliving of very early experience which are permitted by cultural forms may be significant, as when children pass through not only a stage of dispossession by the next younger sibling but stay within the family circle long enough to watch the dispossessor dispossessed (55, 57), or, contrastingly, when very little counterpointed patterning is imposed upon the primary learnings of the first year of life (36).

### PROBLEMS OF CLINICAL IMBALANCE

One of the most frequent questions which psychiatrists ask anthropologists is about the amount of neurosis, the number of psychotics, found in other cultures. While attempts to answer this question do focus upon the point of easiest apparent communication between the clinician, whose ear is attuned to trauma, and the anthropologist, who studies whole societies, it is doubtful whether this is the most fruitful line of communication. Advance in psychodynamics at present is compromised by the circumstance that the greatest discoveries have come from the study of the sick, the traumatized, the mutilated. It is customary to rationalize this circumstance by pointing out that the abnormal case throws into high relief processes which are less easy to identify in the normal. This argument is perfectly defensible, provided that the word "abnormal" is not interpreted in terms of a culture which implicitly identifies the abnormal with the undesirable, the pathological, but instead considers the abnormal as all that is out of the usual—the most intelligent as well as the least, the most gifted and creative as well as the most psychotic and disturbed, person in any given society. But this has not been the case. Within a culture which once lumped together the saint and the insane as equally closely related to God, medicine took a dominant role in continuing to classify together the unusually gifted and the unusually vulnerable, the blessed and the wounded, so that we came to have, in effect, a view of the world in which there were two kinds of people, the "normal," those who managed to make their way through life without revealing such psychotic, neurotic, or somatic disorders labeled "psychosomatic," sufficient to demand the care of the clinician, and those who land in the office or the hospital (60). The artist, the scientist, or a religious leader is likely to be tacitly classified as probably just as sick, really, but with a lucky talent or a lucky orthodoxy which made him, certainly not normal, but economically and socially self-sufficient. By classifying the gifted and the mutilated together, one could ask of the anthropologist whether it was not possible to view whole cultures as more or less neurotic, in perhaps a different sense than in the question of how many neurotics and what kind does a culture produce. It was possible to question seriously whether the Manus were not all compulsive neurotics and whether whole cultures could not develop methods of child rearing, on the one hand, and organizational forms, on the other, within which only neurotic individuals existed. There again, implicitly, the problem came to be of seeing cultures as more or less pathological, with all adjustment lumped together as normal, varying toward the possibility of pathology.

A reconsideration of this whole position seems called for, not only if there is to be optimum communication between psychiatrists and anthropologists theoretically, but also if we are to work together toward a world in which we not only describe and analyze existing cultural paths and attempt to cure those who fail to use them but face the task of constructing, out of our insights, cultures in which human potentialities will have fuller play. To appreciate fully the contribution which the anthropologist, studying a whole culture, can make, it is necessary to hypothesize another specialized discipline comparable to psychiatry, a discipline which would fall within the field of education but which is not found there today. For the word "abnormal" we would substitute the word "special" and define the necessary symbiotic relationships between those who study cultural regularities, the expected path of human development within defined cultural settings, and two disciplines which make detailed, year-long individual studies of special cases of trauma and of blessing. This hypothetical discipline, which would complement the psychiatrist, would concentrate upon, study, and facilitate the creativity of those individuals in whom innate capabilities were present to a very special degree—the child whose faith in life had been reinforced because the death of a sibling had been followed by the birth of a second sibling, in contrast to the child who had experienced the death of his own mother and three foster-mothers; the boy who was reared in a society where the ability to paint was acclaimed in males as well as in females, in contrast to the boy who had a gift for painting but was born in a frontier American town. For it seems worth emphasizing that psychoanalytic theory has not developed merely by consideration of the pathological but by detailed, careful, exceedingly time-consuming attention to particular, individual cases, whose need and circumstances permitted them to enlist a physician's time and care for many hours over several years. Analytic insights are the results of some of the most painstaking, detailed clinical research that has ever been done. Freud, in his great inclusiveness, was interested in both gift and trauma (27), and Alexander (5) has stressed the significance of an ordered division of labor for the release of human creativity. Today insight is heavily focused on the traumatic side, so that it is possible for Kardiner to advance the thesis that "the projective systems of society," by which he means its art, religion, etc., are derived from the *nuclear trauma* common to individuals in that society (45). In actual treatment of the ethnological material, the loving mother or the strong, protective father, good child care as well as bad child care is included; but it is the discrepancies, the contradictions, the discontinuities, of experience which are postulated as the dynamic forces producing the symbolic systems which we call "cultural." Roheim has been less tempted to do this, but his preoccupation in identifying plots which lie beneath particular cultural systems (80, 81) with the particular plots which have been identified as traumatic in our society and his neglect of the whole diffused pattern of human culture, which only in origin or particular version shows the immediate reflection of a particular childhood sequence, have lowered the impact of his conceptions. Jung, while conducting a battle for the recognition of gift and creativity, has again obscured the issue by combining the conception of creativeness with ideas of the horrendous nature of some unconscious processes, this classification again dependent upon our European tradition.

Only by imagining that it would be worth while, both to subject and to observant scientist, to spend as much time studying the very well as the very sick, the very strong as the very weak, the very gifted as well as the individual who fails, can we really dramatize what the problem is. The sick, frustrated, miserable neurotic is willing to sit and detail his free associations within a painful, exacting framework of increasing admission of the unacceptable, to a physician who is specially trained in this exercise of his therapeutic gifts. But the gifted have no such specialized ear, except when they also happen to be sick, so that what detailed material we have on the gifted is inextricably woven with material on the traumata which they had experienced and which now form, as in any personality, part of the whole. Only in the situation where one analyst trains another do we get a hint of what it would be like if one could combine in a teacher psychological skill and the practices peculiar to a creative profession.

At present, however, when psychiatrist and anthropologist work together exchanging insights, the anthropologist's data tend to be skewed. The record of the way in which a people manage to live an ordered life, marry, and reproduce becomes a record of the degrees of distortion which are socially tolerable; and all cultures are seen as elaborations of nuclear traumata, in each of which exorbitant prices are paid for adjustment, on the one hand, or maladjustment, on the other.[3] With such phrasing, attention is directed toward the disease conditions in different cultures with an expectation of finding a high rate of hypertension here, of asthma there, or toward the incidence of identifiable sexual neurosis, or frank psychotic states. The *usual* adjustment in each society is seen as strength, intertwined as it is with penalties, vulnerabilities, possibilities and actualities of breakdown, all of which are then seen as weaknesses. It then becomes possible to use Rorschach categories, based upon such a view, and describe the character of the Ojibwa Indians, living and surviving in a hostile, difficult world, whose character structure shows clear indications that they so regard the world, as intrinsically mutilated personalities (17). If such intensive listening for distortion and for trauma is applied to all societies, without any compensating listening for the fulfilment and blessings which come to each individual in the course of learning to be a human being in his particular culture, many of the issues which it would be helpful to illuminate are blurred. For instance, it is quite possible to regard different cultures on a variety of scales, stressing different values—survival under a set of given conditions, survival under the stress of change, survival at the cost of very heavy maladjustment of the individuals which constitute them, survival with gains of great beauty and heightened function of the individuals who constitute them. But, in order to do this, the culturally usual behavior must be listened to with two ears, trained in the psychodynamics of both trauma and blessing, while the anthropologist pro-

3. Two particularly stimulating attempts to combine cultural theory and the details of particular disease states (15 and 85) both tend in this skewed direction.

vides the data on how a particular society, with a particular set of institutions placed within a group of surrounding societies and related with a given set of technologies to the environment, permits human personality to develop. When this is done, the anthropologist will no longer be seen as the protagonist of the normal or usual, against which the unfavorably pathological is opposed as the only alternative, so that the normal becomes only a more tolerable, less expensive form of trauma.

Once this issue is clearly understood, then the anthropologist can begin to consider—with the psychiatrist's help—cultures as they provide different conditions of growth for their members. It will be possible to show that a culture may present a serious defect, both in the way the young are reared and in its political institutions, as Victor Barnouw, in his study of the Wisconsin Chippewa (6), has suggested that the ease with which these Indians, who had previously lived such an isolated and self-sufficient life, became parasitical upon the white civilization was due to a culture in which dependency needs in the child were aroused and left unsatisfied, because there was no system of political authority which could integrate them. Or the adjustment of the Dobuans to their poverty and meager resources can be seen as a viable form, in which each individual carried a load of hostility, which, while appropriate to the ongoing state of his society, was heavily weighted on the negative side. In contrast to the way in which the Chippewa of Barnouw's description over-welcomed the white man, who filled a need, the Dobuan (13, chap. v; 26; 80) could use the literacy the missionary brought him only to fake documents which would involve his neighbors in deeper embroilment with one another.

But, while using the insights of the psychiatrists to suggest that particular societies might survive and perpetuate their institutions by a form of learning which heavily traumatized every individual born into it, the anthropologist may go on to consider two other cases. The first is a society like Samoa (55, 57, 58), in which a set of social arrangements, a relationship to the environment, and a way of learning existed which did not penalize the culturally adjusted individual. He lived a continuously rewarding life, seeking no goods which he was not able to find, disturbed only by those misfortunes which are the lot of man—illness and death. But for the unusual individual, one gifted beyond his fellows, there was no place. Where the Dobuans had all been so reared as to show a high evidence of trauma, quite viable within their social circumstances, but still readily identifiable, the Samoans were so reared as to obviate trauma in the sense of bad distortions of personality but also, by their insistence on slowness, on never acting beyond one's years, on never bursting out above the usual, were prevented from any use of special gifts in the arts, in religion, in philosophy, or in science.

An even greater complication is introduced when we consider the Manus (25, 64, 65), who show such close resemblances to many emphases in our own culture. They do not, like the Samoans, emphasize a balance between need and fulfilment, between body and outer world, so perfect that almost all aberrant behavior—whether of initial receptivity to trauma or to blessing—is barred out, but, instead, live in a one-sided world in which intelligence, competence, a high standard of living, and an alert, inquiring, interested attitude toward the outer world are maintained by a method of child rearing in which competing tendencies, any desire to listen to one's own heart, to see visions, to find beauty, remain well below the surface. Rorschachs of the Manus would show, undoubtedly, great impoverishment in the fantasy life. Observation of their way of life and study of their institutionalized kinship arrangements show that there are many human potentialities of which they make little. They work with an intensity and drive which accord but ill with life on the Equator. They die young. Yet in a society which offers no competing vision of another way of life from which the Manus, with his pattern of repression, is barred out, attention only to the degree of traumatization would not be a full answer. Rather, Manus may be seen as a culture which has a set of institutions and a method of learning that provide one of the possible fits between human impulses and social forms, when the relationships between all human beings, including mother and child, are construed in terms of intervening material objects, when the attention is directed outward to the observable relations between objects, and human intelligence is given free play to probe into and manipulate such relationships.

The cultures which show a high development of the symbolic life present us with the third problem. If we again consider Bali (10, 11, 52, 53, 54, 57, 59), it may be described as a culture with a delicately balanced relationship between people and the environment in which food and material goods were adequate, warfare and crime at a minimum, and the arts in a high state of development. Carving, painting, puppet-making, the construction of millions of beautifully devised perishable offerings from fruit and flowers, music which filled the air day and night, and dances which, when practiced by little children, were still subject to a highly self-conscious aesthetic standard filled most of their time. The satisfactions which the people derived from all these elaborate forms, whether as critical spectators or as practitioners, were such that they moved lightly, unfatigued, with a dreamy gaiety, through their lives into the next world, believing that a few generations later, unremembered, they would come back into this world again, reincarnated in the same family. Learning was like a dance, and the learning followed the movements of the one who was skilled in the given art; violence and grief were dramatically expressed on the stage but were muted in real life. However, when we examine the way in which the little child learns to be a Balinese, we find a whole series of events which, interpreted within our psychiatric knowledge, seem traumatizing. The child is stimulated to expressions of emotion, and then, just before the climax, the mother turns away, leaving the child at first raging and despairing, later apathetic and sullen, finally committed to a relationship to people which will ever remain distant, wary of too much expressed feeling, yet sensuously rewarding, so that the Balinese has not only tolerance but pleasure in being packed closely together in crowds, body against body. The Balinese who is frightened falls asleep, a soft sleep neither overlimp nor overrigid, but one from which it is hard to wake him. The Balinese who has to wait may curl up in a fetal position—and fall asleep. So acute is his awareness of each part of his body that a man watching a cock fight can be seen to be identifying not with one cock or the other but with the battle, which he re-enacts between his two responsive hands. A whole man may go into trance, or only the hand may be put in trance. Within his own highly elaborate system of time and space, he moves relaxed and graceful; in a totally unknown situation he is unable to act at all. On tests (1) the Balinese respond like schizophrenics, but they are functioning members of their communities.

Any attempt to state Balinese culture in psychodynamic terms challenges all our knowledge both of social forms and of psychodynamics, even though the picture has the advantage of such apparent clinical clarity. One may say that this is a protected society, on an island, far from the main roads of competition and war, with a set of historical institutions well advanced in devices for co-operative and ordered living, such as the village commune with its rotation of duties; a caste system muted to a situation in which the casteless people were also the great majority and the indigenous population; a light feudal rule which did not lay too heavy a hand on the resources of the people; a religious system which lacked any tendency to exclusiveness, dogma, or the centralization of religious authority; highly developed crafts; writing and money and metals sufficient to make exchange and government easy. Add to this an artistic inheritance from peoples whose cultures were more complex and highly developed than they themselves, from India, Southeast Asia, China (32); a religion with a philosophical system much more complicated than their own demands for complexity, so that one has the spectacle not of a people laboriously coping with an attempt to understand the universe— which characterizes most of the known high cultures of the world —but instead standing on tiptoe to see into the unknown through a set of windows already intricately designed by others. Then consider the delicate fit between bodily experience and articulate social form, so that not only is creeping articulately forbidden as animal behavior but infants are carried in such a way that the much greater emphasis on flexion than on extension is such that child specialists here feel that crawling behavior would not appear in any case. Finally, it is possible to identify in Bali, as Gregory Bateson (7) has, a fit between social life and individual value system, in which the social life is seen not as the result of an unsteady balance, in which a political system somehow maintains order through utilizing unrelated and sometimes diametrically opposed individual motivations, but as a higher-order fit, in which the premises of the society and of the individual are one. Or, responding to the question which Loretta Bender[4] has raised, of how many schizophrenics can a society absorb and survive, one might say that Bali had been able to absorb a much higher number of those who would be schizophrenic in other societies, until their special potentialities, seen now as one variant of human nature, had helped develop a social order which was self-perpetuating. To this all children born in Bali were exposed, they, in turn, absorbing, in posture and gesture and capacity to move

4. Discussion by L. Bender at the 1948 annual meeting of the American Orthopsychiatric Association in New York, at the Hotel Commodore, April 14, 1948.

within a highly protected, symbolic system, something of the special gifts, the special vulnerabilities, the special sensitivities of the potentially schizophrenic, fitting in with the phrasing that "schizophrenia is not so much a disease as a way of life." In studying Balinese culture, the details of childhood experience may be seen as a way in which a culture perfectly adapted to the particular constitutional needs of schizoid individuals is communicated to all human children, involving far greater trauma for some than for others, subduing all to a state where they do not threaten the pattern, and developing an insatiable demand for symbolic rather than immediate satisfactions, turning the schizoid hunger for a meaningful pattern into an appetite for the practices of living arts.

A culture may be seen as the historically developed way in which the human potentialities for internally oriented, medially oriented, and externally oriented feeling-thought are regulated, canalized (72), and patterned so that they may be learned, shared, and perpetuated, and individuals who share them may live together in societies. Margaret Lowenfeld's World Test (48) provides a model of the process of fusion in the life of a patient, which occurs for most people in the ordinary course of human development in a coherent culture. The patient builds a three-dimensional world, conforming at least minimally to the time and space relationships on which human adjustment to external objects is based, using culturally provided symbols—small models of cows and crocodiles, lampposts and houses, policemen and cowboys—and so finds his place among the accultured members of his own society.

## Problems of Preventive Psychiatry

Cultural materials provide the practicing analyst with data for enlarging his theoretical concepts and for sharpening his appreciation of the way in which his patients are representative of their cultures or of the two or more cultures through which they have passed. But, while data on homogeneous, beautifully integrated cultures or lopsided, distorted cultures, meager and imperfect cultures, and cultures having emphases strongly contrasting with our own can all provide material to think with, the patient who reaches the consulting room at present is predominantly the product not of the failure of his culture to allow for his particular gifts or to provide him with the appropriate set and sequence of learning experiences but of culture change (23). This is particularly true if we can separate from the whole class of patients who need psychiatric care those whose illness is due to disease, physical trauma, or identifiable physical basis for their condition, and deal only with functional disorders of the type which make the patient suitable for psychoanalytic treatment. It seems important to do this because the bulk of our theory comes at present from the prolonged observation of this particular group of individuals whose disorientations and inappropriate learnings still leave them with the vigor required for an analysis. Every such patient may be looked at anthropologically as representative of the process of the rapid change and disorganization of our present-day society, very often a process which was already expressed in cultural mismating and misrearing of parents and grandparents. A type of childhood conviction of sin which would have been adequately cared for in a religious system in which conviction of sin was a prerequisite of salvation is found associated with education which has destroyed all religious belief and the possibility of religious practice (22); a parental interdiction of masturbation which would have laid the groundwork for a successful life as a witch-burning Puritan father is found to be crippling within the permitted experimental sexual practices of present-day urban life; expectation of lifelong obedience and dependency on father and husband is incompatible with the demand that a woman be able to leave home and find work alone in a distant city.

From painstaking analyses of such cases the psychiatrist obtains the sort of detailed data on contemporary human needs with which he and the anthropologist can work together to make those inventions which will provide a new type of strength to individuals, a strength particularly necessary for a world in which distortion and discrepancy may be expected to increase. The need for these new strengths is likely at present to be expressed by social scientists as a diatribe against one or another of our existing institutions—the family, the church, the wage system —and by psychiatrists as a diatribe against "the use of fear in child rearing," "maternal rejection," etc. When the inadequacy of present individuals to rear children, or even live themselves, in a world they are unprepared for and the inadequacy of the institutions through which they attempt to live are stressed, the whole argument, seen psychologically, tends to revolve around the question of trauma and the removal of circumstances which traumatize rather than around the need to create new institutions suited to a world which has never existed. In the civilizations of the past, in comparisons of homogeneous cultures in the present, we can study the ways in which each culture presents the new-born child with a setting in which some will be specially blessed, some exist in a state regarded as normal for that society, and some will be wounded beyond repair. But it is within the changing culture of the present, armed with the delicate, detailed knowledge of the consulting room, that we can set to work to devise ways not merely for preventing trauma but for developing individuals with new forms of strength. And here a special kind of data can come from the psychiatrist's practice, if he focuses not only on trauma but also upon gaps in the experience of his patients, if he asks what behavior is required of individuals for which they have had not the wrong preparation, not a series of threats where rewards would have been better, not an isolated experience of parental intercourse uncorrected by a dozen other corrective experiences, but no experiences at all.

The model for such gaps can be found in the experience of institutional children, who grow up unable to form stable family connections and, in turn, produce more inmates of institutions. What must be done to provide the growing child with models of behavior which those around him cannot, in the nature of our society, adequately represent? We have plenty of material on how to rear a cheerful little cannibal, for whom a gentle responsive mother would be a very poor preparation; on how to rear an individual who will ask his father's approval for his acts until he dies, for whom parental goads to early independence would be most unsuitable; but we know practically nothing about how to rear individuals who will live in a world which can barely be guessed at, most of the details of which are still unknown. Erikson (23) has pointed out the way in which the need to be ready to move at a moment's notice or stay where one is forever has been built into American character structure over several generations. But the next step will be to devise those steps in child rearing, in feeding, and nursery-school education in counseling agencies spaced throughout the critical periods of life. We need methods of re-educating the grandparent generation so that they, disoriented by children and grandchildren of whose like they have no experience, may not themselves feed back their disorientation and despair into the society.

Self-demand feeding—a practice which has come into modern American life from the combined insights of the psychiatrist, the child psychologist, and the anthropologist—is an example of such a form of scientific co-operation. Self-demand feeding is no return to a primitive past, no reinstatement of a mother-child relationship which has been the bulwark of earlier forms of society. It is a new invention, through which mothers, for the first time in history, are able, with clock and chart, to discover and institutionalize the particular rhythm of each newborn child, so that the child may experience a new form of relationship between its own impulses and the demands of an ordered society. In earlier forms of society, the most loving mother had either to remain in a form of purdah with her child or sometimes to leave it hungry because she had no way of knowing when it would be hungry or, alternately, she had to teach the baby to "want to be fed" at stated intervals. These both were viable ways of rearing children, but they lacked the possibilities for strength presented by self-demand feeding in which the impulses of the child and the exactions of modern scheduled society are fitted together, neither denied at the expense of the other. At present, neither the scheduled baby so common in urban American society nor the permissively, casually unscheduled baby found in the rural lower class is prepared to meet the demands of modern life. The scheduled baby will be too rigid to function fully, the casually indulged too undisciplined. In the child fed by self-demand we hope, not to eliminate a trauma, not to correct a defect, but to fill a gap, a gap in the present methods of child rearing, once adequate and now inadequate.

Preventive psychiatry may be narrowly conceived as getting at problems in an early stage or widely conceived as the psychiatric contribution to a new venture of constructing new cultural forms, from within which individuals of hitherto nonexisting types of strength—and doubtless new vulnerabilities also—will emerge to put into practice our rapidly developing body of insights about human nature.

Social change takes place today on a world stage, and in each country the insights and practices of physician and social scientist are only a part of the whole changing climate of opinion within which men are seeking to come to firmer grips with the forms of their culture. But these insights and practices are nevertheless significant and may, perceptively and responsibly exercised, sometimes be crucial.

## BIBLIOGRAPHY

This bibliography was prepared in May, 1949, and has not been altered except where articles then in manuscript have been subsequently published.

1. ABEL, T. M. "Free Designs of a Limited Scope as a Personality Index," *Character and Personality*, 7:50, 1938.
2. ABEL, T. M. "Is a Psychiatric Interpretation of the German Enigma Necessary?" *Am. Sociol. Rev.*, 10:457, 1945. A good statement of the type of misunderstandings which arise from a translation of the psychiatrist's emphasis on sequence in the single life-history.
3. ABEL, T. M.; BELO, J.; and WOLFENSTEIN, M. "An Analysis of French Projective Tests," in *Some Hypotheses about French Culture*, ed. R. METRAUX ("Columbia University Research in Contemporary Cultures," Document PR 4 [unpublished], 1950), pp. 48–69).
4. ABEL, T. M., and HSU, L. K. "Some Aspects of Personality of Chinese as Revealed by the Rorschach Test," *Rorschach Res. Exchange & J. Project. Techn.*, 13:285, 1949.
5. ALEXANDER, F. *Our Age of Unreason* (rev. ed.; New York: W. W. Norton & Co., 1951).
6. BARNOUW, V. "The Phantasy World of a Chippewa Indian," *Psychiatry*, 12:67, 1949.
7. BATESON, G. "Bali: The Value System of a Steady State," in *Social Structure: Studies Presented to A. R. Radcliffe-Brown*, ed. M. FORTES (Oxford: Clarendon Press, 1949).
8. BATESON, G. *Naven* (Cambridge: At the University Press, 1936). A Study of the Iatmul of New Guinea.
9. BATESON, G. "Social Planning and the Concept of Deutero-Learning," in T. M. NEWCOMB and E. L. HARTLEY (eds.), *Readings in Social Psychology* (New York: Henry Holt & Co., 1947), pp. 121–28.
10. BATESON, G., and MEAD, M. *Balinese Character* ("New York Academy of Science Special Publications," Vol. 2 [New York, 1942]).
11. BELO, J. *Bali: Rangda and Barong* ("American Ethnological Society Monographs," No. 16 [New York: Augustin, 1949]).
12. BENEDICT, L. "A Study of Bagobo Ceremonial, Magic, and Myth," *Ann. New York Acad. Sc.*, 24:1, 1916.
13. BENEDICT, RUTH. *Patterns of Culture* (Boston: Houghton Mifflin Co., 1934).
14. BOGORAS, W. "The Chukchee. II. Religion," *Mem. Am. Mus. Nat. Hist.*, 11:277, 1907.
15. BOOTH, G. C. "Variety in Personality and Its Relation to Health," *Rev. Religion*, pp. 385–412, May, 1946.
16. BRODY, S. An unpublished study of European and American folktale variants, done for modern children's stories.

17. Caudill, W. "Psychological Characteristics of Acculturated Wisconsin Ojibwa Children," *Am. Anthropol.*, 51:409, 1949.
18. Chase, R. (ed.). *The Jack Tales*, illustrated by Berkeley Williams, Jr. (Boston: Houghton Mifflin Co.; Cambridge: Riverside Press, 1943).
19. Devereux, G. "Institutionalized Homosexuality of the Mohave Indians," *Human Biol.*, 9:498, 1937.
20. DuBois, C. *The People of Alor* (Minneapolis: University of Minnesota Press, 1946).
21. Earthy, D. *Valenge Women* (London: Oxford University Press, for the International Institute of African Language and Culture, 1933).
22. Eliot, T. S. *The Cocktail Party* (New York: Harcourt, Brace & Co., Inc., 1950), Act II, Celia's speeches.
23. Erikson, E. "Ego Development and Historical Change," in *The Psychoanalytic Study of the Child*, Vol. 2 (New York: International Universities Press, 1947).
24. Erikson, E. "Observations on the Yurok: Childhood and World Image," *Univ. California Pub. Am. Archaeol. & Ethnol.*, 35:257, 1943.
25. Fortune, R. F. *Manus Religion* (Philadelphia: American Philosophical Society, 1935).
26. Fortune, R. F. *Sorcerers of Dobu* (New York: E. P. Dutton & Co., Inc.; London: Routledge & Kegan Paul, Ltd., 1932).
27. Freud, S. *New Introductory Lectures on Psychoanalysis* (New York: W. W. Norton & Co., Inc., 1933).
28. Freud, S. *Totem and Taboo*, authorized translation with Introduction by A. A. Brill (New York: Moffat, Yard, 1918).
29. Gifford, E. W. "Tongan Society," *B. P. Bishop Mus. Bull.*, No. 61, 1929.
30. Gildersleeve Stories for Children: "Jack and the Beanstalk," "Puss in Boots," "Rumpelstiltskin" (Capitol Record Albums, CD 11).
31. Gorer, G. *The American People* (New York: W. W. Norton & Co., Inc., 1948).
32. Gorer, G. *Bali and Angkor, or Looking at Life and Death* (Boston: Little, Brown & Co., 1936).
33. Gorer, G. "Discussion of 'Comparative Study of Culture and Purposive Cultivation of Democratic Values' by M. Mead," *Science, Philosophy and Religion, Second Symposium* (New York, 1942), pp. 78–81.
34. Gorer, G. "The Life of Kurma," in *Himalayan Village* (London: Michael Joseph, 1938), pp. 387–88.
35. Gorer, G. "Themes in Japanese Culture," *Trans. New York Acad. Sc.*, Ser. II, 5:106, 1943.
36. Gorer, G., and Rickman, J. *The People of Great Russia* (London: Cresset Press, 1949; New York: Chanticleer, 1950). Recent work done under the auspices of the Columbia University Research in Contemporary Cultures on Russia and by R. Metraux and associates on France suggest two contrasting possibilities, in which Great Russians tra-

ditionally seem to have left the stages of childhood between walking and school unelaborated, while the French lay down a basic pattern very early and each later stage adds to its intricacy but does not change its form.

37. GRINNELL, G. *The Cheyenne Indians* (New Haven: Yale University Press, 1923).

38. HENRY, J., and HENRY, Z. "Speech Disturbances in Pilaga Indian Children," *Am. J. Orthopsychiat.*, 10:362, 1940.

39. HENRY, J., and HENRY, Z. *Doll Play of Pilaga Indian Children* ("American Orthopsychiatric Association Research Monographs," No. 4 [New York, 1944]).

40. HENRY, W. E. "The Thematic Apperception Technique in the Study of Culture-Personality Relations," *Genet. Psychol. Monogr.*, No. 35, pp. 5–135, 1947. For examples of protocols see pp. 85–86 and 104.

41. HOSE, C., and McDOUGALL, W. *The Pagan Tribes of Borneo* (London: Macmillan & Co., Ltd., 1912).

42. JOCHELSON, V. "The Koryak. I. Religion and Myths," *Mem. Am. Mus. Nat. Hist.*, 10:13, 1905.

43. JUNOD, H. *Life of a South African Tribe* (2d ed., rev.; London: Macmillan & Co., Ltd., 1927).

44. KARDINER, A. *The Individual and His Society* (New York: Columbia University Press, 1939).

45. KARDINER, A. *The Psychological Frontiers of Society* (New York: Columbia University Press, 1945).

46. LANDES, R. "The Ojibwa of Canada," in *Cooperation and Competition among Primitive Peoples*, ed. M. MEAD (New York: McGraw-Hill Book Co., Inc., 1937), pp. 87–126.

47. LASSWELL, H. D. "Contribution of Freud's Insight Interview to the Social Sciences," *Am. J. Sociol.*, 45:375, 1939.

48. LOWENFELD, M. (ed.). *On the Psychotherapy of Children: A Report on a Conference Held at the Institute of Child Psychology, London, August, 1948, on the Theory and Technique of Direct Objective Therapy* (London and Essex: E. T. Herron, n.d.).

49. MADARIAGA, S. *On Hamlet* (London: Hollis & Carter, 1938).

50. MALINOWSKI, B. *Sex and Repression in Savage Society* (New York: Harcourt, Brace & Co.; London: Kegan Paul, 1927).

51. MALINOWSKI, B. *Sexual Life of Savages in North-western Melanesia* (New York: Liveright; London: Routledge & Kegan Paul, Ltd., 1929). An ethnographic account of courtship, marriage, and family life among the natives of the Trobriand Islands, British New Guinea.

52. McPHEE, C. "Dance in Bali," *Dance Index*, 7:153, 1948.

53. McPHEE, C. "Five Tone Gamelan Music of Bali," *Musical Quart.*, 35:250, 1949.

54. McPHEE, C. *A House in Bali* (New York: John Day Co., Inc., 1947)

55. MEAD, M. "Age Patterning and Personality Development," *Am. J. Orthopsychiat.*, 17:231, 1947.

56. MEAD, M. *And Keep Your Powder Dry* (New York: William Morrow & Co., 1942).

57. MEAD, M. "The Arts in Bali," *Yale Rev.*, 30:335, 1940.

58. MEAD, M. *Coming of Age in Samoa* (New York: William Morrow & Co., 1928). Reprinted in *From the South Seas* (New York: William Morrow & Co., 1939).

59. MEAD, M. "Community Drama—Bali and American," *Am. Scholar*, 11:78, 1941.

60. MEAD, M. "The Concept of Culture and the Psychosomatic Approach," *Psychiatry*, 10:57, 1947. This paper includes a discussion of the "normal."

61. MEAD, M. "Contrasts and Comparisons from Primitive Society," *Ann. Am. Acad. Pol. & Soc. Sc.*, 160:23, 1932.

62. MEAD, MARGARET (ed.). *Cooperation and Competition among Primitive Peoples* (New York: McGraw-Hill Book Co., Inc., 1937). A discussion of one way in which cultures may be grouped as types under the headings of co-operation and competition.

63. MEAD, M. "An Ethnologist's Footnote to 'Totem and Taboo,'" *Psychonanal. Rev.*, 17:297, 1930. Detailed reference for the statements quoted can be found in this article.

64. MEAD, M. *Growing Up in New Guinea* (New York: William Morrow & Co., 1930). Reprinted in *From the South Seas* (New York: William Morrow & Co., 1939).

65. MEAD, M. "An Investigation of the Thought of Primitive Children with Special Reference to Animism," *J. Roy. Anthropol. Inst.*, 62:173, 1932.

66. MEAD, M. "Kinship in the Admiralties," *Anthropol. Papers Am. Mus. Nat. Hist.*, 34:183, 1934.

67. MEAD, M. *Male and Female* (New York: William Morrow & Co., 1949).

68. MEAD, M. "The Mountain Arapesh. I. An Importing Culture," *Anthropol. Papers Am. Mus. Nat. Hist.*, 36:139, 1938; "The Mountain Arapesh. II. Supernaturalism," *ibid.*, 37:317, 1940; "The Mountain Arapesh. III. Socio-economic Life; IV. Diary of Events in Alitoa," *ibid.*, 40:159, 1947; "The Mountain Arapesh. V. The Record of Unabelin with Rorschach Analyses," *ibid.*, 41:289, 1949.

69. MEAD, M. "On the Implications for Anthropology of the Gesell-Ilg Approach to Maturation," *Am. Anthropol.*, 49:69, 1947.

70. MEAD, M. "Psychological Weaning: Childhood and Adolescence," in *Psychosexual Development in Health and Disease*, ed. P. HOCH (New York: Grune & Stratton, Inc., 1949), pp. 124-35.

71. MEAD, M. *Sex and Temperament in Three Primitive Societies* (New York: William Morrow & Co., 1935). Reprinted in *From the South Seas* (New York: William Morrow & Co., 1939), Part I.

72. MURPHY, G. M. *Personality* (New York: Harper & Bros., 1949).

73. OLANSKY, H. "Infant Care and Personality," *Psychol. Bull.*, 46:1, 1949. A good statement of the type of misunderstandings which arise from a translation of the psychiatrist's emphasis on sequence in the single life-history.

74. H.R.H. PRINCE PETER OF GREECE. "Tibetan, Toda, and Tiya Polyandry: A Report on Field Investigation," *Trans. New York Acad. Sc.*, Ser. II, 10:210, 1948.

75. RADCLIFFE-BROWN, A. R. "The Mother's Brother in South Africa," *South African J. Sc.*, 21:542, 1924.
76. RADIN, P. (ed.). *Crashing Thunder: The Autobiography of a Winnebago Indian* (New York: Appleton, 1926), pp. 1–4.
77. REICHARD, G. A. *Social Life of the Navajo Indians* (New York: Columbia University Press, 1928), p. 62.
78. RIVERS, W. H. R. *The Todas* (London: Macmillan & Co., Ltd., 1906).
79. ROHEIM, G. "The Garden of Eden," *Psychoanal. Rev.*, 27:1 and 177, 1940.
80. ROHEIM, G. "Psycho-analysis of Primitive Cultural Types," *Internat. J. Psycho-Analysis*, 13:2, 1932.
81. ROHEIM, G. *The Riddle of the Sphinx* (London: Hogarth Press, 1934).
82. STEWART, K. *Magico-religious Beliefs and Practices in Primitive Societies: A Sociological Analysis of Their Therapeutic Aspects* (Ph.D. thesis, University of London, 1948). The dreams quoted bear the following numbers in the Stewart dream lists: Negrito: 7, 67, 112; Yami: 8, 160, 128; Senoi: 74, 241, 247.
83. THOMPSON, L. "Indian Personality Research" (unpublished manuscript).
84. WOLFENSTEIN, M., and LEITES, N. *Movies: A Psychological Study* (Glencoe, Ill.: Free Press, 1950). These authors have elaborated on the way in which the American father is portrayed in motion pictures.
85. WOLFF, H. G. "Protective Reaction Patterns and Disease," *Ann. Int. Med.*, 27:944, 1947.
86. ZILBOORG, G. "Masculine and Feminine: Some Biological and Cultural Aspects," *Psychiatry*, 7:257, 1944.

# XIV

## CLINICAL PSYCHOLOGY

### David Shakow, Ph.D.

CLINICAL psychology cannot be defined in a simple clear-cut way. If defined too broadly, its scope overlaps considerably with related fields, such as psychiatry; if defined narrowly, it does not cover areas which are at present definitely within the range of activity of clinical psychologists. In a period of remarkable public interest in the general area of mental health, a restricted and rigid definition might also tend to hinder natural growth.

It can, however, be said that clinical psychology is concerned with the psychological adjustment problems of the individual—more specifically, with the determination and evaluation of capacities and characteristics relating to adjustment and the study and application of psychological techniques for improving adjustment. Clinical psychology approaches these problems from the point of view and with the skills of its particular training, just as adjustment problems are approached by other interested disciplines according to their own background and training.

Clinical psychology as a field in its own right had its beginnings in 1896, when Lightner Witmer set up a Psychological Clinic at the University of Pennsylvania (2). This step was taken in the setting of a general psychology which has a "long past" dating from the very beginnings of philosophy, but only a "short history," starting about the third quarter of the nineteenth century, as a field for scientific study. Against a background of academic psychology—a psychology that was almost entirely concerned with *general* laws, particularly those relating to sensation and perception—Witmer applied some of the methods of the laboratory to the problems of the *individual* case. An approximation of what has since become known as the "team" approach in the psychiatric area was early adopted by the Psychological Clinic at the University of Pennsylvania. Physicians, especially neurologists, collaborated with the psychologists at the clinic in

449

the study of cases, and there was an early and continuing use of social workers.

During the period in which the University of Pennsylvania Psychological Clinic was developing, other factors were at work which played roles of varying importance in the growth of clinical psychology. Prodromal signs of the Binet development had appeared earlier, but it was not until 1905, with the publication of the first form of the Binet-Simon test, that the influence of this instrument became marked.

Beginning with the latter part of the nineteenth century and through the early part of the twentieth, a most important development was taking place in the field of psychiatry which had a considerable influence upon the course of clinical psychology. The functional point of view was becoming more and more prominent through the activities of such men as Charcot and Janet, but most particularly of Freud, abroad, and Meyer in this country.

This trend toward a functional point of view led to the development of another type of clinic in the United States. In 1909, William Healy, in association with the Cook County Juvenile Court of Chicago, started a Behavior Clinic for the study of delinquents (6). It is from this development that the child-guidance movement ordinarily dates its origin. Healy had been impressed by Witmer's clinic, but his general approach was in many ways quite different. The approach to the problem that Witmer developed has had an important but limited effect on the development of clinical psychology, determining its pattern only in the early days. On the other hand, Healy's approach has had a more pervasive effect on clinical psychology, especially in its latter phases. Witmer's consistent concern was with educational problems, primarily those of the mentally defective. This emphasis on the intellectual-cognitive aspects of personality naturally led mainly to contact with the educator in the setting of the school or institution for the feeble-minded. Healy's primary emphasis on the affective aspects of personality involved a broader study of the individual and contact with a much greater variety of social agencies and institutions and called for a more profound, dynamic psychology.

A development paralleling the development of these clinics, and one that is of some importance in the history of clinical psychology, was the establishment of psychological laboratories in hospitals for the mentally disordered, beginning as early as 1894 in this country (21). The McLean Hospital, St. Elizabeth's Hospital, the Boston Psychopathic Hospital, and the Worcester State Hospital are among the outstanding early examples. In some respects the work in these institutions followed along more conservative academic, experimental lines. Other aspects of their activities helped to broaden considerably the range of application of test devices. In these centers, too, there was an early association of psychologists with psychiatrists, both more extensive and intensive than that found in the Witmer type of clinic.

From these beginnings the scope of activity of clinical psychologists during the last fifty years has been quite broad. This range includes, besides work in child-guidance agencies, work in psychiatric hospitals, mental hygiene clinics, vocational guidance centers, school systems, student personnel services, prisons, schools for the delinquent, general hospitals, neurological hospitals, hospitals for the tubercular, nursery schools, case-work agencies, schools for the handicapped, and agencies working with the alcoholic and with the aged.

Since, as has already been pointed out, some of the areas covered by psychology are overlapping, whereas some are distinctive, it should be instructive to consider the relations of the psychologist to the other members of the staff in the psychiatric setting.

When the team approach was first put into practice, what happened typically was what generally happens in new developments where the participants are relatively untrained. Simplicity, naïveté, and specialization of the highest degree characterized the organization. The psychiatrist as physician made a physical study of the patient; the social worker went out into the community and conducted a social investigation, which resulted in a social history; the psychologist gave the mental tests. When the physical, social, and mental-test studies were completed, an evaluation conference, attended by all three, was held, and on the basis of the pooled findings the psychiatrist carried out the indicated therapy with the patient. The patient was usually a child, since it was almost exclusively in child-guidance clinics that the team approach was the standard practice. If, in addition to personal therapy, environmental modifications were indicated, the social worker was called upon for this additional activity.

It soon became obvious that others besides the patient proper—

usually the mother—also needed therapy. This task naturally fell to the social worker, since she had already established contact with the outside community. The limited scope of the psychologist's activity was broadened somewhat when it was recognized that certain problems, such as those of speech or reading difficulty, were fundamentally re-educational problems. These were turned over to him as the person best versed in educational procedure. It developed, however, that speech and reading problems were not mere matters of tutoring or habit training but were integrally associated with personality difficulties. Since these problems were already in the psychologist's hands, it was natural for him to continue with them at this broader level, and so the way was opened for the psychologist to work with related problems of general personality therapy. With the gradual broadening of the field of the other members of the team, the psychiatrist extended his own field to include occasional work with the adults in the child patient's environment. Under these circumstances, it was natural for the social worker to feel that age was not a reasonable basis for distinction in her own treatment work, so she began working with children. And the psychologist, on the same general grounds, began to work therapeutically with parents.

Thus what started off as a group whose members each had a very specialized and compartmentalized function became in practice a group of persons having overlapping and sometimes quite similar functions. This overlapping also resulted in the fact that frequently all three members no longer worked on the same case together. Sometimes only one, more frequently two, and, relatively less frequently, all three disciplines were involved in dealing with the same case.

Under these circumstances, what is the division of responsibility which the team situation now calls for? In answering this question, we must recognize that two important factors are involved. The first is the obvious one of the nature of the training provided by each of the disciplines. The second is a factor which is sometimes neglected in formal discussions of the problem but which is of paramount importance in the practical setting. I refer to the personality, interests, and special abilities of the individual staff member. In a field where personality factors play such an important role and where variations in the special background, interests, and abilities of workers are so great, the needs of the patient demand that both these factors be given due consideration.

We can best indicate the division of responsibility and activity among the members of a clinic whose workers are equally well trained in their particular specialties by the consideration of each of the six major functions of a clinic's activity: diagnosis, research, teaching, consultation, community relations, and therapy.

In relation to diagnostic work, each member of the team naturally makes the important diagnostic contributions which arise from the traditional approach of the discipline he represents: the psychiatrist, the medical-psychiatric; the social worker, the social and developmental data, which come from the family background history; the clinical psychologist, the psychological data, which come from psychological tests and situational studies.

In the research sphere each profession will have problems which fall within its own field and will wish to work with these relatively independently. Problems requiring co-ordinated attack are taken care of by representatives of the disciplines involved.

With respect to teaching, each profession under ordinary circumstances takes care of its own group of students and also carries the responsibility for that program of training in its own field which is laid out for the students and staff workers in other fields.

In the sphere of consultation (with representatives of other agencies, professional persons, and parents) each profession naturally takes care of the problems which are most relevant to its major competence. Problems of intellectual status, developmental stages, special abilities, and defects are usually the task of the psychologist; problems of a social and socioeconomic type, the task of the social worker; and problems of psychiatric and psychosomatic character, the task of the psychiatrist.

Community relations, which involve contact with other social agencies, with professional persons—such as ministers, physicians, and teachers—and with the lay public, are best established by each profesion in its own field in so far as lectures and other group contacts are concerned. Presumably any of the members of the staff would be prepared to give talks on the general problems of mental hygiene.

In relation to therapy, all three types of workers concern themselves with one or another of the various forms of psychotherapy, with an understandable concentration of effort by the social workers on cases where the problems are mainly social, by the psychologist where they are mainly educational, and by the psychiatrist where they are primarily psychosomatic.

Although in the six major clinic functions there is participation by all the disciplines, in three of these functions—namely, therapy, research, and community relations—one or another particular discipline is more prepared by training and predominant interest to take the major role.

The leadership in therapy rests in the hands of the psychiatrist because of his medical background, with its social and legally recognized responsibilities for treatment, and because of his great concern with this problem. The leading role in research would generally fall most naturally to the psychologist because of his special preoccupation with this aspect and because of his training, which places emphasis on investigative approaches. Predominant concern with community relations is the obvious responsibility of the social worker because of her extensive community contacts, her wide acquaintance with social organization, and her concern with the social forces in the community.

A clinic organized to take advantage of the different specialized backgrounds of the disciplines involved, as well as of their common skills, and, in addition, to take advantage of the special background and competence of its individual staff members can be said to meet the true meaning of the "team" approach. Such an approach involves a co-ordinated attack based on co-ordinated thinking about the mental hygiene problems of the individual and the community.

I have mentioned the range of activities that the psychologist is involved in as a result of his special training. It would be profitable to examine this training briefly. The last several years have seen much preoccupation with the problem of training in clinical psychology. A great variety of influences both from within and from without the field have caused clinical psychology to call upon its practitioners for competence in three major functions: *diagnosis*, the use of procedures directed to acquiring knowledge about the nature and origin of the psychological conditions under investigation; *research*, the systematic experimental or clinical attack upon specific problems for the advancement of knowledge; and *guidance and therapy*, the study and use of techniques for improving the condition of the person who comes for help. It is toward competence in these three functions that training in psychology is being more and more systematically directed at the present time.

The generally accepted pattern of training of the clinical psychologist is that proposed in the report of the Committee on Training in Clinical Psychology of the American Psychological Association (1). This program is the natural outgrowth of a long series of efforts, arising mainly in field centers (16), to systematize the training which had remained in an unorganized state for a long time. The extensive and more intelligent use of psychology during the second World War and the development of the Veterans Administration (15) and the United States Public Health Service (3) programs gave already going efforts a great impetus and resulted in the adoption of a general program. The pattern followed has been somewhat different from that of psychiatry, in that it has emphasized more the development of existing university departments as central clinical training centers and has encouraged the integration of field training centers into the university programs (5). Although several suggestions for the establishment of special professional schools in clinical psychology have been made, present opinion seems to favor working within the framework of existing university departments of psychology expanded to meet the special needs of clinical psychology.

One of the problems of the past which is being given careful consideration at present involves the recruitment and selection of potentially able clinical psychologists. The importance for clinical work of good personality characteristics as well as high intellectual qualities is receiving recognition (11).

Until psychology becomes fairly well known as a field of vocational choice, it is unlikely that undergraduate prerequisites for clinical psychological training will be made as definite as those now current in medicine. Even then, it is questionable whether rigid prerequisites will ever be established. The desirability of a broad scientific and humanistic background is recognized. This is expected to include an acquaintance with the principles of science, physical, natural and social, and with the principles of logic; an acquaintance with world literature, particularly in the field of biography and character description; and an acquaintance with broad cultural and humanistic fields. Experience with varied human settings such as comes from contacts in factory or field is considered an asset. Only enough of the elementary aspects of psychology are included in the under-graduate program to give the student a real "feel" for the content of psychology.

The actual program of training consists of a graduate-level four-year course which leads to a doctoral degree (1). This is ordinarily followed by five years of experience, at least half of which is spent in a recognized training center. Such a program makes the candidate eligible for the examinations of the American Board of Examiners in Professional Psychology, which issues diplomas of specialization in clinical psychology.

The contributions of the psychologist in the psychiatric setting will be discussed in relation to the three major areas already considered in the description of team activities and training, but mainly in relation to two of them, diagnosis and research.

It is probably fair to say that there is, on the one hand, a tendency on the part of the psychiatrist to pay too much attention to diagnostic contributions from the psychologist and, on the other, not to take these contributions seriously enough. In the field of psychiatry, where diagnosis and judgment depend so much on qualitative bases, it is natural to place rather exaggerated importance on quantitative scores of some aspect or other of the personality when these are made available. On the other hand, owing to the fact that the qualitative observations of the psychologist frequently fall into the same general categories as those of the psychiatrist, there may be a tendency to pay less attention to this aspect of his contribution.

In the diagnostic[1] realm what questions should be put to the psychologist to which he may legitimately be expected to have a reply? Before answering this query, it should be understood that the answers which the psychologist gives should ordinarily be considered to be of suggestive, complementary, or corroborative significance in the context of findings provided by a number of disciplines. Only occasionally can they be considered definitive. Frequently, the covert psychological examination provides data on characteristics and traits which are not elicited by the ordinary overt psychiatric examination.

The psychologist, on the basis of the diagnostic devices which

1. By "diagnostic," the author means, of course, a good deal more than mere "pigeonholing." Diagnosis is here concerned with the origin, nature, and especially the dynamics of the conditions under study and with suggesting hypotheses as to outcome under varying forms of disposition.

he uses, can with varying degrees of completeness and assurance, depending on the problem and the conditions of the examination, provide answers to questions which fall into four major areas: intellectual aspects of the personality, affective-conative aspects of personality, certain aspects of diagnosis, and certain aspects of disposition.

In the intellectual sphere some of the questions may be: At which level of intellectual activity is the patient functioning? What relationship does this level have to his optimal level? What specific intellectual abilities and disabilities does he have?

With respect to the emotional-activity aspects of personality, the questions may be: What are the patient's fundamental traits and characteristics? What are his dominant preoccupations? What are his latent trends? How much do these characteristics aid or hinder the achievement of his intellectual or other capacities?

With respect to diagnosis, such questions may include: What kind and what degree of disturbance does he manifest in intellectual functions generally and in specific functions, such as memory, reasoning, or association? What kind of syndrome do the psychological tests show? What evidences of change in function does he manifest now (e.g., following a course of therapy or a long illness) as compared with his functioning at an earlier period?

With respect to disposition, the questions may be: What educational recommendations can be made? What vocational recommendations are indicated? What are the prognostic possibilities of the use of his capacities in a vocation or in education or in life generally, with or without therapy?

The above are broad questions, the answers to which depend on the use of a variety of psychological procedures. Some of these procedures or devices attempt to obtain information primarily on intellectual functioning, some on emotional functioning.

The essential scientific methods available to both psychiatry and clinical psychology are, of course, naturalistic observation and experiment.[2] The former is the naturalist's standard approach, in which conditions are accepted as given and generalizations are made from selected observations. The latter, on the other hand,

---

2. A more detailed discussion of the investigative methods of the psychologist will be presented later in the context of a consideration of research.

attempts to set up the conditions to be observed, trying in so far as possible to control all variables but one, and then to make generalizations.

In the field of psychology a widely used method has developed which falls somewhere between these two. I have reference to the use of tests. This method resembles the experiment, in that the conditions are set up by the experimenter but the control of the variables is only moderately achieved. Various forms of statistical control have, therefore, to be introduced as substitutes for the experimental controls.

If we compare the methods used by psychiatry and those used by clinical psychology in the diagnostic realm, it appears that the predominant method used in psychiatry is that of naturalistic observation, whereas that of clinical psychology is testing. In the case of psychiatry, one deals mainly with the case history, which consists essentially of observational data obtained vicariously through relatives and acquaintances or from self-observation by the patient. These data are recorded either by the psychiatrist himself or by a social worker. In addition, the psychiatrist makes use of clinical observation, that is, contemporary observations made either by himself or by his surrogates, such as nurses.

The psychologist, although he depends on clinical observation to some extent—I refer to the observation of behavior during the course of the examination—places major dependence on testing procedures. In order to make the tests informative and dependable, three types of controls are set up: pre-examination controls, examination controls, and postexamination controls. These controls are set up in order to reduce the amount of dependence placed on the observer. Not having these controls, psychiatry puts a tremendous burden on the observer as the recording and evaluating instrument. Although the burden on the psychologist still remains great, these control devices help to reduce the amount of this dependence.

Let us examine the various types of control in order. The pre-examination controls involve the standardization of tests, in relation to both material and methods, until satisfactory criteria of adequacy have been met. With few exceptions, acceptable test devices go through a long period of preliminary study and trial before they are finally ready for use. A large body of tentative material is worked through, and final selection of content is made on the basis of the discriminative quality of the items to evaluate the function tested. In addition, considerable experimentation goes on with respect to the manner of presentation of the material, resulting in a standardized set of instructions. By these methods there is achieved at least some reduction in the variables which might be introduced by the observer or examiner into the situation.

The second of these types of control—those established during the examination proper—relates to the problems of "representativeness" and "optimity" of results. It is concerned with the determination of where the patient's present performance places him in relation to his potential present performance and to his fundamental capacity. An attempt is made here to determine how good a sample of the patient's optimum ability, in so far as tests are able to get at these capacity-capability levels, has been obtained during the present examination.

Psychometric determinations, even more than physiological determinations such as oxygen-consumption rate and blood pressure, are affected by the condition of the subject during examination. It is therefore essential to evaluate the adequacy of the examination results. If these are reasonably close to the *optimum* performance of which the subject was capable at *any* time, they may be considered both optimal and representative. If the results obtained are the best which the patient can obtain during the more or less immediate period of the examination (and if, at the same time, they are lower than those he could obtain at the time of his best performance), the results may be considered representative but not optimal. A consideration of the many factors which must be taken into account in arriving at this important judgment will make the distinction between the two clearer.

The factors disturbing representativeness are generally of a temporary nature. Some are under the partial control of the subject: effort, interest, self-confidence. Others are almost entirely outside the subject's control: a psychotic episode (temporary manic, excited, or hallucinatory conditions), an emotional upset, marked anxiety, physical handicap (loss of sensory aids, such as glasses, etc.), passing physical illness (headache, etc.), fatigue, poor test conditions.

The actual quantitative changes produced by these temporary factors, that is, the unrepresentativeness, is to be seen in their effect on mental age in various groups. In a study (19) carried out on a variety of mental disorders, the average additional decrease in mental age level, over and above the effect of the disorder, was found to be about 13 per cent. The decrease varies considerably, however, with the type of mental disorder. Thus in a feeble-minded group having an associated psychosis, the difference was negligible, whereas in chronic alcoholism with psychosis it was about 20 per cent, and in dementia praecox, simple group, about 30 per cent. The importance of taking into account the factor of representativeness is thus clearly indicated.

The optimity of the examination is affected not only by all the factors of a temporary kind mentioned in the discussion of representativeness but also by a group of factors of a relatively permanent nature, such as physical disability (uncorrected deafness, paralysis, etc.), psychotic state of a prolonged type, chronological age beyond approximately forty, and language disability.

A judgment of "unrepresentative" or of "not optimal" is not, of course, automatically made when some or even all of these factors are present. Rather, the examiner should consider the presence of such factors as cues for further investigation. He must then examine them carefully in relation to test performance and evaluate the role which each may have played in affecting the results. It is conceivable, though not actually likely, that many of these interfering factors may be operating and the examination results be evaluated as optimal.

For purposes of illustration, let us take one of the factors—chronological age. Numerous studies (13, 14) have indicated that certain psychological functions begin to show a decline at approximately the age of forty. The curve of function is, of course, based on an *average* tendency in the general population. In some persons the decline comes earlier, in some later. It is important for the examiner to be aware of this contingency in order to evaluate the performance of the particular subject with respect to the possible effect of age on performance. If the evidence, such as a considerably lower proportionate score on immediate memory items as compared with the score on reasoning items and vocabulary, is in the direction of decline, then a lack of optimity is indicated.

In relation to this problem the most difficult factor to evaluate is the effect of mental disorder. As stated earlier, when the patient is in a psychotic or other disturbed episode, the representativeness should be questioned, but when the disordered state is more permanent, the optimity is also questioned. It is obviously difficult to distinguish between, or to set arbitrary limits for, episodes and more permanent states. The examiner must keep in mind the primary purpose of making these judgments, namely, to evaluate fairly the person's psychological *capacity*. At the same time, it is necessary to determine his *functioning* ability, i.e., what he has to work with at the present time. If, from all the evidence available with regard to his psychotic condition, the person's performance today is the best he would be likely to achieve during the approximate period of the next several weeks or more, then the examination is considered representative. A statement to this effect means that, in the opinion of the examiner, the patient is functioning at a level of performance as high as he is likely to attain if examined during the reasonably near future. When the examiner, however, has some basis for believing that the patient could achieve a higher level of performance within such a period of time, he must consider the examination unrepresentative.

The judgment of optimity in relationship to mental disorder is particularly difficult and requires a kind of clinical judgment which only extended clinical experience can provide. The question placed before the examiner here is really: What more or less permanent effects has the disorder had on the psychological functions which prevent the present measure from being as high as the highest which the person would have obtained at some earlier time, i.e., at a period of optimum performance? If there is any evidence in the history or psychiatric record or internal evidence in the test itself that the best performance has not been obtained, the examination is not considered optimal. It must again be stressed here that the presence of mental disorder does not *ipso facto* result in the judgment of "unrepresentative" or "nonoptimal." Occasionally there are cases of even long-standing psychoses in which some of the functions measured by tests appear to be little or not at all affected.

Representativeness is, of the two, the more easily determined. Optimity can to some extent be gauged from internal evidence provided by the tests, but to a greater degree it is determined from the factors mentioned above, together with an evaluation of the educational and vocational achievement and, when available, previous psychometric results.

The third type of control is the postexamination control. This has to do with the problem of norms, relating the performance of the patient to that of other persons in a particular group. With few exceptions, tests are not considered adequate until explicit norms of this kind have been established on certain samples of the population.

There is need for care in sampling the group in order to avoid bias. If we wish to be able to say that X is better or worse than the average, and perhaps even say *how* much better or worse, then we must be sure that our average is a real average and not due to age, sex, race, personality, or occupational or other forms of selection. Complicated statistical methods for selecting adequate standardization groups, which we need not go into here, have been developed. Any group may be used for standardization purposes if it is clearly defined and carefully selected. Usually the norms are based on a variety of samples. To give a few examples, they may be age norms established on persons of different ages or autogenous norms based on racial, handicapped, or diagnostic groups.

Scores obtained by subjects may be expressed in norms in a variety of ways. Norms may be given in terms of age. In this case a statement is made about the score being the equivalent of such and such a chronological age or mental age level (or a derivative of this in terms of I.Q. level). In other cases the norms may be given in terms of centile standing or in quintiles, quartiles, or deciles. We may say, for instance, that a person's score falls into the lowest quartile of those for his age group. In still other cases the norms may be given in terms of standard deviational units, a statistic which is particularly adaptable to the kinds of distributions of functions which are obtained in psychological studies. An individual score could be described as falling one standard deviation above the average score of the group, which would mean that it falls at about the upper 15 per cent mark.

The important point for our purpose, whichever norms are used, is that dependence is not placed on the individual examiner's privately established norms (in other words, his "judgment"), but rather upon objectively obtained criterion data. Any adequate estimate of a subject's psychological capacity must therefore be based on an evaluation in terms of two standards: Where does the person stand in relation to the *group?* Where does he stand in relation to his optimum *self?*

The difference in the predominant emphases of approach of psychiatry and psychology to the problems of the study of the person makes a combined attack by the two disciplines desirable.

Although there is indeed some overlapping in the methods used and in the area covered, the major differences lead to obtaining both complementary and supplementary data with checks and counterchecks. In an area where the difficulty of obtaining dependable data is relatively great and the phenomena dealt with complex and difficult, the need for such control is obvious.

In emphasizing the "objective" character of tests, it is not my intention to minimize the importance of the "subjective" controls. These controls are essential if the greatest advantage is to be gotten from the objective characteristics. Psychological examining is not a matter of machine-tending; it is a complex human relationship calling for all the skills and sensitivities demanded by any situation requiring the establishment and maintenance of rapport. The examiner must recognize when tests are called for and when they should not be used. He needs to know what tests and combinations of tests are required in specific problems, and what their limitations are, as well as their strengths. Besides having an insightful knowledge of the diagnostic and prognostic aspects of his test findings, the examiner must be sensitive to their therapeutic implications. In fact, it is necessary that he have a "therapeutic attitude" in his testing, that is, one which avoids probing and the carrying-out of misplaced therapy. In keeping with good testing procedure and without violating the controls, he must leave the patient better rather than worse for the test experience. The examiner must have a sense of balance between the extremes of rigorous, pedantic exactness and slovenly "guessing." He must recognize that different problems lend themselves to differing degrees of control and that there are times (in certain stages of development of a problem) when a rough negative correlation appears to obtain between psychological significance and degree of control. While always working for reasonably greater control, he must be honest both in designating the degree obtained at the particular time and in admitting ignorance and tentativeness when such are the case. The psychologist must have enough security, on the one hand, not to escape into exactness about the insignificant and, on the other, not to escape into meaningless profundities because he is overcome by the complexity and difficulty of the significant. He must have a sense of responsibility about his test findings—an appreciation of the fact that they make a real difference to a particular individual and to those involved with him. The psychologist must recognize that he carries this responsibility as well as the broader social-scientific one of awareness of the research implications of his findings for advance in a field which needs much further work.

Having considered the general principles of testing, we may now discuss some of the available tests. The degree to which psychological testing has permeated our culture in the last twenty years is striking. There are in existence at least five thousand different tests of a psychological nature. An estimate made recently indicates that in 1944 some sixty million psychological tests were given to twenty million persons. For our purposes it is sufficient to become acquainted with the general categories of tests and to understand something about the most prominent tests used in the psychiatric clinical setting. I shall therefore consider first the problem of the classification of tests.

Tests are designed not only to study different functions, an aspect which we shall take up shortly, but also to study various groups of persons. These may include persons in different age ranges; groups of persons with different kinds of handicaps, such as deafness, blindness, psychosis, and neurosis; groups having special vocational characteristics. Some tests are intended for persons at a high level of functioning, some for persons at a low level; some tests use language as a means of communication, others deliberately avoid the use of language, employing instead other types of symbols or performance. Some tests emphasize underlying capacity, whereas others deliberately attempt to study the achievement or acquired knowledge of the person. Again, some tests emphasize intellectual characteristics, whereas others are primarily devoted to a study of nonintellectual or affective aspects. Some are intended for individual administration, whereas others are intended for groups.

We are here concerned primarily with those tests that attempt to measure characteristics that appear mainly to derive from underlying capacity and from the natural maturation of the organism, rather than with tests that are directed at determining the level of achievement derived from specific training. In the latter category fall those tests which attempt to measure educational achievement, skills in school subjects and vocational fields.

The capacity tests may be divided into four major groups: psychomotor, intelligence, nonintellectual aspects of personality, and special aptitudes.

Psychomotor tests generally deal with simple functions, such as steadiness, speed of tapping, and reaction time. Ordinarily, tests of this kind are little used in the clinical psychiatric setting except when organic functions appear to be affected.

The next major category, tests of intelligence, is one of the most important. This area is, in fact, the most highly developed area of the testing field. Intelligence tests fall into two major types: those dealing with composite aspects of intelligence and those dealing primarily with single aspects of intelligence. Among the former are such tests as the Stanford-Binet (25) and the Terman-Merrill (26)—respectively the 1916 and 1937 revisions of the Binet—and the Wechsler-Bellevue (28). Here also are included group tests of intelligence, such as the Otis Self-administering Test of Mental Ability and the Miller Mental Abilities Test. Among the individual tests falling into the second type of this major category are special tests of such single functions as thinking and memory. Commonly used tests of this kind are the Vigotsky Test (4), a test of conceptual thinking, and the Wells Memory Test (23).

A third category involves those tests dealing with nonintellectual aspects which have loosely been called "personality" tests. These are mainly of two types: questionnaire and projective. The questionnaire type, of which the Thurstone Personality Schedule and the Bernreuter Personality Inventory are good examples, provides descriptive statements with regard to personality and asks the person to identify himself with either the presence or the absence of the attitude or behavior described. The responses are scored according to available norms. In general, tests of this kind have many defects—primarily in that they tend to elicit unconscious halo effects—and have therefore only limited usefulness. The projective tests of personality are among the most important devices available. In recent years they have taken a very prominent place in the batteries of tests used in the clinical setting. The major instruments in this area are the Rorschach Test (12), which emphasizes the formal characteristics of personality, and the Thematic Apperception Test (17), which emphasizes the content aspects. The well-known Word Association Test is one of the earliest forms of projective test.

The last category under this major grouping of capacity tests is the one concerned with tests of special aptitudes. These tests aim to get at underlying aptitudes for special fields, such as art, music, mechanics, medicine, and aviation. The test items are based on an analysis of the major functions necessary for the achievement of particular vocational and avocational goals. The attempt is made to determine potential skill in these fields before the person has had any actual training in them. In the clinical setting these tests are relatively unimportant. Further, the tests themselves have reached only a limited stage of development.[3]

We are now ready to consider some outstanding examples of tests in the intelligence and personality areas.

We may take two examples of the individual intelligence test—the Revised Stanford-Binet Intelligence Scale and the Wechsler-Bellevue Intelligence Scale. In 1916 Terman published the first Stanford Revision of the Binet Test, and in 1937 the further revision here referred to. The test is designed to determine the general level of mental ability of the person tested. It consists of a large number of items arranged from the two-year to the superior adult level. In the case of the younger children, such tasks as building block towers, naming objects, etc., are used; at the higher levels, items involving functions such as reasoning, both verbal and numerical, are employed. Tests of memory are included throughout the scale. The test results are reported in terms of mental age and I.Q. In general, the Stanford-Binet Intelligence Scale is the most valuable for use with children, for whom it was mainly designed.

The Wechsler-Bellevue Intelligence Scale was organized to measure intelligence in adults and adolescents and is given orally to individual subjects. It consists of ten subtests, five of which are primarily verbal and five primarily performance. The verbal tests depend on language both for giving directions and for the responses of the subject. In the performance tests only the oral directions given by the examiner depend upon language. The five verbal tests cover information, comprehension, arithmetical reasoning, memory span for digits, and recognition of similarities. The five performance tests involve arranging pictures in a proper sequence, completing incomplete pictures, imitating a design with blocks, assembling a disassembled object, and learning pairs of associated symbols and digits. An alternate verbal test—vocabulary—aims at obtaining a measure of the person's past learning ability. The Wechsler-Bellevue Scale has been standardized on a large number of children and adults, ranging in age from ten to

3. A detailed discussion on the use of tests in diagnosis is to be found in Rosenzweig (20).

sixty. The results are given in terms of verbal and performance I.Q.'s and a combined I.Q.

The projective tests of personality, in contrast to those we have just discussed, do not require "correct" responses and allow for freedom and spontaneity in answer to the specific stimuli. Since the answers may be considerably elaborated and freedom for the expression of unusual trends is permitted, they are of particular value in the psychiatric setting.

We may now consider two of these tests—the Rorschach Test and the Thematic Apperception Test. The Rorschach Test consists of a set of ink-blots to which the subject is requested to give associations. The scoring of these responses is carried out on the basis of four types of analysis: (*a*) number of responses; (*b*) location of responses: whether a given response is to the whole blot or to only part of it; (*c*) determinants of response: whether form, movement, or color or a combination of these is perceived; (*d*) content of the interpretations: whether human, animal, landscape, etc., was seen. A psychogram is made from these scores which takes the interrelationship of these various kinds of response into account, i.e., the individual record is considered as a whole, not as a set of isolated scores. On the basis of this psychogram, considerable information about fundamental personality characteristics is made available. Intellectual creativity, autism, richness or poverty of associations, capacity for outwardly directed affectivity, egocentricity, capacity for social rapport, degree of control over intellectual processes, adaptability, introversiveness and withdrawal, self-appraisal, stereotypy, aggressiveness, orderliness, conformity—these are some of the characteristics on which the Rorschach may throw light. In addition, the test may be of aid in diagnostic classification, since certain combinations of response types are found empirically in particular personality and diagnostic groups.

The Thematic Apperception Test consists of a series of pictures arranged in separate groups for male and female subjects and for adults and children. The subject is instructed to regard each picture as an illustration and is then requested to tell a story to go with it, identifying the characters, explaining their relationship to one another, and giving the background for the situation and its outcome. The material is recorded verbatim and is then analyzed according to the major themes which are revealed. As far as the subject knows, this is a test of creative imagination.

He ordinarily believes that he is discussing entirely impersonal material; actually, he provides the examiner with considerable information about his own background, preoccupations, and latent trends, including his attitudes, ideals, and needs and his relationships to important persons in his environment. One obtains from the analysis of these data an understanding of the content of the person's thinking, that is, with *what* he is concerned. The Rorschach, on the other hand, primarily provides a statement about the formal characteristics of the personality, that is, *how* the person reacts and expresses his concern. These tests are thus complementary, and therefore the use of both together is a particularly desirable clinical practice.

The attempt to understand the dynamics of the individual maladjusted personality brings into focus the need for relating his problems both to his resources and to his methods of dealing with such problems. What contribution can the psychological examination make to this task?

In the task presented by the integration of data from the various disciplines frequently concerned with the study of a patient—particularly in bridging the gap between extremes provided by psychiatric and physiological-biochemical data—the psychological material is in a favorable position. Its position is strategic because, on the one hand, its more controlled and objective nature makes it adaptable for correlation with physiological and biochemical material and, on the other, its behavioral and higher-level functional nature makes it directly comparable with the psychiatric and social data.

In addition to the final goal of integrating the psychological findings with those of the other disciplines, the psychological program has another aim, that of establishing a unified psychological portrait of the individual patient. This picture is derived from a battery of tests. Certain general principles of the sampling of psychological functions lie behind the selection and administration of a test battery. These principles involve sampling (1) in different areas, (2) for content as well as for formal aspects, (3) by overlapping devices, and, where possible, (4) under conditions of stress as well as under ordinary examination conditions.

In the present consideration of sampling it is unnecessary to go beyond the simple but useful tripartite classification of cognitive, affective, and conative, using these terms in their conventional meanings. Although any device employed inevitably taps all three areas to some degree, certain devices are especially useful for investigating functions predominantly in one or another of these areas.

The same generalization holds for the structural-contentual dichotomy. Some devices are more adequate for investigating the formal or structural aspects of personality, i.e., the *how;* others for exploring the contentual aspects, i.e., the *what.* A general weakness in many investigations of personality, especially in those of a psychometric nature, has been the emphasis on the formal aspects of the personality at the expense of content. Although this one-sided emphasis is understandable and in some respects justifiable, the result of it has been to disregard a most important source of information about personality. Although the realm which one necessarily enters when one becomes involved with content is less objective and quantifiable, the broader understanding of the particular personality which study of this aspect affords is impressive.

The third principle of sampling—the inclusion of overlapping devices—is essential in any attempt to sketch a broad psychological portrait on the basis of necessarily limited sampling. It is a most useful way of increasing the reliability of the personality evaluation. The proper evaluation of personality cannot be achieved through the employment of any single device, and in this connection the importance of a battery of tests cannot be overemphasized. Frequently one device, e.g., the Rorschach, provides the most revealing data for one patient, whereas, for another, one of the other devices, e.g., the Thematic Apperception Test, provides the most dependable and productive material, while the Rorschach results are relatively barren. Whether this is due to differences in the relative sensitivity of persons at various personality levels or to some other cause, the fact remains that no one device is always productive, and even at best no one device is sufficiently broad and dependable to give reasonably complete and reliable data. Only by means of a battery of tests can one approximate a relatively extensive, integrated, and dependable personality analysis.

The fourth principle—testing under stress conditions—is found to be of value in adding significant detail to the picture of the patient. Although it is true that almost any testing situation involves stress to some extent, the concern here is with situations which attempt to place unusual pressure on the subject. Stress—

whether in the sense of distraction, failure, or frustration, whether it be hypothetical or real, personal or impersonal, peripheral or central, or physiological or psychological—is bound to reveal additional characteristics of the person under study. Stress also serves to bring out differences between persons which examination under ordinary conditions would not reveal. The data derived from testing under stress conditions gain from the integration of the separate findings. This is accomplished by disregarding the boundaries of individual tests, by comparing one with another, and by cross-checking for congruences and differences. The aim is to obtain as complete a psychological analysis of the patient as possible—an analysis which covers attitude and intellectual and affective-conative aspects of personality structure and content.

The attitude of the patient is revealed in his involvement with the tasks put before him. His effort, attention, and expenditure of energy, his mood, general co-operativeness, and responsiveness, play roles here. The representativeness and optimity of the results obtained and the handicaps from which the patient suffers that may have affected the test results are also important.

Personality structure is considered from two points of view: intellectual and nonintellectual. In the former the quantitative results, such as M.A., I.Q., and percentile rank, are discussed. The qualitative findings are analyzed with respect to the light they throw on comprehension, judgment, thinking and reasoning, learning, memory, imagery, etc. In the latter, consideration is given to such items as affective responsiveness, anxiety, security, maturity, and goal behavior (venturesomeness as opposed to cautiousness, realism as opposed to unrealism of approach, plasticity as opposed to rigidity, consistency as opposed to variability). An evaluation is made of the subject's reactions to stress situations as they affect these characteristics.

Content is analyzed through a consideration of the major sentiments and complexes revealed by the subject. Particular attention is paid to those which relate to (*a*) family—paternal, maternal, filial, fraternal, and conjugal relationships; (*b*) sex—prenubile and nubile heterosexual attitudes, homosexual and other aberrant attitudes; (*c*) aggression—manner of expression of aggression, whether direct or indirect, externally or internally oriented, punished or unpunished (need for guilt and expiation), and reciprocated or initiated; (*d*) ideals—social and vocational; (*e*) any other sentiments and complexes which appear to be of special importance to the subject.

Following the analysis, a summarizing evaluation may be made, giving a tentative dynamic and structural synthesis derived from the mass of psychological data. This evaluation is available for comparison with the evaluations made by the representatives of the other disciplines.

A condensed case study,[4] that of patient W., has been selected to illustrate the use of a test battery in some of its aspects.

During the examination W. co-operated well, manifesting some degree of interest in each of the variety of tests, but his responses were given in a slow and hesitating manner. Numerous signs of "tension," such as humming, drumming on the chair arm, and occasional laughing, were present.

The patient attained a "superior" intellectual rating. Vocabulary achievement was at the top decile level for adults. The poorest performance was on items involving rote memory and conceptual thinking. In the latter, although he did not actually give evidence of the concrete thinking often associated with schizophrenia, he substituted vague generalizations for true concepts. The results were considered representative of the general state of the patient at the time of the examination, but there was some question as to whether they could be characterized as optimal.

In other formal aspects of personality, there was evidence of marked constriction, as shown by data from the Rorschach Test. Many fissures in the constrictive wall indicated that this manner of defense was not entirely effective. These manifested themselves in various forms of "looseness," e.g., bizarre responses and variation in the quality of responses (initial poor responses which, on second thought, he would replace with good responses). There were, however, several Rorschach Test signs which called for favorable interpretation. Conventionality of response, interpreted as evidence of contact with the environment, was seen in a high number of popular responses. The improvement in the quality of responses on second thought (already mentioned) and some degree of "warmth" as indicated by his color responses were also in his favor. An attempt to attain a higher level of mental activity than he was capable of was manifested both in the Rorschach Test and in a certain pretentiousness which appeared in the Stanford-Binet vocabulary responses.[5] This was also shown in his general manner of expressing himself on the Thematic Apperception Test. His exceptional interest in small details and in human and animal parts shown on the Rorschach Test was also manifested on the Thematic Apperception Test.

In "goal behavior" W.'s outstanding characteristic was one of cautiousness associated with some rigidity. In a motor task, the successive aspi-

4. A more detailed discussion of this case as well as the principles of study here presented will be found elsewhere (24).

5. E.g., "hysterics" is defined by him as: "state of nervous exhaustion associated with persons suffering a mental breakdown due to external harassment."

rations he set for achievement also indicated a cautious approach associated with rigidity.

The effect of placing the patient in stress situations was to create a considerable disturbance of expression in the formal aspects of his personality. In tasks involving goal behavior, after repeated failure he still rigidly maintained the aspiration level adopted during success. With further prolongation of failure, however, the rigidity broke down, and W.'s behavior fluctuated between undue cautiousness and an unrealistic return to the highest aspiration level set during success. This fluctuation may best be interpreted, perhaps, as due to a conflict between an unrealistic reluctance to accept a lowered aspiration level and a realistic need to be cautious in a situation of repeated failure. In a learning situation under stress he showed considerable disturbance; there was a cessation of further learning, even in trials not involving stress.

An analysis of the content in the test material, based mainly on the Thematic Apperception Test, indicated that his major problems revolved around the areas of family, sex, and aggression, all of which appeared to be closely interlinked. The stories revealed considerable conflict with respect to filial relationship. Although benevolent familial attitudes are described in several instances, there seemed to be an inability on the part of a child character ever to accept both parents at one time, or to accept an originally described familial setting as satisfactory. There was a distinct trend for existing family constellations to disintegrate. This occurred in one of three ways: (1) One of the parents (usually the mother) was blamed, and the child accepted living with the other, with whom he went away to another setting. (2) Both parents were eliminated either by death or by being characterized as inadequate in their method of bringing up children. This was followed by the youngster's being adopted, or at least brought up, by somebody else. The surrogate parent was sometimes male and sometimes female. (3) The central character escaped entirely from the family environment to new people and surroundings.

Stories involving the relationship between the sexes were apparently embarrassing to the patient and usually given with some hesitation. In general, they emphasized the distinction which he consistently drew between passion ("carnal" relations) and love. He showed little concern for more permanent love relationships, while temporary love and "carnal" relationships seemed to occur only in connection with primitive or foreign persons.

The aggression expressed in the stories was weak and usually associated with "badness" and ignorance; it appeared only as an attribute of inferior persons. In the main, the central character was the object of assault or the object of unfair treatment. He tended to be passive, suppliant, or bewildered, and when aggression was evidenced it would quickly become attenuated or generalized, e.g., a specific physical attack on the central character was changed into a battle between the power of intelligence and ignorance. The reaction to such aggression was generally one of seeking support and guidance from others to attain strength. Frequently, however, the central character would leave the field entirely as a solution to the problem.

In relation to goals the central characters very consistently showed marked dependence, frequently turning to protective figures to help them out of difficulties. The need for "affiliation" and "succorance" seemed great. The goals were weak, uncertain, conventionalized, and not clearly defined. Only one goal, namely, marrying a "nice girl," was mentioned more than once, but even then quite tentatively and with little force.

Several other trends which seemed to be of importance should be mentioned. There was much preoccupation with details of physiognomy and bodily characteristics. The reference to physical characteristics as indicators of moral and psychological characteristics, usually of a negative type, was frequent. Although this trend was more marked for male figures, it was found also with respect to female figures. In a superior manner, W. described characters as of "low" nature, although they appeared quite clearly to be projections of himself. There was, too, an interest in the general details of the background, some emphasis on the unreality of the pictures, and a sensitivity to the part which the photographer played in their making. Some of the elaborative details of the themas given by W. revealed an underlying suspiciousness.

In summarizing and evaluating the psychological findings, the following points stood out. W. appeared to be a person of superior intelligence who had not quite settled down to a definite way of handling his problems. Three trends were discernible: (1) a realistic, at least superficially socialized, trend which gave evidence of a continuing contact with the environment; (2) a constrictive trend which served to shut out the environment and to permit him to build himself up to a superior status; (3) a loose, unorganized trend, manifesting loss of control. The first trend seemed fairly weak, and the major battle appeared to be between the latter two. The central problems revolved about the relationship between aggression and the familial triangle situation. There was some ground for tentatively suggesting the following hypothesis: Basic to his then existing condition was a marked confusion and bewilderment concerning his relationship with his mother as a source of satisfaction for his unconscious needs, with a resultant turning to the father figure for the satisfaction of these needs. A similar pattern was present in the closely related aggressive trends. Tentative attempts at aggressive expression which had met with rebuff apparently led to bewilderment and to a search for support in some kind of positive action. The various types of solution, however, were not clearly differentiated and seemed to be milling around in a confused mass, none of them having sufficient underlying force to go anywhere in particular. The similarity of this pattern to the earlier description of the formal aspects of W.'s personality is striking.

At the time when the above psychological report, based entirely on independently derived test data, was made, the following material was reported by staff members representing other disciplines.

According to the physicians' statement, W. had been committed to a state hospital in 1941, because of "depressed appearance, extreme apathy and untidiness, a belief that his mind is being read, great thinking difficulty."

The history obtained by the social worker, before the commitment was, in brief, as follows: W., 33 years old, was born in a small town, the youngest of nine siblings, three brothers and five sisters, who appear to be in good physical and mental health. As a small child he was considered unusually cross and shy but was much superior intellectually to the rest of the family. He achieved excellent marks in school and was given piano lessons beginning at the age of 10. His father was a heavy drinker and a domineering person, toward whom W. apparently developed considerable antagonism which he generally covered up. The father died of arteriosclerosis and angina pectoris at the age of 68 when the patient was about 17. The mother, aged 73 at the time of the history, was in good health. W. graduated from an outstanding secondary school with honors and entered a well-known college. The whole family helped him financially with his schooling. This was supplemented by money borrowed from the college and by what he earned through working in one of the dining-rooms and at the post office during the school year and vacations. It is reported that he studied very hard thoughout this whole period and that he had very little outside recreation. He is said to have had a marked feeling of responsibility and to have been sensitive to the pressure exerted by the family. He had feelings of inadequacy and considered himself unable to measure up either to their expectations or to the standards of his college. At various times he stated that the work was very difficult for him and that he never felt that he had an adequate grasp of the situation.

Always considered a quiet, seclusive, introspective type of person, he had but one close friend at college, from whom he drifted when the latter married. He was interested in the piano, which he played fairly well, but he avoided playing for others. One of the informants described him as an "idealist, very hard to talk to" and as having difficulty in expressing his ideas. After graduation, he continued to work in a post office for a short time and then held successive positions in brokerage offices, at a department store, and finally at one of the railroads. He was employed by the department store for three years and did quite well in the cashier's office. He became discontented in the latter department, however, and insisted on being transferred to the merchandising department against the advice of his superiors and colleagues. As was expected, he did not get along well there. He finally left the department store and was given a job as the baggage master of a small railroad station near his home town on the strength of his father's previous good work record for the railroad. It was while he was on this job that he was drafted into the army. The record at the railroad indicated that his adjustment had not been of high quality.

W. had not been considered to be an altogether healthy person. He was slightly deaf; and there was some possibility that he had suffered from convulsions as a baby. At the age of 25 he was involved in a serious automobile accident but suffered no obviously severe injuries.

There is a report that during the 26–27-year age period a "change" occurred in the patient's personality. He became indifferent to the Episcopal church to which he belonged and had formerly attended regularly. W. no longer cared to play the organ as he used to do, and he began worrying about world conditions and became "pessimistic." He grew careless of his personal appearance, was moody, indifferent, and preoccupied, and readily gave up his jobs. He began to "run wild" and became involved in financial difficulties through gambling, especially on horse races. His stated purpose at the time was to try to make money rapidly in order to pay back his school debts. Although abstinent with respect to alcohol before graduation from college, he now became a social drinker, but never to the point of intoxication. At this period, and for the first time in his life, he began to associate with girls. He contracted gonorrhea, for which he was treated but toward which he reacted violently with anxiety and guilt feelings. At about the same time he was going out regularly with a girl whom his family had selected for him and whom they were very desirous that he marry. After three years of association, however, this relationship faded out; the family never knew quite why.

The patient was drafted in one of the first registration groups. After he registered, the family noticed that he was very depressed and unhappy about it and apparently dreaded going into the army. When he was notified to report for the draft he suddenly disappeared without a word to anyone and was not heard from for several weeks. At this time his home town police were notified that W. had been picked up in Florida, in a confused and dazed condition. He was brought back and taken almost immediately into the army, where he was unable to adjust himself to camp routine, repeatedly returning home AWOL. Within a month, more positive symptoms developed, and he was sent to the army station hospital. There he stated that for years he had had peculiar experiences and that people had been reading his mind. He remained at the camp hospital for about four months, when he was transferred to a state hospital.

During this hospital period he was described as preoccupied, emotionally unresponsive, slow, vague, and indefinite in this thinking, and possibly hallucinated. He was tried at various occupations but showed no particular interest in his work and often sat reading a paper rather than working. After 27 months spent at this hospital with relatively little change in condition, he was transferred to another hospital at which he was given the intensive study here described.

The relevant physical and physiological findings reported at this time were a suggestion of hypometabolism, low blood-vitamin level, and a slight degree of "tension" in each of three oral glucose tolerance tests: a control, under stress in a pursuitmeter situation, and under stress in an interview situation.

The outstanding psychiatric data reported were a stiff and rather manneristic attitude, some disturbance in associations, and strange ideas about circumcision and about being used as a test case in a murder trial. He showed some unresponsiveness, fear, irritability, and inappropriate affect. There was reason to believe that he experienced auditory hallucinations. His delusional formations dealt with persecutions, thought influence, and thought transference. He indicated that his heterosexual adjustment was not adequate; that he had attempted intercourse only with prostitutes and that this had not been satisfactory. He reported being strongly attracted to a girl whom he had met while working as baggage master. Actually he had established no contact with her, although she was the subject of many of his fantasies.

One important group of preoccupations centered around telepathy and ideas of influence and reference. He felt that he could project his thoughts into people and that he was used as a transmitting agent. Reports made over the radio, he felt, sometimes referred to him. Thus in a recent broadcast he had heard Lowell Thomas describe a submarine rising to the attack, as a "long, low, flat, extended shape." W. felt that "low," "flat," and "shape" referred to him: "low" because people think he is low morally; "flat" because the people supporting him are flat-broke; and "shape" because he is interested in the shapes of women and not so much in the sentimental side of love.

On the basis of the assembled data the staff made a diagnosis of "Schizophrenia, Other Types." Some staff members, however, emphasized the predominant paranoid content. The prognosis was characterized as "guarded." It was considered poor for "social recovery," but it was believed that after a time he would be able to make a limited adjustment in the community. The staff recommendation was that he remain in the hospital for treatment, which was to consist of psychotherapeutic interviews combined with occupational and vitamin therapy. Further physiological studies were to be carried out, and, if these indicated its desirability, thyroid therapy was to be added.

The major purpose of giving the case report here is the exposition of psychological procedures. It is, therefore, not possible to consider in any detail the integration of psychological findings with those derived from other sources. The report has been concerned primarily with integrating the material obtained from the variety of psychological devices used. The numerous correspondences between the independently obtained psychological data and those obtained through social service investigation and psychiatric study will no doubt have been noted. Even though the latter are necessarily presented in mere outline, the attempt has been made to provide sufficient material to permit appreciation of the manner in which the psychological data corroborate and complement the other data—the combination of which results in a fuller and more sharply focused portrait of a living patient.

So many questions relating to reliability and validity, so many problems relating to manner of presentation and communication, arise in the process of attempting to compress an extensive body of psychological data—data concerned so largely with both present cryptic activity and with inferences respecting past activity—that a report such as the present one must necessarily be made with some hesitation and reservation.

In material of this nature the reliability and validity of any one generalization depends on a synthesis of amassed cues, major and minor, direct and inferential, presentative and symbolic, provided by many disciplines. Generalizations are composed from these varied reflections of the same facet of the personality by the different techniques which attempt to describe it. In the study of W. certain generalizations seemed to have adequate foundations. Unfortunately, even the addition of material which was available but not discussed in this report, material from psychiatric, physiological, social work, and psychological sources, did not permit the further generalizations which the delineation of W.'s portrait required.

Studies of this kind make available to the student of personality a body of data which even the most complete verbal report of psychosomatic events cannot convey. A report such as this one, despite its attempts to supply a systematic framework, is, even so, able only to provide relatively isolated, and at most partially corroborated, samples of behavior. These samples of quantifiable and unquantifiable behavior, taken from different areas, frequently lose their significance because viewed out of context, and they inevitably make such a report inadequate in many respects. The difficulty is enhanced by the many obstacles to facile communication in the sphere of personality. Such problems as are raised by theoretical biases—the attenuation of scientific concepts by common-sense language, the lack of rigorous use of terms, both within psychology and among related disciplines, as well as many other handicaps—are generally acknowledged.

I recognize the existence of the difficulties which undoubtedly give rise to errors or ambiguities in generalization. Despite these handicaps, a field so complex as personality study demands perseverance in the attempt to integrate the independent data obtained from different disciplines. Continued study and research are also needed both in the development of an adequate language and in the fundamental problems of personality uncovered by individual studies. Fairly extensive experience with the types of procedures described here results in the conviction that they contribute considerably to the understanding of the individual personality by laying bare both superficial and more deep-lying personality characteristics and content. Furthermore, they accomplish this task frequently in relatively less time than is required by other methods, and they offer pertinent cues for further investigation of the particular personality both to the psychiatrist and to the psychologist.

Because of the major clinical concern of the volume, I have

tended to emphasize diagnostic aspects. More and more, however, the clinical psychologist is becoming concerned with the pressing and limitless range of research needs in the field of personality. Although the research interest of psychology has always been great, growing out of its background as an academic discipline, the focus of its concern has not been in the area of motivation until recently. However, a marked shift of interest in this direction has taken place in the last several decades. This must largely be ascribed to the remarkably pervasive influence of Freud and his concepts on psychology not only in the area of abnormal behavior but also in the wider areas of personality, learning, and social relations. With the gradual growth of facilities for adequate training in psychology, increasing numbers of persons are entering the field who, in addition to a background in fundamental research, have also the essential attitudes and points of view that derive from clinical experience in diagnosis and therapy and from exposure to the complexities of human motivation that such experience gives. Such a background will, on the one hand, give some assurance of preoccupation with significant problems and, on the other, sufficient concern with rigor in investigation as to lead to studies fitting more obviously into the body of current biological research, broadly conceived.

The methods of investigation used by the psychologist are in essence not different from those generally used in biology. The differences which do exist lie in the problems created by, and the advantages accruing from, work with subjects of greater complexity and having well-developed symbolic functions. We may roughly classify the methods into four groups, even though in actuality they shade off one into the other and are, therefore, not always clearly distinguishable. These are: (1) naturalistic observation, (2) seminaturalistic observation, (3) free laboratory, (4) controlled laboratory.

The first method provides for the study of the organism in a relatively free, natural habitat in which the widest range of stimuli and responses growing out of the particular setting are observed. These observations are made as completely and as accurately as possible, usually by an outside observer. Thus in a hospital setting it may be desirable to study group behavior as it naturally structures itself on the ward or to study the complex therapeutic situation with the free give-and-take of the patient-therapist dyad through the use of devices such as sound movies.

The second method, the seminaturalistic, may be provided for either by a "natural habitat" or by a laboratory situation. In the former, the degree of freedom is somewhat limited as compared with the first group; in the latter, the degree of freedom as compared with the two following groups of laboratory approaches is greater. In either case the stimuli are varied, and the degrees of freedom of response permitted are considerable. Some controls and limitations on the situation are, however, set up in order to direct behavior along certain lines. In the field of test procedures, the analogous device is the projective technique. In the experimental area an investigation directed at studying the susceptibility of schizophrenic subjects to environmental stimulation (18) might be cited in exemplification. In this situation various objects having different degrees of interest-demand character are left around a room into which the patient is introduced. He is told that the examiner will return shortly after he has completed another piece of work. The patient is observed in this relatively "free" situation for a stated period of time, and a detailed record is made of the range and intensity of his preoccupation with the objects and with himself.

In the third type of approach, the free laboratory, although some degree of variation in the stimuli and degree of freedom of response is still maintained, they are considerably reduced as compared with the former two methods. Here specific instructions are given the subject to respond in certain definite ways to stimuli, and recordings may be made of various physiological functions accompanying psychological response. An example of this kind of situation is a variation of the Luria experiment (9), in which the subject is required to respond orally to the stimulus words of a free association test. At the same time he is required to press on a tambour with one hand, and a recording is also made of finger tremor from the other hand and of respiration and galvanic skin response.

The fourth type, the controlled laboratory approach, carries the degree of control still further. Here both the stimulus and the response are quite fixed and limited. Studies of the latent time of the patellar tendon reflex (7) at the lowest psychological level or of reaction time (10) or simple psychomotor learning (8), at a higher level, fall into this category.

It is obvious that the methods of investigation described lend themselves to the accumulation of relevant data for methodological and descriptive purposes as well as for theoretical ones. It is likely that for some time in the future considerable effort will have to be expended by the psychologist in sharpening old tools and devising new ones. The problems in the field are so complex that considerable ingenuity will have to be devoted to this task. The psychologist need not, of course, limit himself to the study of the disordered person. Depending upon the nature and needs of the problem, he may use normal or even animal subjects, setting up, for greater control, situations which nature provides reluctantly or in too complex a setting.

Besides the accurate descriptions of behavior that are, of course, the essential basis for any theoretical development, there are some special problems of description to which the psychologist can make a special contribution. I refer here to objective studies in the evaluation of the effects of therapies or other modifications of behavior. The activity of the psychologist should, however, be mainly directed to the exploration of the fundamental aspects of personality with a view toward developing comprehensive theories of personality. Hypotheses along these lines may be derived directly from experiment or from clinical experience and study, preferably from thoughtful integration of both. The great growth of Freudian hypothesis and theory, based upon years of broad clinical experience and insight, now calls for a period of systematic experimental study in order to consolidate it into the body of psychological knowledge.

The important problems calling for study in the area centering around psychopathology and personality are numerous. They involve both factors of a structural kind and those of a functional nature. Because of the manifold effects of disturbances in the needs upon the ego structure, reflections of these disturbances are found in almost all aspects of the psyche. For this reason, besides the immediate problems of motivation, the areas of receptive and perceptive processes, the mechanisms of response, learning and memory, thinking and imagination, intelligence and social and group behavior call urgently for study, in both their cross-sectional and their longitudinal aspects.

In some of these areas experimental work may be carried out independently by the psychologist. But in most areas collaborative work with psychiatrists, neurologists, physiologists, internists, and other specialists is a necessity in order to obtain the most productive use of the material and to make the most meaningful advances (22).

This chapter can close on no more appropriate note than the above. An acquaintance with the relative states of development of the social sciences when compared with the physical, or even biological, sciences and close knowledge of the development of the sciences concerned with interpersonal relations must force the student to conclude that one of society's greatest present needs is research in this area. In this research each of the disciplines closely or even remotely related to these problems must make its individual, but particularly its joint, contribution to the understanding of the fundamental processes. The increasing cooperation in the day-by-day diagnostic and therapeutic activities should serve the additional function of providing background and experience for some of these joint research efforts.[6]

## BIBLIOGRAPHY

1. AMERICAN PSYCHOLOGICAL ASSOCIATION. "Report of the Committee on Training in Clinical Psychology (D. Shakow, Chairman)," *Am. Psychologist*, 2:539, 1947. Recommended graduate training program in clinical psychology.
2. BROTEMARKLE, R. A. "Clinical Psychology, 1896–1946," *J. Consult. Psychol.*, 11:1, 1947.
3. FELIX, R. H. "Mental Hygiene and Public Health," *Am. J. Orthopsychiat.*, 18:679, 1948.
4. HANFMANN, E., and KASANIN, J. "Conceptual Thinking in Schizophrenia" ("Nervous and Mental Disease Monographs," No. 67 [1942]).
5. HARROWER, M. R. (ed.). *Training in Clinical Psychology: Minutes of the First Conference* (New York: Josiah Macy, Jr., Foundation, 1947).
6. HEALY, W. *The Individual Delinquent* (Boston: Little, Brown & Co., 1915).
7. HUSTON, P. E. "The Reflex Time of the Patellar Tendon Reflex in Normal and Schizophrenic Subjects," *J. Gen. Psychol.*, 13:3, 1935.
8. HUSTON, P. E., and SHAKOW, D. "Learning Capacity in Schizophrenia," *Am. J. Psychiat.*, 12:881, 1949.
9. HUSTON, P. E.; SHAKOW, D.; and ERICKSON, M. H. "A Study of Hypnotically Induced Complexes by Means of the Luria Technique," *J. Gen. Psychol.*, 11:65, 1934.

6. The volume edited by Watson (27) contains a catholic presentation of articles dealing with several of the topics touched upon in the present contribution.

10. Huston, P. E.; Shakow, D.; and Riggs, L. A. "Studies of Motor Function in Schizophrenia. II. Reaction Time," *J. Gen. Psychol.*, 16:39, 1937.
11. Kelly, E. L. "Research in the Selection of Clinical Psychologists," *J. Clin. Psychol.*, 3:39, 1947.
12. Klopfer, B., and Kelley, D. M. *The Rorschach Technique* (Yonkers-on-Hudson, New York: World Book Co., 1942).
13. Miles, W. R. "Age and Human Ability," *Psychol. Rev.*, 40:99, 1933.
14. Miles, W. R. "Psychological Aspects of Aging," in E. V. Cowdry (ed.), *Problems of Aging* (Baltimore: Williams & Wilkins, 1939), chap. xx, pp. 535–71.
15. Miller, J. G. "Clinical Psychology in the Veterans Administration," *Am. Psychologist*, 1:181, 1946.
16. Morrow, H. R. "The Development of Psychological Internship Training," *J. Consult. Psychol.*, 10:165, 1946.
17. Murray, H. A. *Thematic Apperception Test Manual* (Cambridge, Mass.: Harvard University Printing Office, 1943).
18. Rickers-Ovsiankina, M. "Studies on the Personality Structure of Schizophrenic Individuals. I. The Accessibility of Schizophrenics to Environmental Influences," *J. Gen. Psychol.*, 16:153, 1937.
19. Roe, A., and Shakow, D. "Intelligence in Mental Disorder," *Ann. New York Acad. Sc.*, 42:361, 1942.
20. Rosenzweig, S. *Psychodiagnosis* (New York: Grune & Stratton, 1949).
21. Shakow, D. "One Hundred Years of American Psychiatry—a Special Review," *Psychol. Bull.*, 42:423, 1945.
22. Shakow, D. "Psychology and Psychiatry: A Dialogue," *Am. J. Orthopsychiat.*, 19:191, 381, 1949.
23. Shakow, D.; Dolkart, M. B.; and Goldman, R. "The Memory Function in Psychoses of the Aged," *Dis. Nerv. System*, 2:3, 1941.
24. Shakow, D.; Rodnick, E. H.; and Lebeaux, T. "A Psychological Study of a Schizophrenic: Exemplification of a Method," *J. Abnorm. & Social Psychol.*, 40:154, 1945.
25. Terman, L. M. *The Measurement of Intelligence* (Boston: Houghton Mifflin Co., 1916).
26. Terman, L. M., and Merrill, M. A. *Measuring Intelligence* (Boston: Houghton Mifflin Co., 1937).
27. Watson, R. I. *Readings in the Clinical Method in Psychology* (New York: Harper & Bros., 1949).
28. Wechsler, D. *The Measurement of Adult Intelligence* (3d ed.; Baltimore: Williams & Wilkins, 1944).

# XV

## ANIMAL PSYCHOLOGY IN ITS RELATION TO PSYCHIATRY

### David M. Levy, M.D.

THIS chapter will very likely be regarded as the one least relevant to the main subject of this book. The reason for this lies in the attitude of psychiatrists toward studies of animal psychology and in the manner in which these studies have been pursued. Although certain resemblances of animal behavior to our own may be seen, our own behavior is regarded as infinitely more complicated and superior, befitting the higher order of man in the animal scale. The complexity of our order, judged from any one of the products of civilization, seems to set us so far apart from the animal world that, however "human" many animal anecdotes appear to be, most psychiatrists may wonder or be amused but never interested to the point of seriously incorporating such stories into the process of theorizing about human psychology. The same holds true for animal studies that have scientific validity. Though they cannot be assigned to the category of harmless anecdotes full of the flaws of human projections, like stories of infants by proud parents, these studies have never become an integral part of clinical thinking in psychiatry.

The psychiatrist's way of disregarding studies of animal psychology, or at least of keeping them in a separate compartment when formulating theories in psychiatry, does not apply to other fields of medicine. In the study of anatomy, comparisons of animal and human structure are taken for granted. The principles of human physiology have been derived largely from experiments made on animals—for example, studies of the anatomy of the frog, the embryo of the chick, the alimentary functions of the dog, the genetics of the fruit fly, are all integral parts of the study of the human animal. A hormone, crystallized in pure form from the thyroid of sheep, pig, cow, or man, may yield the same chemical product and be readily accepted as such. Yet the same behavior responses of man and animal to almost identical situations are difficult for us to accept as illustrations of a common principle of psychodynamics. We have accepted our kinship with the animal world structurally and biochemically, but we remain isolationist psychologically.

## NATURAL OBSERVATION VERSUS EXPERIMENTATION

Animal psychology became a valid field of scientific study in the latter part of the nineteenth century. Its growth into a scientific discipline involved a long struggle with "nature lovers" and romantic natural historians. It became especially sensitive to all anthropomorphic thinking. The natural historian who mixed together careful observation and careless interpretation was rejected as strongly as the writer of popular books containing a jumble of fact and fable. In the process of liberation from anecdotage, the animal psychologist emulated the experimental biologist and physicist. He narrowed the field of animal studies to precise data verified by measurement and experiment. This purification resulted in a curious situation—that of a discipline in which all knowledge was barred that did not emerge from the laboratory. It might be compared to a field of medicine divested of all clinical knowledge, i.e., knowledge derived from observation and histories of patients at the bedside or in the office. Medical practice would then be limited to the application of that small fraction of medical knowledge which is verified by experiment and by accurate measurement.

Actually, in his day-to-day behavior with animals, the psychologist behaves "clinically" like the physician. He is aware, for example, from his experience with chimpanzees that one of them appears quite irritable, that another is friendly, that a third is quite likely to make a vicious attack on the experimenter. Moreover, his own behavior to the chimpanzees is based on such knowledge, often with the same assurance, depending on how well he "knows" his animals, as that derived from experimental studies. He depends on the kind of knowledge that goes into the making of human attitudes. His experience teaches him that he has every reason to anticipate the behavior of each chimpanzee in the same manner essentially as he learns to anticipate the behavior of a human being. Yet, for his scientific work, he is loath to study the animal outside the conventional system of observation and controls that comprise the criteria of the experiment.

An event that took place in a center for the study of experimental neurosis in animals may illustrate this point more clearly. An investigator was demonstrating to a class of students the effect of an experimentally produced neurosis on the cardio-respiratory functions of a pig. The animal was prepared in the usual Pavlov frame, and the pulse and respiratory tracings, etc., were made visible to the class. The investigator was about to point out the irregularities in the tracings, as he had done on a number of other occasions. To his surprise, however, the tracings were normal. Proof of the experimental neurosis was not demonstrable.

The mystery was solved very quickly, apparently to everyone's satisfaction. One of the students present at the time had taken care of the pig during the previous summer season. He became quite fond of the animal and hosed him often during the hot summer days. The pig apparently noticed him among the other students. He grunted in what was interpreted as an affectionate greeting when the student came close. During the next demonstration and thereafter, when the student was no longer present, the pig performed in the anticipated neurotic manner.

It is interesting that this significant event, as important to the psychiatrist as the experiment itself, was not made the basis of an independent investigation. It contained probably the essential ingredients of the "positive transference" of psychoanalysis and might have aided in a simplification of that concept. Actually, the episode served a purpose in influencing a series of experiments in the center in which it happened. The reactions of a sheep in a Pavlov frame were studied while its lamb was near by. The study of animal attitudes, in this case compounded of maternal feelings, was thus made secondary to a Pavlovian experiment.

## LIMITATIONS OF THEORY AND METHOD

The same episode reveals other restrictions of the animal psychologist. He is often wedded forever to his animal or his instrument. A psychologist who uses the method of Pavlov, for example, feels bound to his apparatus and to the theory of conditioning that seems to be an integral part of it. The apparatus which was first designed to serve the investigator may in the course of time tend to enslave him. The skill developed in learning to master the new instrument or the theory out of which it evolved may become a controlling interest. The investigator's thoroughness, his erudition, which encompasses the literature accumulated by colleagues working with the same device, even his profundity when he is capable of plumbing the depths, may serve finally to restrict his vision. In the extreme instance the investigator can understand nothing until it passes through the special machinery of his familiar world, translated into his specific language, concepts, and methodology. The resistance to new points of view is readily understandable when it involves a modification of technical skills and a system of thinking that represents, besides a life-long habit, a source of security and self-esteem.

The gradually diminishing returns from the special tool and special theory is a problem that applies to the entire domain of science. It is an important problem, particularly in a young science, whose development is easily retarded by rigidities, and in a psychological science, whose area is so vast that the temptation always arises to secure a firm foothold, however narrow the field.

## INFLUENCE OF PSYCHOANALYSIS ON ANIMAL PSYCHOLOGY

In recent decades, animal psychology has had sufficient impact from other disciplines to shake its complacency with traditional formulas and subject matter. Of the various influences that have widened the scope of animal psychology, most pertinent for psychodynamics is the influence of Freud. This is revealed specifically in the selection of experiments that deal with his theories and generally in the utilization of psychoanalytic concepts.

Experiments in animal psychology have been concerned with testing hypotheses. Rats, for example, have been used to demonstrate the principle of regression (26). When the floor (a steel grill) on which the rats rested was charged with an electric current, they learned to absorb the shock by sitting on their hind legs. In the next stage of this experiment, the rats learned to turn off the current by pressing a pedal. When this habit was established, it took precedence over the previous habit. That is, whenever the rats felt the electrical shock, they did not sit on their hind legs. Instead, they pressed the pedal which eliminated the painful current entirely. Pressure on the pedal was presumably a superior, as it was also a later, form of adjustment than the earlier one of merely reducing the pain by sitting hunched up in a certain way. The pedal was now charged with electricity. The rats, accustomed to relieve their distress by pressing the pedal, had another shock to contend with. Thereupon, they went back to sitting on their hind legs, their first method of contending with an electrical floor. In other words, according to the experimenter, by surrendering a later and superior method for an earlier and inferior one, they illustrated the principle of regression. The superior method was still available to them, regardless of the charged pedal. A second group of rats, who had never learned the sitting-down method, continued to press it even when it became charged, and so cut off the current.

This experiment is a good example of a large number of similar efforts. It may be used as an illustration of the problem involved in the attempt to capture a concept, derived from theorizing about human behavior as it is revealed through free verbalization often vaguely defined, and to pin the concept down to a neat experiment. In the process the concept is given sharp definition. It is then tested out through the behavior of animals in a controlled situation, so designed that the concept can be translated into activity which belongs exclusively to the concept as newly defined. The activity which tests the operation of the concept is bound within a framework which it is hoped will demarcate it from the other concepts and so free it from the myriad of relationships with which it was originally perceived in the psychoanalytic situation.

When the experimenter finds that the concept is "valid," he is still at a loss. He wonders if it is the real thing. In the experiment with rats, the investigator called the assumed regression an "analogue" of regression. After all, regression in humans refers to historical regression—a return, in response to a difficulty, to an earlier and inferior mode of adjustment at one time considered appropriate—for example, the return to bedwetting on the part of the older child following the birth of the baby. But is that in principle the behavior of the rat who had learned only two ways of dealing with an electrical floor? Given any two methods of equal or different values, would the rat use the first method if the second were blocked; and if he knew only one method, would he not more likely persist in it, there being nothing else to do? The regressive behavior of the child is one of a variety of possible responses. When the baby comes, if the older child is presumably jealous and feels the loss of love and attention, he may attack it, hit at its crib, talk about it in a derogatory manner, show off, refuse to notice it, or use an opposite tack and show it excessive affection and admiration. Furthermore, the situation in the case of the child is usually said to be a "natural" one; that is, it is the sort of thing that commonly happens. The situation in the case of the rats is "artificial." It is the sort of thing that does not happen to rats in their natural state.

The concept of regression, though simpler than most other concepts in psychoanalysis, also remained a problem. The notion of using an earlier and inferior method of adaptation is simple enough. As a dynamic process, however, it is more difficult to comprehend. Is regression a return to a well-organized mode of behavior, typical of an earlier stage (and also reinforced by "fixation" through erotic determinants, according to the original definition), or is it a disorganization? In the supposed regressive behavior of some schizophrenics, investigators have found no evidence of a throwback behavior, since all evidence of the behavior manifested was never previously observed. Is disorganization that has the appearance of regressive behavior to be differentiated from true regression? Also, is it fair to apply the term "regression" to a previous mode of behavior that has nothing to do with erotic elements?

The experimenter was well aware of the conceptual difficulties in his experiments with rats. Yet, like so many others, he preferred to use a device which was a poor fit for the concept he tried to test. There are numerous examples of regressive behavior in animals to be observed clinically, as in humans. They appear to be identical modes of response. Actually, the situation of the older child and the new baby is repeated time and again with the pet dog and the new baby. The most recent example that comes to mind is the return to wetting the floor on the part of a well-trained dachshund when a baby was adopted. The dog displayed the usual repertoire of responses observed on such occasions. He growled at the baby, though he never attacked it; he barked more than usual; he showed off his few tricks repeatedly; he tugged at his mistress' skirts when she fondled the baby. He went through such capers for about six weeks and thereafter "accepted" the situation.

Systematic clinical studies of animal behavior, besides adding to our knowledge, would render superfluous a number of animal experiments designed to "test the claims" of psychoanalysis and to discover mechanisms readily discerned through observation of spontaneous behavior. Such studies would also aid experimental procedures by indicating those areas in which controlled observations would be most necessary and fruitful.

## Special Advantage of Experimental as Compared with Clinical Studies

Examples of the manner in which the experiment aids the clinical investigator may be cited. The first is concerned with the influence of special events in infancy on adult behavior. In this experiment a number of rats was subjected to periods of hunger in infancy. To test the effect of this experience in adult life, the amount of food they hoarded was measured. Some of the rats who had experienced the state of hunger in infancy hoarded much more than the others.

The investigator stated that his experiment was devised in order to get controlled evidence concerning the claims of psychoanalysis that experiences during infancy can affect adult behavior (9). Such claims are shared by psychiatrists generally, child psychologists, educators, and a variety of investigators in other disciplines. They are easily verified by the study of case records in any number of schools and clinics. In one sense, therefore, like the previous experiment, an attempt was made to verify the obvious. Further, the main line of sequence, infantile starvation to increased adult hoarding, is not necessarily a test of the claims that "experiences during infancy affect adult behavior." Suppose there were no difference in regard to adult hoarding among the control and experimental rats. One could then conclude only that the experience of starvation in the infancy of the rats was not followed by a particular type of behavior (hoarding) in adult life.

The experiment was selected for this chapter, not as verification, but as an illustration of its particular advantage over clinical studies. The starvation period can be controlled. You can place it any day you wish. You can starve the rat much or little. You can control various aspects of the experience in a manner which renders your conclusions more definite, sure, and accessible than those derived from untangling a pattern out of the web of human behavior.

The experience of starvation, though equal in terms of diminution of food and span of time, was initiated at different ages. It was started in one group of infant rats when they were 24 days old and in another when they were 32 days old. Only the 24-day group manifested excessive hoarding. The 32-day group hoarded no more than the controls. Evidently, response to the particular experience of starvation was significantly altered by a difference of 8 days of age.

To test differences in hoarding in adult life, all the animals, experimental and control, were subjected to a preliminary period of partial starvation. They were given just enough food for subsistence for 5 days, in order to stimulate them to collect the pellets of food, the number of which constituted the measure of hoarding. The preliminary period of starvation was necessary because rats who are well fed have little or no propensity to hoard.

The experiment offers a good illustration of "operational" value. The starvation period can be produced at any time in the life of the animal, so that the period of susceptibility in infancy can be accurately determined. We know in the group of animals studied that, in terms of hoarding, starvation must be experienced before 32 days of age to have an effect in adult life. But how severe must the starvation be? The experimental tool allows a measure of the experience in terms of food privation applied as a single experience or as one of a series or in a variety of combinations. What is the minimal experience of starvation that will have an effect on adult hoarding at the most susceptible age? How severe must the experience be at the least susceptible age to have an effect? There is involved the problem of susceptibility in terms also of individual differences of personality. That would require, besides genetic studies, the kind of clinical observations that are made in humans.

There remain the large variety of "traumata" to be studied in the same manner as starvation. The investigator referred to observations that thirst alone, as well as hunger, was followed by an increase in hoarding. Would fear-provoking experiences in infancy or later have a similar effect? Is hoarding a general rather than a specific tension-relieving outlet? We know that it is rendered excessive by more than one type of experience.

### Psychological Vulnerability

The points raised in the previous paragraph indicate the special advantage of experimental procedures over clinical observations in the solution of problems requiring precise control. Their application to problems in human behavior is quite direct. The evaluation of a disturbing event in infancy on the individual personality requires, besides knowledge of particulars, knowledge also of general laws of special susceptibility in terms of developmental age and of the type of external agent. What difference does it make if event A (a fright, a period of separation from the mother, a change to a new place of residence, or an experience of starvation) occurs when a child is aged 3 months, 9 months, 2 years, 3 years? Holding the age factor constant, what difference does the type of experience make? It is in this area that so much of value can be learned for preventive psychiatry.

Carefully compiled case studies furnish details that may approximate an experimental situation. It has been found (18), for example, that presumably normal children who undergo surgical procedures at the age of 12–24 months are much more likely to have subsequent emotional difficulties than when operated on after that age. It has been found also that the 12–24-month group manifest such difficulties in the form of rather uncomplicated anxiety symptoms (fears, phobias, and increased dependency) as compared with older groups, whose anxieties when they occur are more likely to be complicated by aggressive behavior. The age factor (12–24 months) appears to be more significant than any other factor investigated (dependency on the mother, special experiences, etc.). In terms of available data, susceptibility is very high in the second year of life (involving the majority of children at that age), fairly high in the third year of life (involving a third), and of decreasing magnitude in later years. Similar studies for the first year of life are not at hand.

The special vulnerability of the organism to a variety of disturbances of function, emotional and physiological, may follow the same general principle in a number of animal species. Each type of disturbance may have its own particular mode of function, aside from the individual unique response. But the uniqueness of response requires full study. However emotionally vulnerable to an operation an infant may be at 18 months, a study of his response to that procedure cannot be understood as an individual experience without knowledge of his personality, which includes all his typical modes of behavior, and also the specific history of his emotional growth. The same applies to animals.

The specific influence of psychoanalysis on animal psychology has been illustrated in two sets of experiments. In the first, the main difficulty for the experimenter was to place the animal in a situation comparable to one in humans. In the second, the difficulty was easily solved, since the task was simply to prove that an event in infancy has an effect in adult life and was therefore readily applicable to animals. On the whole, psychoanalysis has had more influence on the concepts of the animal psychologist than on his specific experiments. This influence bears fruit eventually in experimentation, but the direct connection with the psychoanalytic concept, out of which the experiment emerged, is often lost and may even be unknown to the investigator. A large number of experiments in frustration, for example, though initiated by psychoanalytic concepts, have, in the course of time, become imbedded in the method and the language of the experimenter and are regarded as an offshoot of findings originating in the laboratory. The psychoanalyst who reads the literature and listens to papers by experimental animal psychologists, even by those apparently opposed to psychoanalytic concepts or unaware of them, meets many familiar Freudian ideas. They are seen particularly in experiments and discussions of drives, needs, goals, motivation, conflict, frustration, shame, anxiety, sex, aggression, and regression.

## Experimental Neurosis

The field of activity in animal psychology most directly related to psychopathology owes its origin to Pavlov (28). He observed various mental states of immobility in dogs that were by-products, so to speak, of salivary conditioning experiments. An accident was probably more effective than any other factor in stimulating the experimenter's interest in the animal's abnormal mental states. Pavlov's dogs were subjected to a severe experiment, unaccounted for in the series listed in the laboratory notebooks. Their kennels were suddenly submerged by a rapidly rising flood. During their exhausting struggles to escape drowning by swimming in trapped space, there were flashes of lightning and a variety of explosive sounds near and far—rushing water, falling timber, claps of thunder. For some months after their rescue, they showed, besides the effects of exhaustion, generally depressive states and abnormal reflexes of the kind now made so familiar to us in the numerous studies of "experimental neurosis." Though the dogs recovered in time from their state of shock and became to all outward appearance as normal as they had been before, when one of them was tested by the sight of a trickle of water flowing under a door the acute anxiety state followed immediately.

Reproduction of abnormal mental states was accomplished in the experimental situation by repeatedly imposing a task on the dog beyond his power of discrimination. The abnormal emotional states which resulted were measured in the usual Pavlovian manner, through their physiological expression in pulse frequency, blood pressure, salivary flow, etc. Not all dogs can be made "neurotic" by the methods employed. Though a constitutional difference may be taken for granted, there is still much to be learned about the significance of the experience for the individual animal. Liddell (20) has indicated a number of the difficulties involved. He states that the setting in which conditioning experiments ordinarily take place is itself a traumatic situation. The animal is in a state of tension, no matter how simple the task, because of the degree of restraint involved in controlling its movement and withstanding the monotony of repeated stimuli, as long as the experiment goes on. The animal's relation to the experimenter, Liddell states, must also be considered. Let us assume that the dog's relationship to the experimenter is such that he is very eager to succeed in performing his task. He is then, theoretically, more likely to develop an experimental neurosis, because he will more likely persist in attempting a discrimination that is beyond him. The reverse would also follow. The less "goal-directed," the less likely will the dog be to be caught in the trap of straining all efforts to do the impossible. Why does the experiment have to be repeated a number of times to produce the neurosis? Because the animal presumably is able to dissipate the effects in some manner, most likely by releasing pent-up energy through running about and sleeping it off. If the interval of time between the experiment is too long, the neurosis does not take place. Hence the repetitions must be so placed in time that the dog's own curative functions are not allowed to go on to completion. The process is thus analogous to accumulation of tensions in a person who can hardly overcome the emotional effects of one crisis before he finds himself in another and then another, until he breaks down.

The experimental neurosis as conceived by Pavlov may be regarded as a functional disturbance originating in the cortex of an animal, strongly goal-directed, probably constitutionally predisposed, and in a situation involving physical and emotional strain. Pavlov was interested primarily in the instrument of discrimination, the cortex, as a mechanism rather than in the animal as a motivated organism. The experiment is not analogous to the flood, whether one accepts or rejects the theory that the focus of the disturbance in the former lies in the problem of discriminating two closely matched stimuli. In the flood there was no problem of that sort. There was no need to discriminate. There was one obvious danger and a desperate attempt to escape it. Furthermore, the escape was successful. The animals were saved and recovered their ability to respond to conditioning experiments. True, a reminder of the experience—the sight of water dripping under the door—precipitated anxiety. The anxiety remained latent. It was not manifested in the experiment after recovery. Unlike the experimental neurosis which produces a more or less chronic and generalized dysfunction, the experience of the flood operated to produce anxiety only when a sample of the original event (that operated quite like a "symbol") was brought to the consciousness of the animal. In contrast with the experimental neurosis, which is analogous to schizophrenia, the experience of the flood resulted in a phobia.

## Clinical Neurosis and Psychopathology

Generally, in animals as in humans, one fear-provoking or painful experience may carry potent reminders for a long time. The monkey who coughed and spluttered and ran when a lighted cigarette was brought near his nose acted the same way later when a piece of cigarette paper was brought near. A hen, once frightened by the sight of a guinea pig, always avoided the room in which the event occurred, in spite of inducements of heaps of grain. The locality of a disturbing event has particular significance. The place where danger threatens evidently must be well remembered if the animal is to survive. Response to the single threatening event, often so excessively traumatic to the human psyche, is well revealed as a basic adaptation in animal studies.

The biologist, Whitman (33), made an interesting experiment and an interesting deduction relating to this subject. During the mother bird's absence, he displaced one of her eggs, putting it on the rim of her nest. In the case of the robin there was immediate abandonment. In the case of the pigeon there was quite a different response. The pigeon worked the egg back to its original position and continued its brooding. The robin's response was an immediate instinctive reaction to change in a familiar visual configuration. A wild bird must act in stereotyped fashion. The locus of its nest, its structure, its relation to the immediate environment, are selected with an eye to safety. The bird is alerted to every detail of its habitat. The slightest alteration is a danger signal. There is no time to investigate. The solution is flight. Unlike the robin, the pigeon was domesticated. Its sense of danger was lulled. Safety means time and opportunity for selection. The pigeon could afford the time for more learning, for more plasticity, therefore, of instinctive behavior. How Whitman's observations hold for all bird species, I do not know, but the principle that modifiability of "instinctive" behavior is facilitated by security and diminished by danger, though not absolute, appears to be well founded. That it applies to a response as fundamental as reaction to a site of danger indicates that many "innate" responses are plastic. Memory of place applies also to pleasurable and exciting experiences. The memory of safety areas are also important for survival. The significance of such place memories in human psychology is well illustrated in clinical histories, often strikingly in dreams.

In relation to the psychoses, animal psychology has furnished chiefly "analogues" of hypnosis, catalepsy, and catatonia. Thus far they have contributed little to our understanding of psychotic states.

Reactive depressions in animals appear to be of a different order (31). They are not "analogues." They contain essentially the same type of depressive response to the loss of a loved object as we observe in humans. The mourning of a dog for his departed master is a familiar example. The story of Cupid, a young *Rhesus* monkey, has become a classic example of emotional turmoil arising out of "marital" difficulties. The response finally took the form of an agitated depression. The account contains all the elements of conflict, guilt, privation, devotion, masochism, and love. Cupid was first attached to an older female, with whom he lived monogamously for three years. She was then taken away. A simple depression ensued. He was given a young female, to whom he adjusted after an initial period of hostility. Some time after the new relationship had been established, apparently with success, he was led past the cage of his first female. Their eyes met. She shrieked excitedly. Cupid's psychosis followed immediately. He bit himself repeatedly and severely, causing deep lacerations. He became restless and agitated. He would not eat. He withdrew all contact from his second female and his human attendants. After some time, the psychologist restored the first mate. The change was favorable. The older female fondled

Cupid, nursed him devotedly, and gradually "calmed his nerves."
Fourteen months elapsed before he recovered.

The organic and toxic psychoses of animals, though similar in
their essential pathology to those of humans, have not been investigated from the point of view of psychodynamics. The variations in the response of dogs to hydrophobia, of horses to loco
weed, of cattle to snakeroot, etc., have not been explored, except
as symptoms of brain pathology.

Mental deficiencies occur in animals as well as in men and can
be classified according to etiology in the same manner; for example, developmental defects, prenatal infections, inherited
amentia, etc. Mentally defective animals have been studied almost exclusively in zoos. Presumably they do not survive in a
state of nature.

## Some Basic Studies in Psychodynamics

For the rest of this chapter I propose to list a number of basic
studies in psychodynamics, in which the investigation of animal
behavior may play an essential role, or indeed might have done so
already if we had integrated available knowledge. The list proposed is not intended to cover the field. It includes examples
derived partly out of my own attempts to solve problems arising
in psychiatric work with children by means of animal studies
and partly out of ideas that stem from current interests and discussions with colleagues in psychoanalysis and animal psychology.

### 1. PRIMARY NEEDS

Among primary needs are included all innate needs of the
organism, whatever function they subserve—chemical, physiological, emotional, social, etc.

An example of a chemical need is the need of calcium. Hens
deprived of calcium appear to go on a frantic search for it. They
will peck at buttons and other hard objects. When supplied with
calcium after being starved of it, they will eat about the same
amount, whether it is exposed to their view or concealed in other
food. How do they know what they need? How do they know
when their need is satisfied?

These problems have not been solved, but the theories, which
represent tentative answers, and the lines of inquiry apply to
humans as well as animals. In a state of tension arising from a
chemical imbalance, the animal is restless and searches in a man-

ner that appears to be somewhat guided. When the appropriate food is found, it is ingested until the animal is "satisfied," in other words, until the internal environment is in equilibrium. The release of tension is concomitant with the inner chemical balance.

The usual need of food is felt specifically as hunger, and the physiological gastric mechanism that first initiates the feeling has been thoroughly investigated. The need of calcium and other special mineral foods or hormones is not felt specifically like hunger and thirst. It is felt more vaguely as discomfort or restlessness or a general anxious state.

Sucking is apparently an innate physiological need (13). The mammalian fetus has been exercising mouth and neck muscles repeatedly in preparation for sucking and swallowing. As in the case of many other needs, once the process of satisfying a sucking need is initiated, it goes on to a point of satiety, of fulfilment. If that point is not reached when a feeding is finished at breast or bottle, the lips remain tense. Babies or puppies who have been deprived of sucking activity too soon can sometimes be observed making sucking movements after breast or bottle has been withdrawn. When the sucking phase of the feeding act in repeated feedings remains incomplete, then finger-sucking or some other substitute form of sucking is bound to follow.

A clinical study has been made of the average daily sucking time of 30 babies of 7 months of age (29). The group contained 15 babies who were finger-suckers and 15 who had never developed that habit. When the average number of minutes of sucking time per day for each of the 30 infants was arranged from high to low, not one case of finger-sucking occurred at the high end of the scale (130 or more). Every infant whose average time was at the low end of the scale (70 or less) was a finger-sucker.

The relation of diminished sucking time and substitute sucking activities has been verified experimentally in dogs. Observations of calves, kittens, and monkeys show similar findings.

The need of pecking in chickens illustrates the same principle as the need of sucking. Chicks reared on a wire floor, with the same amount of food available as an adjoining control group, develop the habit of feather-pulling. Chicks who are on the wire have no opportunity to satisfy their pecking needs on the wooden flood of the henhouse or on the ground (14, 15).

Body movement is another functional need that follows the general pattern of physiologic needs in terms of periodicity, cyclic curve of energy discharge, end-point, and specific evidence of incompleteness (16). In a number of vertebrate species it has been found that, when the animal is confined for a long period of time in a space too small to allow locomotion, it develops head tics (e.g., weaving tic of horses, head tic of bears, head shakes of chickens). Similar head tics have been observed in infants confined too long in cribs.

When space is inadequate to satisfy movement need but large enough to allow locomotion (as in cages at the zoo), stereotyped movements develop. The result of restraint of movement for short periods of time is a temporary movement excess, as in dogs who are released after a period of restraint at the leash or children at recess after a period of restraint in the classroom. Observations of an infant in the creeping stage and later in the walking stage, who was confined in a playpen all day except for two periods of 45 minutes, revealed excessive motor activity during the intervals of free movement.

The physiological needs are closely related to developmental age. The need of body movement, for example, is greater in the second half-year of life than in the first. The needs increase in their early stages with successive fulfilments. Thus the need of movement is greater after a child has experienced freedom of movement.

It may follow also that restraint of a need before it has attained fulfilment (as, for example, in the continuous restraint of American Indian babies in the cradle board) may diminish a need. In the case of the pecking need, when chicks are prevented from fulfilling it and are fed from a dropper the first two weeks of life, the need is lost. Without prolonged efforts on the part of the psychologist to restore it, the chicks would die (4). Needs cannot survive *in vacuo*. The outer and inner environments are concomitant parts of their function. Each need has its own history, its peculiar pattern, its range of modifiability. Each requires special investigation.

Emotional needs have not been studied in animals so thoroughly as have physiological needs, for the reason that they are usually not regarded as primary needs. In the animal's attempt to initiate and complete the act that represents the operation of a need, emotional factors are considered as an integral part of the process at every stage. The need of a feeling, however—as a more or less specific source of tension and striving—is difficult to comprehend as clearly as the more tangible concept of a need of food or sex. In the category of needs, the need of sex is envisaged primarily as a physiological need, however deflected, diminished, or exaggerated it may become through emotional influence. The feeling appropriate to the need of sex, like the need of food, involves specific physiological activity. The animal's need of social relationship, if such a need exists in primary form, as implied in the concepts of social or herd instinct, would be an example of a primary emotional need. The need of maternal love, as a primary emotional need, has been studied clinically in children. Case studies of children deprived of maternal love, though not deprived of the usual nursing care, protection, and training, reveal specific personality difficulties. They include symptoms of "primary affect hunger"—basically an excessive craving for love through close personal relationships, with derivative symptoms, and in a smaller number of cases an apparent loss or diminution of the need for love, with resultant lack of response to emotional influence (the "deprived psychopath"). Emotional ties appear to be a primary need and probably a basic component of other needs involving mutual relationships—sexual, maternal, or social. The need for love appears also to follow the law of certain physiologic needs in terms of excess and diminution.

Experiments on emotional needs of animals have hardly begun. They would reach the core of this problem more successfully than would clinical studies. The case of an emotionally deprived dog has been cited in the literature (19).

### 2. MATERNAL DRIVE

In the maternal activities of birds and mammals, including humans, the same basic factors are manifest: namely, contact (warmth), care (feeding, cleaning), protection, and training. The maternal drive, as measured in animals, is stronger than thirst, hunger, or sex. In experimental studies of the strength of drives, the barrier that had to be crossed to attain the goal to which the drive was directed was an electrified grill with a measurable charge (32). How humans would respond to a similar experiment is not known, though it would seem safe to conclude from clinical data that in a certain percentage of mothers the results would be the same. There is evidently a range in the strength of the maternal drive, a normal distribution curve, in humans as in animals (34).

### 3. AGGRESSION AND DOMINATION

The classical research on the peck-order in chickens was followed by a series of investigations which demonstrated a general principle of domination among vertebrates (30). The peck-order, the rule whereby a rigid caste system develops in a community of animals (so that animal A always maintains ascendancy over animal B, animal B over animal C, and so on down the line) is not inflexible. There are many variations of the original formula, though the principle remains. In a barnyard of 60 hens who have lived together for several months, every hen knows exactly which one is above it and which below it. However this type of social organization has come about, it makes for a more static, stable, and apparently advantageous adjustment.

When two monkeys, strangers to each other, are put together in a cage, one becomes boss over the other, often in a minute's time. They size each other up. It is literally size that usually determines the result, though strength, agility, persistence, or bluff in any of their combinations may determine the outcome (23).

The dominating tendency of human beings, as an innate biosocial response, requires further exploration in the light of these studies. Our usual explanations of aggressive domination in humans are in terms of competitive strivings for maternal love (as in sibling rivalry); compensatory aggression because of anticipated rebuff or anticipated unconscious accusations in social relationships; compensatory aggression based on feelings of inadequacy; as a reaction against submissive, dependent attitudes, etc. They may be appropriate to the data of a given case and yet fail to take into consideration what may prove to be basic biological drives.

Analogous to the behavior of animals is our own "sizing-up" of a new acquaintance and that large variety of human reactions to the stranger—boys ganging up on a newcomer, the primitive's fear of witchcraft in the neighboring village, the suspicion of or even the tentative or ceremonious approach to the new neighbor.

The hens' reaction to a strange hen, even one of their own breed, is to attack it after a minute or two of "sizing it up" (1). The newcomer's personality changes under one's eyes within a short time. Regardless of her previous relationship to other hens, she becomes an outcast. She avoids all places in the henhouse where hens are crowded together. She keeps away from the trough and pecks from the floor. She appears furtive and apprehensive. She keeps isolated from the others. She walks slowly or makes sudden runs as though always in danger. The fury of pecks in the first half-hour of her new residence gradually subsides. Within 10 days to 2 weeks she appears "blended"; it is hard to tell her behavior from the rest.

Little chicks are friendly to each other. The strange chick is not pecked, though for a while it avoids the others and tries desperately to get back home. At about 6 weeks of age, the chicks act like the grown-ups and attack strange chicks very quickly. The reaction appears to be an innate response of anxiety in the presence of the unfamiliar that comes after a period of maturation, followed—in the case of unfamiliar chicks—by an attack.

Aggression in animals, as in humans, is capable of a high degree of modification and a large variety of manifestations. A wounded dog, treated by its master, may visibly curb its "reflex" tendency to bite when its painful leg is moved. As in humans also, a dog may express its frustration through release of aggression. One of my dogs, up to his sixth or seventh year of life, would bite at a bush when I refused to throw a ball for him to fetch. Thereafter, his response to the same type of frustrating situation was patient waiting or insistent barking. Some animals have modified their aggression more successfully than man. The howler monkeys, for example, hardly ever assault one another. Their aggression takes the form of vocalization.

Dominant behavior, as an attempt to satisfy a need for social status, has been so interpreted in chimpanzees and other animals (35).

### 4. AGGRESSION AND SEX

Though all drives require some form of aggression to fulfil their object (using the term "aggression" to include all varieties of self-assertive behavior), a higher magnitude is required whenever the drive involves the play of an ascendant role. The sexual drive, in its relation to social ascendancy and submission, is clearly depicted in a number of animal studies. Among chimpanzees (35), for example, it appears that the female, when highly aggressive as compared with her mate, limits her period of copulation to her few days of ovulation. When submissive to her mate, she yields to his sex demands all through the menstrual cycle, including the period of bleeding. When females are ascendant in the scale of domination, they may appear to struggle against surrender to their own sexual needs because sexual submission to the male may be followed by loss of a dominant position previously held over him. Many animals utilize sexual activity at times as an act of sheer dominance.

### 5. NEGATIVISM

The period of human infancy, starting around 15–18 months of age and proceeding to about 4½ years of age, has been called the "first adolescence." Indeed, the resemblance to the age of puberty is quite striking. The "striving for independence," the "I'll do it myself" of the first adolescence, is frequently manifested in negativistic behavior (as also in the puberty adolescence). Animals may show similar transformation when they grow beyond the earliest dependency period. Resistant or negativistic behavior appears to be a protective barrier against excessive demands on the organism, a protection also against superior force. It is used also as a weapon of hostility, in the form of spite, revenge, and domination. Negativistic phenomena are seen in psychiatry as "normal" stubbornness, as compulsive behavior, and, in its extreme form, as manifestations of catatonia. Various forms of repetitive behavior, the "fixated responses" of animals, belong to this category.

In certain experiments in which rats had learned to jump over a barrier to butt their way through the correct one of two hard paper doors which swung open onto a cubicle containing food, both doors were fixed so that all ensuing efforts were unsuccessful (21, 22). Whichever door the rats tried to enter, they were forced to make the jumps, and they were "frustrated." Under these conditions a variety of reactions occurred, including "a fixed reaction" in a certain small percentage of the animals. Within the "fixated" group, for example, some rats would jump only to the right door and never to the left, even after the left door was later opened and the food in that cubicle exposed. Such fixed reactions may have a basic element in common with a number of compulsive negativistic reactions of humans.

### SUMMARY

Principles of motivation and social behavior may be derived from the study of various species of animals that are applicable to all animal life, including man. Such investigations need not be based on any special interest in human beings or be pursued with a view to clinical application. Nevertheless, they may eventually yield laws more fundamental to human behavior than studies geared to specific theories of human motivation. Studies of the sexual behavior of animals, in which the chemical, neural, psychologic, and genetic components can be investigated separately, may represent one of a number of examples.

In the field of medicine, in anatomy, physiology, psychology, or genetics, those animal studies will be favored that have a direct bearing on current problems. It is worthy of note, however, that animal psychology has its own domain and is not simply an ancillary field of human psychology. In this chapter we have been considering more particularly that segment of the field of animal psychology that has direct application to problems in human behavior.

The advantages of experimental studies of animal behavior have been discussed, in part, with reference to the control of variables. The strength of the stimulus, the precise moment of its application, its duration, etc., can be controlled in a manner which, if successful, results in a definite answer to the question which the experiment was set up to solve. A "critical period" in regard to an experience of hunger or thirst or psychic trauma can be placed in time at any chosen moment of the infantile period. The age of greatest vulnerability for a given type of psychic trauma, if age is itself an independent variable, can be demarcated from the pattern of factors—social relationship, past experience, special susceptibility—with which the event is interwoven. The clinician who insists that any significant experience in the life of his patient represents a unique and irreducible complexity, impervious to scientific research, usually overlooks the fact that his own thinking is based on the hypothesis that the significant experience, however complex, is reducible to simpler components that have wide application. His inference that a patient has responded excessively or peculiarly to a common type of frustration involves the assumption of norms of experience and quantitative deviations from such norms, as well as norms of response and their deviations. The experiment, as a crucial test of hypothesis, can be made to serve the psychiatrist in his psychoanalytic thinking, as it does in his physiological thinking.

The psychological experiment in animal behavior that is designed to add to our knowledge of emotional life has special problems of its own. Animal psychologists are more concerned today with the complexities of relationship, such as between animal and experimenter, and with the individual experience and emotional state of their animal subjects. Greater ingeniousness, subtlety, and variety of experimental procedures are required in experiments of this nature, but the principles of control and precision remain.

The value of the experiment, however well designed in a technical sense, is diminished or even vitiated if the concepts which form its hypothesis are not sharply defined. One of the values of the animal experiment is, indeed, the clear definition of terms. A behavior that is to be observed and measured must be defined precisely. Some experimenters, interested in a psychic mechanism like identification, for example, would not consider it a proper subject for investigation because its meaning is vague. They would prefer to wait until clinical thinking has arrived at a more precise formulation. The problem is sometimes met by investigating certain kinds of behavior patterns that are included in the meaning of a complex term and then redefining the term to mean what the experimenter means by it, or by retaining the complex term and defining the behavior as one of its meanings, or by devising a new term. The temptation for the experimenter to devise a term whose meaning is restricted to his field of operation is a strong one, and in time a new vocabulary arises that deepens the cleavage between clinician and experimenter. It is true that mutual benefits are also derived, as the attempt to make definitions in terms of observable behavior helps to dispel vagaries and dulness of perception.

Besides the advantages of focusing the field of study through control of variables, of quantification, and clear definition, animal studies, either experimental or of the natural history type of observation, offer a corrective to fantastic theories of human motivation. The genesis of behavior in situations identical for humans and animals, to which both respond in the same way, do not require explanations that involve symbolic thinking uniquely human. Animal studies have a sobering influence on theories of human behavior in other respects. They follow more closely the law of parsimony in scientific thinking. The temptation to construct a complicated theory when a simpler one will do is less likely to occur. In tracing through the influence of an early event on later behavior, the animal psychologist enables us to learn whether in a similar quest in human behavior we have relied unnecessarily on the assumption of the highest intellectual function. Animal psychologists are more mindful of developmental levels in their explanation of behavior. They are less likely to explain the behavior of a 3-week-old pup on the basis of adaptations that are not evident until some months later. This type of error is especially prevalent in certain psychoanalytic theories of infancy, in which ideas are ascribed to the infant years before he has reached the level of maturation necessary for their attainment.

A proof of the universality of a human motivational pattern or drive or need is its existence in all human cultures regardless of their diversity. That is proof, at least, of generality in the human species. Animal studies would indicate how far the generality extends among all living creatures. Anthropological studies supply the test of diversity of human motivations, as well as the test of what is uniquely human. Animal studies serve to determine similarities and differences in motivational patterns of human behavior and that of other species.

Finally, for all those who, like Freud, believe in the biologic roots of behavior, animal studies, like the studies of young children, offer the basic data on which theories of motivation must rest. If the primary needs and drives of all mammals are the same, the basic question in the theory of human motivation is a biologic one.

### BIBLIOGRAPHY

1. ALLEE, W. C.* *The Social Life of Animals* (New York: W. W. Norton & Co., Inc., 1938).
2. BEACH, F. A.* *Hormones and Behavior* (New York: Paul B. Hoeber, 1947).
3. BRÜCKNER, G. H.: "Untersuchungen zur Tiersoziologie, insbesondere zur Auflösung der Familie," *Ztschr. f. Psychol.*, 128:1, 1933.
4. BIRD, C. "Maturation and Practices: Their Effects upon the Feeding Reaction of Chicks," *J. Comp. Psychol.*, 16:343, 1933.
5. CARPENTER, C. R. "A Field Study of the Behavior and Social Relations of Howling Monkeys," *Comp. Psychol. Monogr.*, Vol. 10, 1934.
6. COLLIAS, U. "Aggressive Behavior among Vertebrate Animals," *J. Physiol. Zoöl.*, 17:83, 1944.
7. DARLING, F. F.* *A Herd of Red Deer* (London: Oxford University Press, 1937).
8. GANTT, W. H.* *Experimental Basis for Neurotic Behavior* (New York: Paul B. Hoeber, 1944).

* Recommended reading.

9. Hunt, J. McV. "The Effects of Infant Feeding-Frustration upon Adult Hoarding in the Albino Rat," *J. Abnorm. & Social Psychol.*, 36:338, 1941.

10. Katz, David.* *Animals and Men* (New York: Longmans, Green & Co., 1937).

11. Kellogg, W. N., and Kellogg, L. A.* *The Ape and the Child* (New York: McGraw-Hill Book Co., 1933).

12. Kohler, W.* *The Mentality of Apes* (New York: Harcourt, Brace & Co., 1925).

13. Levy, D. M. "Experiments on the Sucking Reflex and Social Behavior of Dogs," *Am. J. Orthopsychiat.*, 4:203, 1934.

14. Levy, D. M. "On Instinct Satiation: An Experiment on the Pecking Behavior of Chickens," *J. Gen. Psychol.*, 18:327, 1938.

15. Levy, D. M. "A Note on Pecking in Chickens," *Psychoanalyt. Quart.*, 4:612, 1935.

16. Levy, D. M. "On the Problem of Movement Restraint," *Am. J. Orthopsychiat.*, 14:644, 1945.

17. Levy, D. M. "Primary Affect Hunger," *Am. J. Psychiat.*, 94:643, 1937.

18. Levy, D. M. "Psychic Trauma of Operations in Children," *Am. J. Dis. Child.*, 69:7, 1945.

19. Levy, D. M. "Psychopathic Personality and Crime," *J. Ed. Soc.*, 16:99, 1942–43.

20. Liddell, H. S. "The Alteration of Instinctual Processes through the Influence of Conditioned Reflexes," *Psychosom. Med.*, 4:390, 1942.

21. Maier, N. R. F. "Abnormal Fixations," *Am. Psychologist*, 1:462, 1946 (abstr.).

22. Maier, N. R. F., and Klee, J. B. "Studies of Abnormal Behavior in the Rat. VII," *J. Exper. Psychol.*, 29:380, 1941.

23. Maslow, A. H. "Dominance-Quality and Social Behavior in Infra-human Primates," *J. Social Psychol.*, 11:313, 1940.

24. Masserman, J. H. "Psychobiologic Dynamisms in Behavior," *Psychiatry*, 5:341, 1942.

25. Moss, F. A. (ed.).* *Comparative Psychology* (New York: Prentice-Hall, 1946).

26. Mowrer, O. H. "An Experimental Analogue of 'Regression' with Incidental Observations on 'Reaction Formation,'" *J. Abnorm. & Social Psychol.*, 35:56, 1940.

27. Noble, R. C.* *The Nature of the Beast* (New York: Doubleday, Doran & Co., 1945).

28. Pavlov, I. P.* *Conditioned Reflexes* (London: Oxford University Press, 1927).

29. Roberts, Ena. "Thumb and Finger Sucking in Relation to Feeding in Early Infancy," *Am. J. Dis. Child.*, 68:7, 1944.

30. Schjelderup-Ebbe, J. "Beiträge zur Soziolpsychologie des Haushuhns," *Ztsch. f. Psychol.*, 88:225, 1922.

31. Tinkelpaugh, O. L. "The Self-mutilation of a Male Macacus Rhesus Monkey," *J. Mammal.*, 9:293, 1928.

32. WARDEN, C. J.* *Animal Motivation: Experimental Studies in the Albino Rat* (New York: Columbia University Press, 1931).

33. WHITMAN, C. O.* *Biological Lectures, 1898* (from the Marine Biological Laboratory, Woods Hole, Mass.) (Boston, 1899).

34. WIESNER, B. P., and SHEARD, N. M.* *Maternal Behavior in the Rat* (London: Oliver & Boyd, 1933).

35. YERKES, R. M.* *Chimpanzees* (New Haven: Yale University Press, 1943).

36. ZUCKERMAN, S.* *The Social Life of Monkeys and Apes* (New York: Harcourt, Brace & Co., 1932).

# XVI

## A REVIEW OF THE INFLUENCE OF PSYCHO-ANALYSIS ON CURRENT THOUGHT

### Henry W. Brosin, M.D.

THE system of ideas worked out and presented to the world by one man, Sigmund Freud (1856–1939), has exercised so profound and far-reaching an influence on the minds of men that it may well be ranked among the great new ideas which, like Darwin's theory of evolution, have shaped the course of history. There is today hardly an activity in the biological and social sciences that has not been deeply affected by Freud's thinking.

### Precursors of Freud

Occasional critics, both friendly and unfriendly, find pleasure in reporting authors who, in one way or another, anticipated Freud. It is generally assumed that even the great original thinkers made their discoveries with the materials and methods at hand and that the history of the development of these makes more understandable the discoveries under discussion. Perhaps such histories also contributed to an understanding of the dissemination of ideas; certainly, in Freud's case the magnitude and violence of the resistances shown to ideas which in piecemeal form had been present for at least two thousand years is an illuminating insight into man's rejection of knowledge about the irrational side of his nature.

The difficulty of accurately assigning priorities to scientific discoveries is well known. Darwin had Wallace, both men's theories growing out of work by Lyell, Lamarck, Buffon; Leibnitz had Newton; and many another innovator found that he had precursors and contemporaries who had anticipated him. Freud spoke of this in "One of the Difficulties of Psychoanalysis" (49), when he pointed out that the Pythagoreans and Aristarchus of Samos in the third century b.c. had already anticipated the great discovery of Copernicus. He specifically mentions as another example the "collaborators and predecessors" of Darwin. He then

508

credits philosophers, principally Schopenhauer, as the thinkers who most nearly anticipated him regarding the concept of an unconscious. In Reik's book *From Thirty Years with Freud* (123) he also states that Goethe and Nietzsche come closest to his views. In the *New Introductory Lectures*, when speaking of the conflict between the erotic and the death instincts, Freud answers a fancied reproach that this is the philosophy of Schopenhauer, with the defense:

> But, Ladies and Gentlemen, why should not a bold thinker have divined something that a sober and painstaking investigation of details subsequently confirms? And after all, everything has been said already, and many people said the same thing before Schopenhauer. And besides, what we have said is not even true Schopenhauer. We do not assert that death is the only aim of life; we do not overlook the presence of life by the side of death [47, p. 147].

In *An Autobiographical Study*, Freud points out that he never abandoned patient observation for speculation:

> Even when I have moved away from observation, I have carefully avoided any contact with philosophy proper. This avoidance has been greatly facilitated by constitutional incapacity. I was always open to the ideas of G. T. Fechner and have followed that thinker upon many important points. The large extent to which psycho-analysis coincides with the philosophy of Schopenhauer—not only did he assert the dominance of the emotions and the supreme importance of sexuality but he was even aware of the mechanism of repression—is not to be traced to my acquaintance with his teaching. I read Schopenhauer very late in my life. Nietzsche, another philosopher whose guesses and intuitions often agree in the most astonishing way with the laborious findings of psycho-analysis, was for a long time avoided by me on that very account [40, pp. 109–10].

One gets a brief glimpse of the magnitude of Freud's achievement when scanning even a partial list of artists and philosophers who have had ideas similar to Freud's. The wide range and depth of his subject matter and his vision will be apparent when we see how many far-reaching universals he was able to abstract from his relatively small sample in Vienna, universals which the finest minds in the history of thought pursued with difficulty and with only partial success.

Before examining the more remote writers who may be of importance to Freud's thinking, it should be mentioned that he thought of his teachers, Brücke, Meynert, Exner, Fleischl-Marxow, and Breuer, as important influences. Through them he absorbed the biological orientation he never abandoned. Bernfeld's

(10) excellent description of Freud's student days during 1873–91 is quite revealing. His obligation to Charcot, Liebault, Bernheim, and Binet has been generously recorded, and his independence of Janet has been sharply asserted.

M. Dorer (30) claims that through Freud's professional associates Freud became familiar with the theories of Herbart, Fauerbach, and Comte, which she says were fashionable during his student days. She tells an interesting but not convincing story, since in the end it would appear that Freud learned almost everything from someone else if one interprets broadly enough. This applies to her analysis of Freud's dependence on Meynert and the latter's tie to W. Griesinger, who had adopted Herbartian psychology. This study of sources leads one to numerous writers, including Augustine as the first to see the unconscious (although he called it the *memoria*), Plato (Charmides), Shakespeare, Dante, Dostoevski, Cervantes, Thomas Aquinas, Montaigne, the French moralists, the Encyclopedists, and the German Romantics. It would appear that Freud, by looking intensively at one patient at a time, over many years, was able to provide a unifying theory which had not previously been available. Obviously, these ideas were latent in many minds but needed Freud to make them explicit.

In his *The Interpretation of Dreams* (45) there are over fifty references to authors since Aristotle, of which a few had glimpses of the psychoanalytic views on the problem. References to a few special authors will show the widespread distribution. Theodor Lipps (43, 50) and Josef Popper-Lynkeus (46) receive special mention by Freud. Various writers have claimed that Freud learned about dream interpretation from the Talmud and the Bible, but this thesis has not been developed and deserves only passing mention. Therapeutic application of dream interpretation is well illustrated in the treatment of King Perdicas by Hippocrates (died 346 B.C.) (20). Aristophanes' (423 B.C.) *The Clouds* (5) has a passage which shows appreciation of free association while lying on a couch, and the need to deal with resistances. Juan Luis Vives, a Spanish philosopher (1492–1540), who was called "the father of modern psychology" by the English philosopher, Foster Watson (141), is described by Gregory Zilboorg as the forerunner of Freud because Vives described psychological associations with emotional origins, the egoistic drives of man, and insight into the true nature of jealousy. "Vives was not only the father of modern, empirical psychology, but the true forerunner of the dynamic psychology of the twentieth century" (150, p. 194).

Free association was also conceived by Frances Galton (56) before 1883 and was utilized by the novelist Édouard Dujardin in *Les Lauriers sont coupés* in 1887 (31). Karl Böhm (67), a Hungarian philosopher, and Carl Gustav Carus (58), born in Leipzig in 1789, are described as anticipating Freudian concepts at some points about the unconscious, sleep, and dreams. Georg Christoph Lichtenberg is cited as a "clandestine psychoanalyst of the 18th Century" (79). In addition to the numerous references to older authors in *The Interpretation of Dreams*, Freud (45) mentions Meringer and Mayer's purely descriptive attempts in 1895 to study slips of the tongue as philological events and concludes that their explanation is "peculiarly inadequate." In 1920, Freud (48) commented upon several reputed predecessors who had utilized the method of free association—J. J. Garth Wilkinson (1857), Schiller (1788), and Ludwig Börne (1823). Freud disclaims any influence from the first two, although he mentioned Schiller's recommendations in the first edition of *The Interpretation of Dreams* (1900). He grants the possibility that Börne's essay, "The Art of Becoming an Original Writer in Three Days," may have influenced him in developing the method of free association. He had been fond of and remembered other essays in the same volume read when he was fourteen years old, and the memories of these kept recurring to him over a long period of years. On rereading the essays, "he [Freud] was particularly astonished to find expressed in the advice to the original writer some opinions which he himself had always cherished and vindicated. For instance: 'A disgraceful cowardliness in regard to thinking holds us all back. The censorship of governments is less oppressive than the censorship exercised by public opinion over our intellectual productions.' [Moreover there is a reference here to a 'censorship,' which reappears in psychoanalysis as the dream censorship.] 'It is not lack of intellect but lack of character that prevents most writers from being better than they are. . . . Sincerity is the source of all genius, and men would be cleverer if they were more moral. . . .'

"Thus it seems not impossible that this hint may have brought to light the fragment of cryptomnesia which in so many cases may be suspected to lie behind apparent originality" (48).

British writers also cited as precursors are Mary Everest Boole (32), wife of the famous mathematician; Erasmus Darwin (28) on birth anxiety; Sir Henry Maine, the "father of comparative jurisprudence," and his pupil Alexander McLennan (87); Timothy Bright (18) who recognized guilt in depressions; Sir W. C. Ellis, M.D. (34); and Hughlings Jackson (45, p. 511).

An American, Andrew J. Ingersoll (1818–93), is credited by A. A. Brill (19) as having had shrewd insights worthy of comparison with Freud. Herman Melville, in the opening paragraph of *Moby Dick*, shows his understanding of aggression as a motivation for depressions. Oliver W. Holmes, Sr., in his novels has a number of suggestive ideas which have been studied by C. P. Oberndorf. Many others could be cited: I. Kant, J. Braid, Feuchtersleben, Wetterstraud, Hering, André Gide, Bergson, E. Mach, Leibnitz, De Biran, Eduard von Hartmann, and Samuel Butler, but no further purpose would be served. R. Dalbiez (27), in an ambitious two-volume work which claims to distinguish between a legitimate psychoanalytic scientific method and an unwarranted Freudian doctrine, has numerous historical references of interest.

Spinoza (1632–77) is the philosopher who deserves much more attention because he anticipated many of our modern thinkers. More specifically, B. Alexander (1) points out that Spinoza's ideal for humanity is identical with Freud's therapeutic goal, namely, the rule of intellect over emotions. In the compactly written five books of the *Ethics*, Spinoza, like Freud, essays the foundation of a synthetic psychology, in which the total picture of a living man is more important than dissection of individual elements, such as perceptions. Freud's conception of "health" is the equivalent of Spinoza's freedom, virtue, bliss, or happiness. These coincidences are not merely verbal tricks, for we find in both writers an interest in the same operations. While Spinoza did not outline the concept of an unconscious as such, he discusses its operation in the sections on memory in terms familiar to Freudians by linking it directly to the affective life of men. The concept of repression is clearly described in Part III (Proposition 12). He also described ambivalence and the dynamic transformations of the "affects" (Parts III and IV). His strict adherence to the principle of psychological determinism and the pleasure-pain principle, together with the expositions on striving for insight and the goal of preserving the personality, adequate and inadequate ideas, and frustration as a source of aggression will be easily recognized by students of Freud. It is curious, as B. Alexander (1) points out, that Freudians have not explored the relations between Spinoza and Freud more thoroughly; for example, it seems probable that the "conatus" of Spinoza is similar to the libido theory (9, 121, 136).

## INFLUENCE OF PSYCHOANALYSIS ON PSYCHIATRY

The magnitude of the influence of psychoanalysis on psychiatry is remarkable, since the number of those who have declared themselves officially as followers of Freud is barely more than a handful; the total membership of the International Psychoanalytic Association in 1937 was 564; the membership in the American Psychoanalytic Association in 1950 was only 446. It becomes even more astonishing when it is recalled that even today the great majority of psychiatrists all over the world are in public or private institutional practice, primarily concerned with the care of psychotic patients.

Before 1900 very few psychiatrists were in private practice for the primary purpose of psychotherapy. Few were able or were permitted by circumstances to carry out intensive, long-term psychotherapy with individual patients suffering from psychoses, severe neuroses, or psychosomatic disorders. Few, therefore, could gather the specialized data which are essential to provide a foundation for theories of perception, learning, memory, and motivation and to expand the frontiers of psychiatry. Although Webster (1941) defines psychiatry as "the medical specialty that deals with mental disorders" and although most laymen believe that psychiatrists are primarily engaged in individual psychotherapy, an actual survey does not support this belief. For example, in the "Review of Psychiatric Progress, 1946" (124) the seventeen topics discussed in review articles range from heredity and eugenics to occupational therapy and psychiatric education; yet they include no reviews of psychotherapy, group therapy, drug therapy, hypnoanalysis, or psychoanalysis. The problems of general psychiatry, centering largely around the institutional care of psychotic patients, continue to dominate the field, to the neglect of individual psychotherapy of nonpsychotic patients. To be sure, the social and financial burden caused by institutionalized patients is enormous and deserves major attention. But it is also true that the number of ambulatory patients who require psychiatric care has grown to unprecedented proportions, and they, too, deserve consideration. The fact that, at present, private practice is highly attractive has induced a considerable number of young men to specialize in this area. However, the current practice of general psychiatry remains grossly heterogeneous. It has been well described by N. D. C. Lewis:

> Present day psychiatry is an odd mixture of internal medicine, neurology, psychology, clinical testing, "psychosurgery" and various drug assaults on the personality, mental hygiene, philosophical speculation and the pseudoscientific diagnoses applied by those who operate on the margins of the speciality [88, p. 1].

While both psychiatry and psychoanalysis are intimately connected with the study of thinking, acting, and feeling, particularly of people with emotional difficulties, the difference between the two disciplines will perhaps become clearer if we remember that Freud saw general psychiatry as the gross anatomy of human behavior, psychoanalysis as its microscopic anatomy (43).

General psychiatry is also concerned with other subjects, such as descriptive psychiatry and phenomenology, heredity and eugenics, neuropathology, biochemistry, endocrinology, electroencephalography, epilepsy, neurosyphilis, toxic-organic disorders including alcoholism, geriatrics, mental deficiency, psychometrics, psychosurgery, physiological treatment of the neuroses and psychoses, family care, industrial psychiatry, and many others which are of only incidental interest to psychoanalysis. On the other hand, general psychiatry has only secondary interest in many technical problems of experimental psychology, education, penology, sociology, social psychology and social anthropology, economics, mythology, language, literature, aesthetics, and other interests of normal man which are of primary importance to psychoanalysis.

Psychoanalysis has been variously defined as follows:

1. A research and therapeutic method discovered by Freud.

2. The body of facts discovered by this method.

3. The theories arising from these facts, especially those concerned with the unconscious, with repression, substitution mechanisms, instincts, infantile sexuality, resistance, dream interpretation, transference, and countertransference.

4. The interpretation of facts from other sources in the light of these theories.

5. An attitude toward human behavior (a Weltanschauung).

6. A unified psychology of human behavior, normal and abnormal, including the development of the personality.

Further definitions of psychoanalysis may be found in this book as well as elsewhere, but considerable semantic skill is required to avoid misunderstanding. This difficulty must also be kept in mind while studying the ways in which psychoanalysis has influenced psychiatry. Another, and not the least, of the barriers to tracing these influences is the strange fact that many persons deny the origin of their ideas because the concepts of psychoanalysis have become commonplace. To explain how this came about is a necessary part of our task here.

An examination of psychiatric books and journals published before 1900 and of non-Freudian literature published before 1920 quickly reveals their limitations. They contain innumerable detailed descriptions of human behavior but no explanation of *how* people become mentally ill because of their emotional conflicts. These descriptions, separating various reaction types, furnish an essential preliminary step toward further accurate investigation. But little or no attention was given to the possibility that a patient's depressive or obsessional state could be the inevitable consequence of his psychological turmoil. Because such severe clinical states seemed foreign to ordinary human behavior, the belief prevailed that they must be due to some defect in the organic physiological apparatus, much like those clinical states caused by toxic drugs, general paresis, or epidemic encephalitis.

Like the seven blind men describing the elephant, the early authors reported innumerable clinical fragments but failed to discover their unified meaning and thus made the total problem only the more unintelligible. Much time can be spent, for example, in charting accurately the 24-hour sleep rhythms of a patient and observing meticulously how sleep disturbances can be influenced by various sedatives. Such information, however, collected without references to the underlying causes, represents a waste of scholarship. It is good energy spent in collecting trivia. This information acquires meaning only when the sleep data and the drug barriers are understood as an index of the underlying struggle of the patients' self-esteem with acute self-criticism, remorse, guilt, ambitions, and the like. If, in addition, the physician can explain this meaning to the patient in a manner which can with reasonable surety either increase or decrease the patient's favorable response to sedatives, then and not until then has he demonstrated a superior insight into the patient's problems and increased his own power to help (146). To add another example, descriptions of eccentric gestures and bizarre posturing may help identify categories of behavior, and such categories may at times be useful in prognosis or in the choice of the most desirable means of treatment.

In pre-Freudian writing it was only rarely understood that such queer actions were intelligible, specific symbols of distracted thinking and feeling. Furthermore—and this is of the utmost importance—these ego-alien actions, as well as normal behavior, can be understood in terms of ordinary, everyday concepts and common-sense logic if we understand that current motivations grow out of internal and external pressures and the development of the patient since his birth. Once the various internal and external forces are so understoood, a co-ordinated developmental sequence can be discerned which gives the clue to many of the mysteries of psychoses, perversions, neuroses, criminality, and other expressions of a disturbed person. Irrational behavior was found in many instances to be intelligible in terms of developmental anomalies, conflicts, fixations, regressions, and similar psychological transformations, without the need to postulate some unknown organic process the presence of which could not be demonstrated.

While Freud and some of his students did not believe that *all* behavior was psychogenically determined, especially in the psychoses, they opened a wide field for intensive study by their observation and free association techniques which are of unparalleled value in eliciting direct information from patients. But the language developed to describe this broad area of observation was new and strange, and many critics were at first unable to see the value of the new concepts. Today, however, there is general agreement among psychiatrists and psychologists that the Freudian model of the ego and of its growth through experience, the Freudian theory of the genetic-dynamic evolution of the personality, and his hypotheses concerning the unitary principles of dreams, delusions, hallucinations, aberrant conduct, and symptom formation are the best available. Painstaking clinical and experimental verification by experts in experimental and social psychology, social anthropology, and similar disciplines has shown the original, daring observations of Freud to be accurate, and his tentative concepts to be extremely useful.

Revisionists, whatever their background, are now paying tribute to one or another of his basic theories, especially that of an active unconscious, for it was this theory which opened up a field heretofore unknown to science and only inadequately described by poets and philosophers, the field called by Spinoza "of human bondage or of the strength of the emotions." It was this theory which made it possible to study and understand the therapeutic properties of love and the destructive properties of hate, to analyze motivations, and to enter the unknown terrain where memories operate almost unchanged throughout a man's lifetime. The world of symptoms, character disorders, dreams, and kindred phenomena now become intelligible and thereby slowly but surely accessible to a more rigorous examination by criteria and methods outside psychoanalysis proper.

Psychiatrists, stimulated by these techniques, especially dream interpretation and the observation of strictly determined recurrent action patterns, began to make freer use of their imagination, to see more deeply into their patients without flinching, to give voice to the distress they saw without surrendering their ideal of an orderly and systematic investigation of human behavior. Unlike earlier static models of central nervous system activity and unlike the limited activities of a hypothetical laboratory man, these new dynamic views made sense in explaining the relation of a man to his family and the family as a meaningful unit in society. Psychic determinism and the pleasure-pain principle made equally good sense when applied to groups. Freud, far from being a teacher of the anarchic, demonstrated order and significance in a universe which all too often seems chaotic and arbitrary. He gave man a chance to study himself in ways which were not known before, and thereby the opportunity to plan and carry out measures which will bring closer his heart's desire.

Yet all these techniques, even if reasonably well perfected for rearing healthy children adaptable to the needs of the twentieth century (including perhaps even the ability to find ways to live in peace), will not tell us what our goals are or should be. To understand our goals, we need the incessant efforts at reinterpretation of the best people in the culture, by whatever ideal "the best" are defined (Plato, Buddha, Lao-tse, Christ). Although Freud is called the "Darwin of the mind" for filling in the evolutionary gap and although his theories may be used as data in constructing new designs for co-operative enterprise, it is by no means an ethical system which he developed.

The revolutionary changes in attitudes toward mental diseases and in the methods of investigating them due to Freud's influence received further support from other major contributions to the concepts of psychological determinism. These contributions become more clear when contrasted with the work of one of the leading pre-Freudian thinkers, Emil Kraepelin (1855–1926). Though a gifted clinician and experimentalist, especially in physiological psychology, Kraepelin did not understand the psychological dynamics which influence the unique, individual man. Utilizing the methods highly approved in his time, "the Era of Systems," he collected innumerable data from thousands of life-histories to determine what they had in common; but he failed to emphasize sufficiently the crucial fact that content was of more importance than appearance and that many psychological states in one man can be altered. He was interested in the form, the external appearance, of the illness, not the content of the patients' preoccupations. Convinced of the organic causation of mental disease, he tried to apply the clinical methods of the eighteenth and nineteenth centuries. Kraepelin's studies were enormously popular with biological scientists, because they supported the belief that mental diseases would be amenable to study and treatment, much like physical trauma and the infectious diseases. Although Kraepelin had many critics among contemporary general psychiatrists, it was not generally recognized that he had to overlook many facts because they did not fit into his system.

The revisions of Eugen Bleuler (1857–1939) and Adolf Meyer (1866–1950) showed much more awareness of psychological determinants in most mental disorders and of the importance of total central nervous system activity. After them has come a large and growing literature substantiating the thesis that psychiatry, including psychoanalysis, has a firm place in medicine in the area now called "psychosomatic medicine." The rich clinical material now becoming available through the detailed correlation of psychological observation and physiological activity as seen in gastrointestinal, circulatory, nutritional-metabolic, and endocrine functions presages the day when physicians can investigate "total function" much more meticulously than is possible today. General psychiatry and psychoanalysis, as well as medicine and surgery, are both expanding widely because psychotic mechanisms are now being described which were not envisioned several decades ago. The psychiatric components in organic disease and their role in complicating convalescence are under sharper scrutiny than ever before, and consequently there is today a greater promise of benefit to the patient.

Another contribution of psychoanalysis to psychiatry and allied disciplines is the far-reaching study of the effect of the observer-therapist upon the patient (*rapport*, transference) and of the reverse relationship (countertransference) in a long-continued therapeutic association. Astronomers, physicists, and psychologists have struggled with numerous practical difficulties presented in experiments by the introduction of errors through the operations of the observer, but psychoanalytic technique compels a uniquely searching inquiry into the subtle interactions between two persons in an intimate experimental situation. Operations which heretofore unaccountably altered the execution of experiments could for the first time be identified and explained as resulting from the unconscious attitudes of either person or from an interaction between them. Furthermore, it is now appreciated that even the original choice of experiments by the scientist may contain an undefined bias which is significant in terms of unconscious operations (17).

Thus psychoanalysis has furnished new experimental methods and has recorded verifiable material, which enable both biological and social scientists to gain new insights into the classical problems of their fields, insights which cannot be overlooked in future conceptualization. Cross-fertilization and "feed-back" mechanisms are now at work among all disciplines; and we may expect that the next half-century will see advances that justify the hope that man can improve his self-understanding and self-control sufficiently to prevent racial suicide.

### METHODS OF INFLUENCE

Psychoanalysis has influenced psychiatry directly through the usual channels of professional communication: meetings, textbooks, journals, and monographs. At the same time, it has had an even greater impact upon popular thought through the media of mass communication, such as popular magazines, newspapers, radio, movies, and literature. The realization that mental disorders can be understood in common-sense terms and be successfully treated created a growing demand by the public for psychoanalytic therapy, which encouraged many younger psychiatrists to study psychoanalysis seriously as the most comprehensive way to help sick people. This general interest in psychotherapy has altered older standards of medical and nonmedical practice and presages a generation of more skilled practitioners. While the total effect of widespread public pressures on psychiatrists is difficult to assess, the pressures will probably continue to exert a most powerful influence upon psychotherapists, most of whom will find themselves unwittingly employing Freudian concepts learned from nonmedical or even popular sources.

The demands of society on medicine vary with the acuteness and magnitude of the social problems. In primitive settings, traumatic surgery, care of infectious diseases, and obstetrics were primary requirements. In our complex urban culture, with its conflicts, society demands a more inclusive system of therapy, one which makes understandable and treats the less obvious traumata. This social need is undoubtedly a factor in the current public interest in psychiatry. A second factor which leads the public toward what may be called "psychological thinking" can be seen in the development of scientific thought since Darwin, which views man as a biological organism and, as such, bound firmly to his environment. If emotional disturbances are caused by an environment that we can control, it follows that the disturbances can be prevented or cured. Finally, the emotional crisis precipitated by the two world wars accelerated the need for therapy and made possible propaganda directed to the general public.

Attitudes toward human mentality are colored by group opinions (mores) of ancient origin and powerful influence which offer dogged resistance to new hypotheses that make men uncomfortable. Examples of such hypotheses—and such resistance—cited by Freud are the Copernican revolution, which took from man his anthropocentric orientation, and the Darwinian hypothesis, which asserted that man was an animal, akin to other animals, thereby adding "biological humiliation to the cosmological insult" (49). Unless we can view the development of these intellectual upheavals in depth and over a considerable span of time, it is difficult to avoid errors. Although the goal of science is to obtain data the validity of which is independent of their origins, it is necessary to examine the genesis of an idea in order to understand its proper place in current affairs.

Psychoanalysis grew up in the era of expansion of science, receiving much support from it and also supporting science, in turn, by feeding back leading concepts. The gains now being consolidated, especially in the social sciences, form a bulwark which should make unnecessary any retreat from the pragmatic position to an "idealistic" one, even though there is evidence that exponents of "idealism" are growing in influence in the postwar period (Toynbee, Sartre, Kafka, Kierkegaard). Freud pointed out that special resistances against psychoanalysis were to be expected because it brings man face to face with the dread fact that his most highly prized function of thinking is partly a result of basic body needs, developing biologically under the influence of an external environment (49). Because the subject matter of psychoanalysis is the irrational in man, many critics mistakenly claim that the methods and data are also nonlogical. Freud is at the same time accused of being a mechanistic materialist without regard for the spiritual in man and, paradoxically, accused also of being the proponent of a subjective, nonmechanistic, irrational system. Both these views will be refuted as the data accumulate to even more impressive proportions and as corroborative evidence is supplied from the biological and social sciences.

Alexander summarizes this picturesque conflict in *Our Age of Unreason:*

Undoubtedly Freud's life work, psychoanalysis, arose from the same opposition [as Shaw, Wilde, Sorel, Pareto, Nordau] to the self-deceptive ideology of the Victorian era, but his writings represented a fundamentally different attitude. The Viennese giant had the courage not only to explore the irrational and asocial emotional forces of man's unconscious, but also to devise a method by which they could be brought under rational control. To Pareto, the origin of rationalization was unknown. He did not see that a person is impelled to rationalize, i.e., to conceal his asocial tendencies from himself and others because of an inclination within himself to disallow such tendencies. This social drift within the personality cannot be disregarded, for it alone makes social life and the improvement of human relations possible. Social progress can be achieved only by strengthening this social self and extending its rule over the destructive emotional forces. Freud's theory is wholly antithetic to Pareto's in its confidence that human nature can be influenced and modified. He insisted that as anatomy and physiology helped combat disease, so a knowledge of the unconscious facilitates the cure of mental disorders by influencing personality. This opens up the possibility of a peaceful cooperation between men. Freud took the first step toward converting the ideal of the Greeks and of Locke, the rule of reason, into a scientific reality. The evolution of philosophic thought from Locke to Pareto completed a cycle from reason to unreason. Freud began a new cycle on a more realistic and scientific level. He was determined that reason should rule again and that its reign should be established by the scientific study of personality, which will lead eventually to its mastery [3, p. 111].

An improvement in general living conditions will also produce the leisure and security necessary to examine the evidence for unconscious operations in daily living. A people fighting a war or engrossed in major materialistic expansion is not primarily interested in psychological operations, even though these are basic to their eventual survival and success. Alexander quotes the maxim: "First live; then philosophize" (3, p. 7) as a summary of the philosophy of our pioneer civilization.

In view of the cataclysms that have struck many of the convictions and faiths by which we live, it is difficult to attempt at this time a more comprehensive evaluation of the influence of psychoanalysis upon psychiatry. Most observers are too close to the events to give an objectively critical opinion.

Since psychiatrists pursue different functions, they tend to form different groups around kindred interests. This leads to unfortunate professional fragmentation and intellectual isolation. It will require much tolerance to counteract this tendency to isolation, especially between the organically minded and the psychologically minded, and also between the different schools among the psychologically minded. But we need the clash of opinions to stimulate the more vital activities in a field of thought. Controversy is the life of science. Clinicians progress more rapidly if they check their methods and results with one another and, so far as possible, with basic scientists in both the biological and the social sciences. Three examples among many will illustrate the need for intra- and interdisciplinary communication.

Alcoholism is a complex personality disorder requiring many data to permit even preliminary generalizations. Numerous workers are studying it from widely varying points of view; yet their publications reflect little cross-examination. For various reasons, psychoanalysts have not distinguished themselves in the treatment of alcoholics, yet their reports on the psychodynamics and treatment of alcoholism are highly informative, suggesting that better techniques may be developed (26, 93). Even if orthodox analytic techniques are relatively too expensive or too slow, it is worth while to study analytically the effective group-therapy methods—including the well-known Alcoholics Anonymous and the new groups for drug addicts and obese persons.

Analysts have long been chided for their lack of interest in psychoses, yet considerable insights in this field have come from the beginnings made by Freud, Jung, Bleuler, Abraham, Ferenczi,

Tausk, Jones, and Rank. In 1928, Rickman published a monograph, *Development of Psychoanalytical Theories of Psychoses, 1893–1926* (125), with 495 titles. There have been many more titles since 1928, yet some current articles show only a primitive grasp of the analytic concepts which are useful in treating such patients.

Until World War I, neither neurologists nor psychiatrists had developed a systematic psychological treatment of persons with head injuries or other types of cortical deficit. Patients from World War II gave considerable impetus to this field, yet the admittedly small but important offerings of the analysts Ferenczi and Hollós, Hartmann, Jelliffe, Schilder, and others have not been adequately utilized for the purpose of studying ego functions in these clinical experimental settings. We must hope that analysts will study intensively and systematically the effects on the ego of shock treatment, lobotomy, and topectomy and will make data available for further explorations.

### Evidence of Psychoanalytic Influence

Freud and his pupils, including those who, like Jung, Adler, Stekel, Rank, and Horney, still retain some Freudian concepts, are a powerful source of ideas in the main stream of twentieth-century psychological progress. But we can also note tangible evidence of the spread of Freudianism in various other ways (74, 77, 143).

Inspection of a university library reveals seven journals, English and German, devoted entirely to psychoanalysis, while thirty-seven journals in neurology and psychiatry and sixty journals in psychology carry articles on psychoanalysis. The number of separate titles listed in *Psychological Abstracts* under the heading "Psychoanalysis" has averaged over one hundred per year since it began in 1927. Thirty-nine textbooks of psychiatry, written by nonanalysts, without exception carry sections or chapters on Freudian theory and practice. Up to now there has been no generally accepted, formal textbook of psychoanalytic psychiatry, although there are many books which serve this function, among them the writings of the well-known older Freudians. Newer texts written by nonanalysts carry much more psychoanalytic material than did their predecessors.

A few quotations from non-Freudian textbook authors will illustrate the esteem in which psychoanalysis is held:

Using this method [psychoanalysis] he [Freud] and his followers worked out the beginnings, at least, of a new system of psychology, which has not only had a profound effect upon psychiatry, but upon all contemporary thought as well. Today even those psychiatrists who do not accept psychoanalysis in its entirety make constant use of its concepts, and all of us, even without knowing it, use many of the ideas and the insights it has given us [110, p. 6].

No attempt is made in this book to conform to the tenets or the terminology of any one school of psychology. . . . It is only fair, however, to say that as far as its basic principles are concerned modern medical psychology owes infinitely more to Freud than to anyone else, and it is impossible to give even the simplest definitions, whatever one's viewpoint, without abundant borrowing of his conceptions and his very phrases [148, p. 36].

It was largely due to Freud and his students that modern psychiatry began to recognize the importance of understanding a patient from a psychological point of view. . . . We are confronted with the interesting speculations and observations of Freud and his followers as the most important school of psychopathology at the present day. . . . Freud has profoundly influenced the treatment of mental disorders by psychological procedures. His fundamental technique of mental analysis was an important contribution to psychotherapy. But his theoretical interpretations never grow out of a sound statistical procedure and amount to nothing more than suggestions for future scientific investigations [106, pp. 1, 33, 55].

Contributions of psychoanalysis have been of considerable importance. Even those who bitterly oppose the theory will usually admit that it has done much to stimulate study and that it has contributed much to psychopathology. Many of the mental mechanisms and much of the terminology which we use today have arisen from psychoanalysis. It has had its effect on literature, drama, art, science and religion. Probably its chief contribution has been to increase the understanding of the importance of early life in the development of personality [94, p. 228].

Similar tributes are found in most of the other texts, including seven texts on "abnormal psychology" written by nonmedical men. An examination of more than sixty-five general books on psychiatry (exclusive of textbooks) reveals that less than five had minimal references to psychoanalysis and only two had none.

More important as an index of the growth of psychoanalysis is the increased number of publications. There are only five psychoanalytic journals printed in English, but *fundamental* psychoanalytic work has been published in eighty-six different medical and psychiatric journals in the United States and Europe, as cited by O. Fenichel in his *Psychoanalytic Theory of Neuroses*. Most writers agree that the quantity of publications about psychoanalysis is increasingly prodigious, although occasionally someone predicts a sudden demise.

Both Americans and Europeans have commented upon the decreased activity among Freudians on the Continent since the war, but it must be remembered that most of this group were forced to migrate. The 1937 membership of the International Psychoanalytic Association is presented in the accompanying tabulation, to give the reader some concrete idea of the number of analysts in Europe before the migrations.

### 1937 INTERNATIONAL PSYCHOANALYTIC ASSOCIATION

| | | | |
|---|---:|---|---:|
| Unattached (United States) | 11 | Holland | 38 |
| Boston | 26 | Norway-Denmark | 8 |
| Chicago | 35 | Paris | 44 |
| New York | 76 | Switzerland | 23 |
| Philadelphia | 9 | Japan | 14 |
| Topeka | 15 | Sweden-Finland | 7 |
| Washington-Baltimore | 24 | Tokyo | 9 |
| Britain | 92 | Vienna | 29 |
| Israel | 17 | | |
| India | 56 | Total (18 societies) | 564 |
| Hungary | 31 | | |

Between 1910 and 1937 there were fifteen psychoanalytic societies in Europe and Asia with a regular membership of 278. There were four in the United States with a membership of 126. Now there are thirteen societies in the United States, with every prospect of more to come. To younger analysts it will be amusing to read that, before the June 4, 1920, annual meeting in New York City, some members wanted to dissolve the American Psychoanalytic Association because it had outlived its chief usefulness as a propaganda organization. It had then but 20 members, several of whom lived a long distance from New York.

The current United States membership of the American Psychoanalytic Association is less than 500. There are about 225 training analysts and 650 candidates in training (113). The total membership of the International Psychoanalytic Association was reported at the last meeting in 1949 at Zurich to be about 800 (126). If the emphasis on quality rather than on quantity of candidates continues, it is unlikely that there will ever be enough psychoanalysts to do the necessary psychotherapy in the United States. Consequently, we need not be surprised if laymen will attempt to supply this urgent need. Artists, philanthropists, industrialists, critics and journalists, scientists not in the field of psychiatry or psychology, social workers, motion-picture producers and directors, teachers, and a host of others have accomplished much in helping the educated layman understand something about the irrational in man.

Another tangible sign of increasing recognition of psychoanalysis by the medical profession and by psychiatrists was the creation, in 1933, of a psychoanalytic section in the American Psychiatric Association, which has a membership of over 6,000. This section has always been extremely popular, reflecting the active interest of many American psychiatrists in psychoanalysis (73, 133, 134).

The recent spread of psychoanalytic influence through the armed services is another important fact. Representatives of the American Psychoanalytic Association, under the chairmanship of Richard Frank, of New York City, are compiling a book describing the war services of about forty-seven analysts and listing their bibliographies (114). The splendid service record of many analysts is gratifying. The story of psychiatry in the Army is well told in the book *Psychiatry in a Troubled World*, by W. C. Menninger (102). He gives a general survey of all psychiatric activities during the last war, as he saw them in the Army, and a survey of the importance of psychiatry to the community. Menninger was chief consultant in neuropsychiatry to the Surgeon-General, United States Army, and attained the rank of brigadier general. While his book does not emphasize the importance of psychoanalytic views in the Army, it is evident that a more dynamic approach was fostered throughout the war by all the armed services. The work of John Murray as head of the Air Forces psychiatry and of Roy R. Grinker in one of the chief Army Air Forces treatment centers is also well known. Many of the young men serving under analytically trained psychiatrists were encouraged to continue their training on demobilization, so that the analytic institutes were flooded with applications after 1945. A number of psychiatrists who were regular Army, Navy, and Air Forces officers became interested in psychoanalysis and are now completing their training. These men will undoubtedly exercise a large influence in the future. The armed services now have a training program in which some of their career officers are permitted three years in which to get psychoanalytic training with official support, after they have demonstrated their competence and interest following several years of service.

In view of this general growth, it is regrettable that there are many projects in the planning phases of the federal government in which psychoanalysts have still not joined with teams of other scientists for the purpose of improving the operations of the various departments. Unfortunately, it is extremely difficult to obtain the services of a psychoanalyst in these projects. In a sense, the situation is reversed since the day Freud complained so bitterly of his isolation, for now there are many openings in important positions, but analysts cannot be obtained, owing principally to the public demand for their services in practice.

Government services other than the armed forces also show tremendous interest in psychoanalytic psychiatry. The United States Public Health Service, through fellowships, is encouraging psychoanalytic training, and, like the armed services, is providing training for their senior staff officers in this field. The Veterans Administration likewise is expending enormous sums on training for psychiatrists and is doing everything possible to support training in psychoanalytic psychiatry. Probably the largest training program in psychiatry ever conceived is being carried on at the Winter General Veterans Administration Hospital at Topeka, Kansas, under Karl Menninger, where 125 residents were in training during 1946–49.

It is interesting to note that in the planning division of various other government and allied services, such as the National Research Council, the National Military Establishment, and the Atomic Energy Commission, a fair number of analysts are on the consultation boards. Since less than 8 per cent of the members of the American Psychiatric Association are analysts, it is apparent that analysts are doing their share of public service. But in terms of the total need there is still a regrettable shortage.

Unfortunately, no detailed report on the influence of psychoanalysis or psychoanalytic psychiatry in industry can be given. We have had few specialists in this field. Only one book, *Human Leadership in Industry*, by a lay businessman, Samuel A. Lewisohn (89), is definitely based upon psychoanalytic principles. A cursory acquaintance, however, indicates that the impact is felt here as well as elsewhere, and at least in one prominent school, Cornell University, there is a psychoanalytically oriented psychiatrist at the head of the School of Industrial and Labor Relations.

The growing influence of psychoanalysis upon the medical profession is tangible. Currently more than thirty-four medical schools have analysts as teachers on their faculties, and more would be so employed if they were available. Unfortunately, only schools in large cities, principally in the northern part of the country, have been able to secure analysts. It is unfortunate also that current university salaries are too low to induce more of the leading analysts to be full-time investigators, scholars, and teachers. Many advances could be made in the next generation if more analysts were to devote themselves wholly to investigation and teaching. The recognition accorded to analysts at the present time is much greater than had been envisaged by Freud. Doctors-to-be are now getting an incomparably better introduction to psychoanalysis than did those of twenty years ago.

Medical schools in cities with psychoanalytic institutes are making use of them to further the training of their residents. In 1945, the Department of Psychiatry of Columbia University College of Physicians and Surgeons, under Nolan D. C. Lewis, created a subdivision concerned with special residency and psychoanalytic training for psychosomatic medicine. In 1949 a similar group was started at Long Island College of Medicine under H. W. Potter. These projects are being carried on successfully with a number of leading psychoanalysts on the senior staff. These are the only universities which can afford large-scale training of this kind, but a number of other universities (Harvard, Cincinnati, Pennsylvania, Johns Hopkins, Illinois, Chicago, Pittsburgh) created senior staff positions for psychoanalytically trained psychiatrists, to work intimately with departments of medicine. These men may or may not have a service of their own, but they work in close co-operation with the department of medicine and function principally in that department. Leading teaching hospitals, like Mount Sinai in New York, Michael Reese in Chicago, and Mount Sinai in San Francisco, have strong psychoanalytic staffs, while others, such as the Mayo Clinic, are acquiring them (113, 134). M. R. Kaufman found that 70 per cent of all members of the American Psychoanalytic Association are teaching in medical schools and hospitals, schools for social work, and allied fields. Eighteen per cent are engaged exclusively as teachers in psychoanalytic institutes and training centers, and only 12 per cent are not engaged in any teaching (73, p. 2; 72, p. 1).

In Chicago, the universities of Illinois and Chicago and the Michael Reese Hospital, in co-operation with the Institute for Psychoanalysis, have formed the Associated Psychiatric Faculties of Chicago. It is hoped that eventually this organization will provide means to help physicians obtain training in psychoanalytic psychiatry at all levels, including regular residencies, the training of medical specialists other than psychiatrists in pscyhoanalytic and psychiatric techniques, and aid research specialists, such as psychologists, biochemists, and physiologists, who want psychoanalytic training.

Although there is lack of unanimity among medical social workers and psychiatric social workers about all their working techniques, most psychiatric social workers favor psychoanalytic psychiatry and look to it for guidance. The reports by Marion Kenworthy (62, 63) and her colleagues are a good survey of current thinking in this growing field (72).

Not much can be said about the influence of psychoanalytic practice upon psychiatric nursing and, perhaps even more important, upon general nursing, but this influence is certain to make itself felt. In the best psychiatric hospitals, which unfortunately are extremely expensive, we have excellent examples of psychoanalytic principles governing nursing practice, by co-ordinating ordinary activity with psychological and other therapies, such as bibliotherapy, recreational therapy, occupational therapy, and hydrotherapy (100, 101).

## PRESENT OUTLOOK

In the middle of the twentieth century, after fifty years' maturation, one can speculate that there is a definite prospect that a stable psychoanalytic psychiatry will become the dominant teaching and therapeutic method, although there will be numerous alterations in vocabulary and presentation of material. The essential Freudian contributions will remain, however much they may be disguised in restatement. With impetus from these ideas, there will be much more widespread psychotherapy in all fields of human relations, including preventive care for normal people, as well as for psychotics, people with character disorders, and criminals. On the one hand, the therapeutic practice of psychoanalysis will, in the United States, be closely allied to medicine, especially with the new drive furnished by the common interest in the psychosomatic approach, while, on the other hand, psychoanalysis will be not be submerged by medicine. Psychiatric social workers, clinical and experimental psychologists, educators of all types, industrial counselors, vocational and religious leaders, artists, philosophers, and scholars in all fields of the social sciences will continue to expand the independent use of Freudian concepts in their work. It is quite likely that after a preliminary period of learning, we can look forward to strong experimentation by clinical psychologists which will be of genuine value in the elucidation of problems in memory, learning, emotions, and clinical states.

The fear expressed by numerous Freudians that the technical level of understanding and skill in management of personality problems arising in the unconscious will decline markedly because of diversion of interest in the analyst is not unfounded. Not everyone who tries can be a really good psychoanalyst, nor will all those who have the potentiality work at it persistently enough to succeed. The temptation remains powerful to make psychoanalysis more acceptable to many classes of people, in order to obtain intellectual, social, and financial support. The urgent need to care for more patients will generate a constant pressure to do more superficial therapy, resulting in the neglect of thoroughgoing analysis. The widespread interests of current analysts guarantee an active growth, free from provincialism, but it will probably be some years before there emerges better theoretical synthesis than that stated by Freud. Perhaps we will have a diffuse phase due to the diversity of interests, during which the wisdom of Freud apparently will be in abeyance. The obscurities caused by this manifold unco-ordinated activity may cause the parent-organizations to crystallize in order to maintain their identity, but we can believe with Hanns Sachs (127) that the best in Freud will reappear.

The tribute paid Freud by Thomas Mann (96, 97), one of Europe's leading living man of letters, augurs well for the continued growth of psychoanalysis and its influence upon psychiatry, not only directly but also indirectly through all phases of human relationships. After several generations of familiarity, we can expect much less resistance from people in general and consequently less need of defensiveness on the part of analysts.

### INFLUENCE OF PSYCHOANALYSIS ON PSYCHOLOGY

Our survey of the influence of psychoanalysis would be incomplete without noting its effect on the basic science of psychology. It is probable that the feed-back from psychology to psychiatry in the next half-century will be one of the outstanding features of their mutual development. It would be a stupendous task to attempt a critical survey of the contents of approximately sixty psychological journals now being published in English. But we can present the views of a few psychologists who have attempted summaries. Articles and books by Moore (105, 106), Brown (22), Flugel (36), Miller (103), Misbach (104), Murray (108), and Rapaport (115–20) will serve as introductions to the student. Moore states explicitly how little academic psychology has contributed to clinical problems or to psychiatry, even though men like Kraepelin and Theodor Ziehen based their careers upon an attempt to establish a basic science of psychology for the purpose of furthering psychiatry. As early as 1914, Adolf Meyer at Johns Hopkins gave a beginning course in psychology to medical students, for a time in collaboration with such notable psychologists as John B. Watson and Knight Dunlap.

For the most part, general and experimental psychologists have not collaborated freely with analysts, but there is evidence that this relationship is improving. The possibility of solving both theoretical and practical differences between experimental psychology and psychoanalysis is illustrated, not too successfully, by the report of Sears (133, 134) on over one hundred projects of objective studies of psychoanalytic concepts, and another survey on similar studies of the analytic process itself and of aggression and substitution mechanisms. Shakow (135) has examined some of the ways in which clinical psychologists and psychiatrists may work together in order to overcome the barriers which were outlined by Freud in *The Question of Lay Analysis* (51).

Rapaport (118) has attempted to clarify psychoanalytic conceptions of the thought-processes and of ego function. He minimizes misinterpretation of psychoanalytic terms by using specific quotations from Freud, for example, Freud's use of the word "ideation" for the product of the primary thought process. The differences between the primary ("ideation") and secondary ("thinking") processes are seen as differences in delays in gratification and are described genetically, topographically, structurally, and economically. Rapaport states: "From the biological point of view thinking is experimental action with small amounts of energy. Thinking explores the possible pathways of action to find the one of least resistance, least danger, and greatest directness, while preserving almost intact the energy necessary for motor action. This formulation integrates the biological advantage of thinking into the psychoanalytic theory of thinking" (118, p. 168).

Another important series of studies of psychoanalytic psychology are those of Hartmann, Kris, and Loewenstein (64, 65, 66, 80, 81, 92); *Childhood and Society* (35) by Erikson includes theoretical and practical contributions on the growth of the ego. For educators and therapists *Love Is Not Enough* (13) by Bettelheim and *Mental Hygiene in Teaching* (122) by Redl and Wattenberg furnish concrete descriptions of the treatment of emotionally disturbed children by utilizing principles of dynamic psychology. The writings of Robert Waelder on paranoid ideas (140) bring into focus the strengths and weaknesses of various older theories dealing with this subject which will help the clinician as well as the theoretician.

The papers by Bronfenbrenner, Bruner, Frenkel-Brunswik, Hilgard, Klein, and Miller presented at the University of Texas Clinical Psychology Symposium on Perception will be of special interest to psychoanalysts, for these workers present evidence that the psychology of personality has received strong impetus from psychoanalytic findings and theories (15). It is well documented that the relationship of motivation, drives, needs, and irrational impulses to studies of perception may be used as a basic approach to an understanding of interpersonal relations. The acceptance of many psychoanalytic theories by psychologists is increasing. Bronfenbrenner attempts an integrated theory of personality by utilizing the views of K. Lewin, Freud, Rank, McDougall, and Sullivan. The Duke University symposium, published as *Perception and Personality*, edited by Bruner and Krech (23), adds additional information to this new large development in the experimental study of perception. It seems that this field is capturing the interest of psychologists as a leading frontier somewhat as did intelligence testing after 1916 and projective techniques after 1940.

Misbach (104) points out that psychoanalytic psychology has done much to expand the horizons of academic psychology but has not contributed significantly toward a solution of the systematic problems which usually concern academic psychology. It is also notable that academic psychology has not contributed much to, or modified, the scope of psychoanalysis, with such exceptions as the influence of W. Köhler on T. M. French. Misbach attempts a systematic review of the principal themes of the two disciplines and finds two major positions with respect to the leading ideas in theories of learning. Leeper (85) has characterized these as "peripheralist" versus "centralist." The writings of Hull, especially in *Principles of Behavior* (69), are the best presentations of the peripheralist position, and the works of the Gestaltists, such as Köhler and Koffka, are used as the best exposition of the centralists. It is clear that the psychoanalytic ideas have much more in common with the centralist position. Misbach thinks it unnecessary for psychologists to attack many of the Freudian ideas concerning maturational stages of instinctual development or the related theory of polymorphous infantile sexuality. He is more concerned with examining the area of ego psychology, used in the broadest sense to designate organized behavior. He discusses the various types of etiologic traumata, such as associated or coincidental events, seduction in childhood, frustration, and emotional atmosphere, and then raises the question of whether there is a psychoanalytic theory of learning. An answer is attempted by stating that the theory of learning must be based upon evidence concerning factors found to be necessary, not merely sometimes apparently operative, in learning. By searching the hypotheses of "the wreckage produced by the fantasy theory," he finds that Freud did have a solution which has not been recognized or has been underestimated. Freud created, virtually *de novo*, the first naturalistic system of dynamic psychology, and he did so under the heavy handicap of the mechanistic philosophy of the nineteenth century:

> The clue for solution is Freud's final definition of the ego as organization, or system, and as the locus of learning. As has yet to be shown more fully, no matter in what direction the origin of fixation is pursued, ego or pre-ego organization is found to be prior to and the basis of the fixation-process. It is merely a restatement of the priority of organization or structure to point out that closure, or insight, is found to be always and necessarily operative. This fact which, considering its dramatic first discovery in the operation of fantasies, should have been remembered has been often overlooked, presumably because of uncertainty as to its theoretical significance [104, p. 149].

Misbach concludes:

> To a considerable extent we are indebted to psychoanalysis, to Gestalt theory and to related developments in psychology for the understandings which have thus far been achieved. We are also much indebted to philosophy, and to accumulated educational and other social experience. But the need remains great indeed for improved educational practices and implementing general principle for learning theory. No matter how convenient for scientific rigor a fragmentary principle may be, it would seem

the part of wisdom not to sacrifice a comprehensive bio-social view in our quest for guiding theory [104, p. 155].

A graphic summary by a psychologist-physician, H. A. Murray, is of interest:

In the short history of abnormal psychology there is no one to compare to Freud. His contribution covers more than half the field; and today a therapist who attempts to get along without him is as helpless as a blind man fumbling here and there where others pick their way with some assurance. For it was Freud who distinguished the pathogenic forces in neurotic illness and showed how their signs could be discovered among involuntary processes: dreams, fantasies, free associations, absent-minded actions, slips of speech and writing, gestures and emotions, wit and laughter, unwarranted interpretations, behavior that is rationalized, accidents, creative art. Since inhibited tendencies are universal among men the methods and theories Freud devised for the understanding of neurotics are just as useful though not so indispensable to the student of normal— especially super-normal—individuals. Thus, by revealing the vast realm that an over-rationalistic psychology had neglected, Freud pushed back the margins of obscurity. The enlargement of consciousness, *that* was Freud's best gift to man [108, p. 136].

INFLUENCE OF PSYCHOANALYSIS ON SOCIOLOGY

Since Freud wrote *Totem and Taboo* (1912) (52), *Group Psychology and the Analysis of the Ego* (1921) (44), *The Future of an Illusion* (1927) (42), and *Civilization and Its Discontents* (1930) (41), sociologists have been enormously stimulated to examine the family as a sociological unit by studying the emotional ties among its members and their relation to the psychodynamics of larger groups. Burgess and Locke's book, *The Family* (1945) (24), describing the transition from an institution to companionship, illustrates some of the methodological problems. Because human experiences studied by psychoanalysts all occur in a social context, psychoanalysis is a part of social psychology and to some students seems to belong much more among the social than among the biological sciences. The progressive demonstration of environmental factors in the formation of personality and personality disorders had increased the points of contact between psychiatry and sociology, and this is reflected in many sociological publications. On the other hand, the writings of such psychiatrists as Plant (112), Schilder (129, 130), Fromm-Reichmann (54), and Sullivan (138) are samples of psychiatric interest in this growth. It is of speculative interest that Sullivan's writings are "reminiscent of the social thought of Cooley, Dewey and Mead" (33). We will cite only one author among several who shows convincingly that sociology and psychiatry have many problems in common and that a special name, "social psychiatry," is being used to designate the growing specialized knowledge of this field. Dunham's (33) comprehensive study is well documented to show the overlapping areas of experimental interest. He believes the leading research areas for social psychiatry to be (1) ecology and statistics, (2) personality and culture, (3) caste and class, and (4) interpersonal relations. The latter includes the subheads: (*a*) personality organization, (*b*) social interaction relationship, (*c*) behavioral consequences, and (*d*) sociometric developments. Four specific problem areas which interest workers in both disciplines are mentioned: (1) follow-up of mental patients discharged from mental hospitals; (2) contrasting family psychologies in various societies; (3) sociological studies of the development of mentally disturbed children, including schizophrenics; and (4) institutional studies, utilizing newer techniques from psychoanalysis, sociometry, and social psychology (33).

### The Influence of Psychoanalysis upon Anthropology

In no field are the productive working relationships more fruitful than those between anthropology and psychoanalysis. The pioneering efforts of Franz Boas, Ruth Benedict, Margaret Mead, G. Róheim, and Edward Sapir, supported by the work of C. Kluckhohn, G. Bateson, G. Devereux, E. Erikson, R. Linton, A. Kardiner, C. DuBois, E. Fromm, F. Alexander, and Dorothea Leighton, give promise of a flourishing collaboration from which will come a synthesis rather than a juxtaposition. Psychiatrists will benefit from the work of anthropologists in the search for concrete evidence of the causes of mental disorders. It is worth noting that after Freud's opening of the field with *Totem and Taboo* in 1912 (52), other analysts, notably Reik, Rank, and Róheim (144), and, in the United States, Brill, Coriat, Brown, and Hamburger, have published significant observations about nonliterate groups. In justice to Kraepelin and others, it should be mentioned that they also began the study of a comparative psychiatry, although without attaining the success of the current workers. Kluckhohn, in an exceptionally good review illustrating the diverse forces at work and the tremendous changes made through Freud's innovations, pays this tribute:

A presentation of this subject matter will be simplified if it is pointed out at the outset that American anthropologists have been influenced almost exclusively by psychoanalytic psychiatry.... Certainly from the study of anthropological literature one gets an overwhelming impression that it is only psychoanalytic writers who are extensively read by anthropologists in this country. One would be hard pressed to discover five citations to nonanalytic psychiatrists, with the exception of Rorschach....

Although a few American anthropologists have shown some interest in the problems of perception and of intelligence tests, academic psychology has had a surprising minimum of influence upon anthropology. Almost the only concept of any wide currency which has been taken over from academic psychology is that of the sentiment (which came mainly via Radcliffe-Brown and other British anthropologists). The influence of the Gestalt psychology upon Benedict and others may also be noted. With these qualifications, it must be said that American anthropology, for good or for ill, has seemed to find only in psychoanalysis the bases for a workable social psychology.

The generalization may be narrowed by noting that we need say little of the older psychiatries which originated in, but diverged from, Freudian psychoanalysis. Jung is talked about by anthropologists fairly occasionally, and one sees references to his work, especially to the personality types, now and then. Radin discussed the implications of Jung's theories for ethnology and predicted that Jung would have a greater influence than any of the scientific group. This prediction has thus far notably failed of justification. Jung's systematic influence in this country in contrast to Great Britain seems to have been restricted to one psychiatrist who used ethnological data and published in anthropological media. Of Rank there is barely casual mention, and in the professional literature I have discovered but three incidental references to Adler. The so-called "Neo-Freudians" (Horney, Kardiner, Fromm, and others) have, as is well known, been highly influential in anthropological circles during the past few years [75, pp. 589–90].

There is not uniform agreement among analysts or anthropologists about these projects, but the main direction seems clear, in spite of strong resistance by more orthodox anthropologists (2, 128). Occasionally an analyst may not support some of the theories of an analytically minded anthropologist (99). This rejection was aided, however, says Kluckhohn, by analysts' "ignorance or failure to discriminate"; and he shows how this came about. He lists propositions on which all anthropologists agree, and he expresses the hope that psychiatrists will use them to avoid offending the anthropologists' sensibilities. These propositions include such items as " 'primitive' societies must not be lumped together. ... Psychiatrists must cease to equate 'primitive' with 'childlike' or 'archaic.' ... The anecdotal approach is worthless. ... Cultures must be regarded as wholes, having organization as well as content. . . . The premises of theoretical arguments must be congruent with anthropological theorems. . . . The psychiatrists must acquire a fuller control of the relevant anthropological literature than they have commonly shown in the past. There must be less uncritical use of data, as well as less snatching of data out of context" (75, pp. 614–15).

The following gains have been made by the psychoanalytically oriented anthropologists: (1) In the techniques of field research, a completely new conception of the number and character of informants needed has come as much from psychiatry, especially through Sapir (128), as from sampling theory in statistics; and (2) new topics have been added to theoretical anthropology. Psychiatry is primarily responsible for the granting of full recognition to interpretative studies of the individual in culture, culture and personality, child socialization, transmission of culture through child training, the abnormal or deviant person, life-histories, culture and motivation, origin of culture in a new sense, new attack on configurational analysis (to what degree can we understand the plot or theme of a culture by reference to the recurrent traumatic situations to which the child is subjected in the family situation?) and to a different approach to psychosomatic problems, such as the relationship of disease pictures to culturally determined forms of character structure.

It is worth pointing out that anthropologists are much more sophisticated now about their interpersonal relationship with their subjects since they have learned more about how interview techniques enable them to get anxiety-protected material, even if this has not been well written up. "Under the impact of psychiatry, anthropology has come to recognize the incompleteness of the question and answer method. The need for passive interviews, for controlled observations, even for simple experiments, for personal documents, dreams, fantasies of individuals, and other informal materials is now seen by a large number of field workers" (75, p. 616).

New conceptual tools have been added, including such concepts as ambivalence, identification, and latent content. The great value of such new interpretations in "family behavior, religion, clowns and formalized joking, suicide, narcotics, and alcoholism," is being more and more recognized. "In conclusion, it may be noted that anthropologists have altered many of their postulates. The whole thinking about the individual informant as a cultural specimen has been sharply refashioned. The false antinomy of 'the individual vs. society' is gradually being abandoned. Assumptions as to the relative proportions of irrational, nonrational, and rational elements in human behavior have been revised; although this last trend was independently forced upon anthropology by its own materials, the trend was given increased momentum by pressure from psychiatry" (75, p. 617).

## THE INFLUENCE OF PSYCHOANALYSIS ON ECONOMICS

In surveying the concrete evidence of the growth of psychoanalytic influence, we have selected illustrations from basic fields where this influence is maximal and of the utmost importance for future growth. We will now discuss the spread of psychoanalysis into areas which are relatively remote but which are of interest to the general reader. To call attention to a few of the major positions in these areas will be of service to the reader as well as do justice to Freud.

The connection between both classical and Marxist economics and psychoanalysis may appear tenuous until it is recalled that all are concerned with human relationships. Unlike sociologists and social anthropologists, most economists make a sturdy attempt to minimize the human factors in their investigations, even though Adam Smith (1723–90), one of the founders of modern economics, wrote extensively on the "moral sense." He described its evolution from the "instinct of sympathy" by means of mechanisms that psychoanalysts would call identification and incorporation into a series of functions not unlike the Freudian superego (*Theory of Moral Sentiments* [1759]). This ethical theory is said to be in internal harmony with Smith's famous economic treatise "Wealth of Nations" (1776), even though it apparently is contradicted in part by that treatise. Reconciliation of the differences between his ethical and economic position is possible, and in the course of lectures including both views, Smith expressed the hope that a freely acting evolutionary process would result in a large measure of social harmony between ethics and economics, although he did not foresee the many barriers to this highly desirable state.

A highly gifted modern economist, Thorstein Veblen (1857–1929), who is still considered unorthodox, saw distinctly these problems of a psychological basis of economic theory and also the inadequacy of current economic theory which operates with an insufficient psychology. Independent of Freud, he saw the draw-backs of older psychological assumptions and favored a new de-terministic outlook. Veblen did not believe that superficial mod-ernization of the psychological elements in social theory would be enough to permit total social theory to maintain a stable iden-tity. His proposed solutions are compared interestingly, if not too successfully, with Freud's by Schneider (132).

Some of the most lively debates about socioeconomic implica-tions of Freudian theory have been carried on by writers inter-ested in Marxism. The opinions offered vary widely regarding the relationships between psychoanalysis and dialectical material-ism. Experts in the latter field are not agreed on the place of psy-chology in socioeconomic theory. While most of them hold to the primacy of economic determinism or to the thesis that the methods by which men make their living is the crucial factor, some are not so adamant as others in excluding all other genetic, sociological, or anthropological views concerning the formation of personality and culture. Freud's own statements are of interest for comparison with his critics. While he modestly disclaims any competence in this field, he offers his lay opinion that other forces are important in the historical process, e.g., social differ-ences arising from original differences between early tribes and races; psychologically the "amount of constitutional aggressive-ness and also the degree of cohesion within the horde, and mate-rial factors, such as the possession of better weapons, decided the victory. . . . The strength of Marxism obviously does not lie in its view of history or in the prophecies about the future which it bases upon that view, but in its clear insight into the determining influence which is exerted by the economic conditions of man upon his intellectual, ethical and artistic reactions. A whole col-lection of correlations and causal sequences were thus discovered, which had hitherto been almost completely disregarded. But it cannot be assumed that economic motives are the only ones which determine the behavior of men in society" (47, pp. 242, 243).

Pannekoek's early exposition of "Society and Mind in Marxian Philosophy" (111) is a sober statement probably acceptable to many psychiatrists. By distinguishing between a crude material-ism and historical dialectical materialism, he shows that there is a definite place for a strictly deterministic psychology in socio-economic theory. Customs, traditions, and family folklore and practices are viewed as real events which exert concrete, specific influence upon personality growth. Apparently the concept of an active unconscious is accepted by him with insistence that a person's ideas are the result of his whole experience, past and present, with the citation from Marx that consciousness is determined by the activity of a man in the real world.

This relatively early appraisal was followed by articles more or less critical of Freud from R. Osborn (109), F. H. Bartlett (6, 7, 8), J. Wortis (147), and J. Marmor (98), and defenses by J. F. Brown (22), D. Rapaport (117), J. T. Stone (137), J. Furst (55), and L. Schneider (132). While the details of this involved controversy cannot be recounted here, the summary by Stone will serve as a useful introduction to the inquiring student. Lawrence Kubie (82), writing of the relation of psychoanalysis to political reforms, also cites a reference to "Lenin's caustic criticism of certain types of blind radicalism (86)." With increased understanding in either camp of the concepts and methods employed by the other, there will be a more accurate definition and appropriate discussion of the real issues.

Perhaps examples from another field will furnish perspective. The fallacy of the either-or position in facing the heredity-environment or mind-body dichotomies will be evident from the following statements by R. W. Gerard, in answer to the question of what determines the sex of an organism:

> The answer will be different quantitatively from case to case, probably all the way from 99% to 1%. You recall that heredity "completely" determines sex; two X chromosomes give a female and one a male. But let me also remind you that environment "completely" determines sex; frog eggs that normally develop into 50% males and 50% females, can be diverted to 100% male or 100% female by changing the concentration of salt in the solution in which they are kept [57, p. 163].

Human relationships provide a deceptive field for quick generalizations and uneasy certitudes, which are in need of sound evidence. From this evidence will evolve a firm basis for opinions about biological determinants and their constant interaction with environmental processes. Facts, not strident humorless debate, will be the final criteria.

### Influence of Psychoanalysis on Religion

Freud in his two essays, *The Future of an Illusion* (1927) (42) and *Civilization and Its Discontents* (1930) (41), established a position which is of importance to the over-all picture of the growth and development of psychoanalysis. Briefly, Freud describes religion as a man-made system of relations based upon his infantile fears. Obviously, this opinion conflicted with established religion, causing much discussion of this problem, especially after the end of World War II. It is impossible in a brief space to give an adequate synopsis or even a thorough bibliography of the problem, but a few pointers show the major importance of the teachings of Freud in this field (29, 90, 91, 149). From a collection of essays by a number of experts in various fields, entitled *Psychiatry and Religion* (91), one can get an understanding of some of the basic questions from the point of view of this group of men who are representative of a good part of the population. Joshua Liebman and his colleagues saw the importance of psychoanalysis, although they felt that its teachings did not go far enough, because they did not really deal with the problem of an ethical and religious orientation. No attempt will be made in this summary to reconcile the various differences, since the problem is far too complex for a brief analysis. Suffice it to say that Rabbi Liebman, after a close scrutiny, the result of which can be seen in his book, *Peace of Mind*, decided that "wherever religion and psychiatry can work together to take a broken, disunited, disordered personality and bring unity into it, there an act of religion is being performed" (90). The moderate position taken by E. Fromm (53) may be of interest in this connection.

To those unacquainted with the current writings on this subject, it may seem paradoxical that so-called "materialistic" psychiatrists can discuss, on a practical working basis, problems common to them and to the minister and priest. The solutions at the present time seem numerous and are not being automatically rejected by practical therapists as poor substitutes for either a materialistic philosophy or an adherence to an orthodox religion, even though skeptics on both sides are not convinced. Some of the most severe critics of psychoanalysis come from orthodox groups; yet within these same circles are scholars with a sympathetic interest, as at the Department of Psychology of the University of Montreal. The brilliant summary of Reik (123) will fascinate those who feel that the churches are trying to put psychoanalysis into their service to the detriment of analysis. Much tolerance and more study will be needed to resolve these classic tribulations of mankind.

Not only the Protestant and Hebrew churches have shown an

interest in the development in psychiatry with its new insights into their pastoral obligations. There has been splendid co-operation between psychiatrists and Catholic institutions in a number of cities in the United States. All this quiet, healthy, and considerable growth is not always understood, in view of a few trends to the contrary. Without debating the virtues of the position of the most vocal critics, we can state that a number of distinguished Catholic psychoanalysts and psychiatrists did not agree with them and issued public replies. Perhaps more significantly, the national Catholic weekly, *Commonweal*, published a strong editorial stating that Catholics need not reject analysis (95). This challenging editorial, written by a Catholic working with the Veterans Administration, defends what he considers good in the Freudian theory while reserving the right to criticize what he thinks is poor. It is interesting that he strongly supports the fact and the importance of the unconscious and the Freudian descriptions of such mechanisms as projection. He states "Freudians can teach much regarding the entire role of family figures in the upbringing of a child. They have studied these matters intensely, whereas our ascetical literature echoes the monastic viewpoint of life in the religious community" (95). He makes the point that psychoanalysis is not a threat to family life but rather the most thorough preparation for parenthood in this age of anxiety.

It is probable that all resident psychiatrists will have the increasing obligation of a bowing acquaintance with these questions, however remote they may seem to them after long training in physical methods.

The reading lists cited in a handbook for pastors, *Problems in Religion and Life* (16), written by a leading educator in this field, Anton T. Boisen, who has worked for many years at the Elgin State Hospital, Illinois, will furnish the beginning student with a splendid introduction. Boisen has a select bibliography in the areas of principles of social inquiries, psychology, sociology, social surveys, social psychology and personality, social philosophy, psychology of religion, sociology of religion, religious education, and psychopathology, including delinquency and child guidance, psychotherapy and counseling, and social work. The texts are, by and large, the standard writings acceptable in any medical school and university in the country. Special attention is called to the work of George A. Coe, *Psychology of Religion*

(25), since this is probably one of the best presentations of the field and will help the student gain basic orientation. A recent book which is finding favor with residents is *Freud and Christianity* by R. S. Lee (84). This minister, vicar of St. Mary the Virgin, the mother-church of the University of Oxford, has a splendid knowledge of Freudian literature and, in a manner parallel to that of Liebman and Harry Emerson Fosdick (37, 38), strives to reconcile Freudian teaching with Christianity, maintaining that psychoanalysis is useful in understanding the teachings of Christ. This book has the advantage of being easy to read, although some complex aspects of the relation of Freudian psychology to Christian ethics are discussed.

It is a question, of course, whether many of the problems dealt with by psychoanalysis are more religious than medical. The recent growth in popularity in Europe of some Jungian doctrines, including a new diagnosis, viz., that of "existential" neuroses, has not influenced the bulk of American psychiatrists or ministers up to this time. It is interesting, however, that the proposition arises in the troubled postwar period and that numerous solutions are being offered. To most physicians the "existential" neuroses are reactive or situational processes, firmly rooted in the biological hypotheses already described. It is worth while to recall at this time that studies on this had been made earlier. Flournoy, a Swiss who occupied the first chair of psychology of religion in the Faculty of Science at the University of Geneva, recognized both the biological postulates and the presence of the unconscious as a source of piety. Such outstanding scholars of the psychology of religion as Neeser, Bergner, and Maeder also support this position.

### INFLUENCE OF PSYCHOANALYSIS ON LITERATURE

For many years psychiatrists have been interested in the artist, the nature of his productivity, and the art process, while writers have always been interested in human relationships, especially the intense feelings, which are also the subject of study by the psychiatrist. Since the first decade of the twentieth century, there has been apparent a tremendous impetus toward psychoanalysis, so that in one form or another its presence is noticeable in the majority of contemporary writers and hence in the general reading population. This fact underlines the difficulty in tracing influences, since many psychologists, psychiatrists, and other scholars are subjected to these ideas without being aware of it. The dissemination of Freudian ideas among authors is described at length by Hoffman (68), who turns the spotlight in the general discussion upon James Joyce of Ireland, D. H. Lawrence of England, Sherwood Anderson and Waldo Frank of the United States, Franz Kafka of Czechoslovakia, and Thomas Mann of Germany. The bibliography of over three hundred articles and books makes this an excellent introductory volume because of its clarity and economy. The student will not be satisfied with Hoffman's interpretations at many points, but the multiplicity of references will enable him to go on with his own explorations with greater ease.

The exposition of Conrad Aiken as contrasted with D. H. Lawrence will be of considerable value to the beginner. Hoffman prints part of a letter from Aiken which is worth quoting:

> For me, [Freud] still fits admirably in such philosophic order as I find necessary—a belief in the evolution of consciousness, awareness, as our prime gift and obligation, and a Socratic desire to get on with it at all costs [68, p. 288].

Aiken makes the point that he was profoundly influenced by Freud:

> ... but so has everybody, whether they are aware of it or not. However, I decided very early, I think as early as 1912, that Freud, and his co-workers and rivals and followers, were making the most important contribution of the century to the understanding of man and his consciousness; accordingly I made it my business to learn as much from them as I could [68, p. 280].

Ludwig Lewisohn also has his place, especially for his defense of monogamy in the novel *Stephen Escott* (1928). It should be pointed out that Lewisohn, in spite of his admiration for Freud, makes it very clear that he thinks psychoanalysis can help only individuals and has very little chance of helping the mass, because knowledge and science are insufficient for this purpose. Like the Marxists, he thinks that something more is necessary to remedy the ills of society, but, instead of the Marxists' economic revolution, Lewisohn advocates an ethical rehabilitation. He is strongly concerned with the problem of Jewish culture for this purpose. He believes that Jews bring to scientific discipline a cultural vision and spiritual awareness which comes from their race. Freud, as we know, did not believe that the analyst can transcend the limits of his science and was against both Jung and our own J. J. Putnam, of Harvard, for trying to make more out of analysis than he thought it could be. These men have something in common with those Catholics who see in psychoanalysis useful tools for individual therapy but who also are quick to point out that religion has higher purposes than individual therapy. It is interesting that in a sense the criticism of Freud here is that analytic practice does not go far enough, whereas many writers, especially psychologists, complain because it does not go anywhere at all. Some analysts with a broader social point of view advocate studying larger social units and their influence on the individual ego.

Other writers who are important in the study of psychoanalysis are Thomas Mann, Henry Miller, Dylan Thomas (the young Welsh poet, who writes in the vein of Joyce or Waldo Frank), Graham Greene, Joseph Freeman, and Arthur Koestler, but this by no means exhausts the list. These writers furnish evidence that the Freudian hypotheses have infiltrated deeply into our culture.

Hoffman, after his extensive book-length examination, makes the following judgment:

The great debt which modern writing owes to psychoanalysis has been recognized by creative artist and critic alike. In no other period of literary history has there been so great an interplay between aesthetic endeavor and scientific research. For this and many other reasons, it has been of great advantage to explore the meaning of that exchange of disciplines. But one must not yield to the temptation to exclude other important influences upon our age, or to neglect the importance of the aesthetic position itself. I should like, therefore, to suggest briefly in a final chapter that Freud shares his position with a number of other important and influential men and to summarize his relationship with them and with the thought and culture of the twentieth century [68, p. 308].

In this patternless pattern of our twentieth century Freud occupies a peculiar position. He is professedly and avowedly a scientist. But his science deals with the very sources of irrationality—or, if you prefer, with the areas of man's affective life which have most definitely been excluded from rational and traditional consideration. Having reopened the debate on the actual motives of behavior of all types, he has had repeatedly to assert that his discoveries and conjectures do not warrant either ungrounded pessimism or unrestrained irrationality. We should return with renewed confidence to the scientific instruments of reason, he tells us; the constructive work of the ego must go on. License and imprudence may set back its work, or nullify it, with dangerous consequences for society and the human soul. Science has dispelled many illusions, Freud says; but the worst illusion of all is that the renunciation of science and of the reason is either good or safe. Our survey of the career of Freudianism in the twentieth century ought by now to have demonstrated to us that Freud's caution has seldom been observed, that he has himself been accused of sponsoring and favoring the very attitude he has condemned [68, pp. 312–13].

Though a number of studies of the relation between psychoanalysis and art have been made, the complexities are far from being understood. Daniel E. Schneider's *The Psychoanalyst and the Artist* (131) makes a tentative exploration into the nature of genius, its development and essential attributes, its dangers and advantages. Using basic concepts of Freud, Schneider attempts to develop a theory of aesthetics. There are sample discussions of the various resolutions of the oedipal conflict in Sophocles' plays, Delacroix's *Journal*, the paintings of Chagall, Picasso, and Van Gogh, two plays by Arthur Miller, and Shakespeare's *Macbeth*.

Lionel Trilling in *The Liberal Imagination* (139) includes an essay on "Freud and Literature" and one on "Art and Neurosis" which delimit the value of Freudian interpretation of works of art and negate the thesis that all artists are "sick" but give full credit to Freud's conception of the structure of the mind. He states:

For, of all mental systems, the Freudian psychology is the one which makes poetry indigenous to the very constitution of the mind. Indeed, the mind, as Freud sees it, is in the greater part of its tendency exactly a poetry-making organ. This puts the case too strongly, no doubt, for it seems to make the working of the unconscious mind equivalent to poetry itself, forgetting that between the unconscious mind and the finished poem there supervene the social intention and the formal control of the conscious mind. Yet the statement has at least the virtue of counterbalancing the belief, so commonly expressed or implied, that the very opposite is true, and that poetry is a kind of beneficent aberration of the mind's right course.

Freud has not merely naturalized poetry; he has discovered its status as a pioneer settler, and he sees it as a method of thought. Often enough he tries to show how, as a method of thought, it is unreliable and ineffective for conquering reality; yet he himself is forced to use it in the very shaping of his own science, as when he speaks of the topography of the mind and tells us with a kind of defiant apology that the metaphors of space relationship which he is using are really most inexact since the mind is not a thing of space at all, but that there is no other way of conceiving the difficult idea except by metaphor. In the eighteenth century Vico spoke of the metaphorical, imagistic language of the early stages of culture; it was left to Freud to discover how, in a scientific age, we still feel and think in figurative formations, and to create, what psychoanalysis is, a science of tropes, of metaphor and its variants, synecdoche and metonomy.

Freud showed, too, how the mind, in one of its parts, could work without logic, yet not without that directing purpose, that control of intent from which, perhaps it might be said, logic springs. For the unconscious mind works without the syntactical conjunctions which are logic's essence. It recognizes no *because,* no *therefore,* no *but;* such ideas as similarity, agreement, and community are expressed in dreams imagistically by compressing the elements into a unity. The unconscious mind in its struggle with the conscious always turns from the general to the concrete and finds the tangible trifle more congenial than the large abstraction. Freud discovered in the very organization of the mind those mechanisms by which art makes its effects, such devices as the condensations of meanings and the displacement of accent [139, pp. 52–43].

This brief survey does not permit the inclusion of philosophers, but a work by Langer, *Philosophy in a New Key: A Study in the Symbolism of Reason, Rite, and Art* (83) has numerous ideas which suggest a kinship with Freudian concepts, although there is no specific effort to demonstrate this relation. Her insistence that the "new key" (symbolic transformation) in philosophy is really *new* and that it changes the questions in philosophy deserves further examination. In this book, as in some others mentioned earlier, we catch glimpses of the philosophy and psychology of the future.

## BIBLIOGRAPHY

1.  ALEXANDER, B. "Spinoza und die Psychoanalyse," *Almanach der Psychoanalyse für das Jahr 1928,* pp. 94–103.
2.  ALEXANDER, F. "The Educative Influence of Personality Factors in the Environment," *Suppl. Ed. Monogr.,* No. 54, pp. 29–47, 1942.
3.  ALEXANDER, F. *Our Age of Unreason* (New York: J. B. Lippincott Co., 1942).
4.  ALLPORT, G. W. *The Individual and his Religion: A Psychological Interpretation* (New York: Macmillan Co., 1950).
5.  ARISTOPHANES. *Comedies,* Vol. 1 (London: G. Bell, 1908).
6.  BARTLETT, F. H. "The Limitations of Freud," *Sci. & Soc.,* 3:64, 1939.
7.  BARTLETT, F. H. "Recent Trends in Psychoanalysis," *Sci. & Soc.,* 9:214, 1945.
8.  BARTLETT, F. H. *Sigmund Freud: A Marxian Essay* (London: Gollancz, 1938).
9.  BERNARD, W. "Freud and Spinoza," *Psychiatry,* 9:99, 1946; also in *Yearbook of Psychoanalysis,* 3:31, 1947.
10. BERNFELD, S. "Freud's Earliest Theories and the School of Helmholtz," *Psychoanalyt. Quart.,* 13:341, 1944; also in *Yearbook of Psychoanalysis,* 1:31, 1945.
11. BERNFELD, S. "Sigmund Freud, M.D., 1882–1885," *Internat. J. Psycho-Analysis,* 32:204, 1951.
12. BERNFELD, S. "Sozialismus und Psychoanalyse," *Sozial. Arzt,* Vol. 2, Nos. 2/3; abstr. by O. FENICHEL in *Imago,* 14:385, 1928.

13. BETTELHEIM, B. *Love Is Not Enough* (Glencoe, Ill.: Free Press, 1950).
14. BISCHLER, W. "Schopenhauer and Freud: A Comparison," *Psychoanalyt. Quart.*, 8:88, 1939.
15. BLAKE, R. R., and RAMSEY, G. V. *Perception: An Approach to Personality* (New York: Ronald Press Co., 1951).
16. BOISEN, A. T. *Problems in Religion and Life* (New York: Abingdon-Cokesbury Press, 1946).
17. BRIDGMAN, P. W. *The Logic of Modern Physics* (New York: Macmillan Co., 1927) (*re* Faraday, p. 44).
18. BRIGHT, T. *A Treatise of Melancholia* (London, 1586).
19. BRILL, A. A. "An American Precursor of Freud," *Bull. New York Acad. Med.*, 16:631, 1940.
20. BRILL, A. A. "Anticipations and Corroborations of the Freudian Concepts from Non-analytic Sources," *Am. J. Psychiat.*, 92:1127, 1936.
21. BRILL, A. A. "Josef Popper-Lynkeus: Translator's Prologue to Dreaming like Waking," *Yearbook of Psychoanalysis*, 4:27, 1948.
22. BROWN, J. F. "Freud's Influence on American Psychology," *Psychoanalyt. Quart.*, 9:283, 1940.
23. BRUNER, J. S., and KRECH, D. *Perception and Personality: A Symposium* (Durham, N.C.: Duke University Press, 1949).
24. BURGESS, E. W., and LOCKE, H. J. *The Family: From Institution to Companionship* (New York: American Book Co., 1945).
25. COE, G. A. *The Psychology of Religion* (Chicago: University of Chicago Press, 1916).
26. CROWLEY, R. M. "Psychoanalytic Literature on Drug Addiction and Alcoholism," *Psychoanalyt. Rev.*, 26:39, 1939.
27. DALBIEZ, R. *Psychoanalytical Method and the Doctrine of Freud* (New York: Longmans, Green & Co., 1941).
28. DARWIN, ERASMUS. *Zoonomia*, 1:148, 1794.
29. DAY, F. "The Future of Psychoanalysis and Religion," *Psychoanalyt. Quart.*, 13:84, 1944.
30. DORER, M. *Historische Grundlagen der Psychoanalyse* (Leipzig: F. Meiner, 1932).
31. DUJARDIN, E. *Les Lauriers sont coupés* (Paris: Librairie de la "Revue Indépendante," 1887).
32. DUMMER, E. S. (ed.). *The Unconscious: A Symposium* (New York: A. Knopf, 1928).
33. DUNHAM, H. W. "Social Psychiatry," *Am. Sociol. Rev.*, 13:183, 1948.
34. ELLIS, SIR W. C. *A Treatise on the Nature, Symptoms, Causes, and Treatment of Insanity, with Practical Observations on Lunatic Asylums, and a Description of the Pauper Lunatic Asylum for the County of Middlesex, at Hanwall, with a Detailed Account of Its Management* (London: Samuel Holdsworth, 1838), pp. 193–204.
35. ERIKSON, E. H. *Childhood and Society* (New York: W. W. Norton & Co., 1950).

36. FLUGEL, J. C. "Psychoanalysis: Its Status and Promise," in *Psychologies of 1930* (Worcester, Mass.: Clark University Press, 1930), pp. 374–94.

37. FOSDICK, H. E. *On Being a Real Person* (New York: Harper & Bros., 1943).

38. FOSDICK, H. E. "On Being Fit To Live With," in *Sermon on Postwar Christianity* (New York: Harper & Bros., 1948).

39. FREUD, S. *Aus den Anfängen der Psychoanalyse: Briefe an Wilhelm Fliess, Abhandlungen und Notizen aus den Jahren 1887–1902* (London: Imago Publishing Co., 1950).

40. FREUD, S. *An Autobiographical Study* (London: Hogarth Press, 1936).

41. FREUD, S. *Civilization and Its Discontents* (London: Hogarth Press, 1946).

42. FREUD, S. *The Future of an Illusion* (New York: Liveright Publishing Corp., 1949).

43. FREUD, S. *A General Introduction to Psycho-analysis* (New York: Boni & Liveright, 1935), pp. 217–27.

44. FREUD, S. *Group Psychology and the Analysis of the Ego* (London: Hogarth Press, 1922).

45. FREUD, S. "The Interpretation of Dreams," in *The Basic Writings of Sigmund Freud* (New York: Modern Library, 1938), pp. 179–549.

46. FREUD, S. "My Contact with Josef Popper-Lynkeus," *Internat. J. Psycho-Analysis*, 23:85, 1942.

47. FREUD, S. *New Introductory Lectures on Psychoanalysis* (New York: W. W. Norton & Co., 1933).

48. FREUD, S. "A Note on the Prehistory of the Technique of Analysis, 1920," in *Collected Papers*, 5 (London: Hogarth Press, 1950), 101–4.

49. FREUD, S. "One of the Difficulties of Psycho-analysis," in *Collected Papers*, 4 (London: Hogarth Press, 1925), 347–56.

50. FREUD, S. "An Outline of Psycho-analysis," *Internat. J. Psycho-Analysis*, 21:27, 1940.

51. FREUD, S. *The Question of Lay Analysis* (New York: W. W. Norton & Co., 1950).

52. FREUD, S. *Totem and Taboo*, in *Basic Writings of Sigmund Freud* (New York: Modern Library, 1938).

53. FROMM, ERICH. *Psychoanalysis and Religion* (New Haven: Yale University Press, 1950).

54. FROMM-REICHMANN, F. "Remarks on the Philosophy of Mental Disorder," *Psychiatry*, 9:293, 1946.

55. FURST, J. B. "Psychoanalysis Today," *New Masses*, 57:13, October 30; 13–15, November 6, 1945.

56. GALTON, SIR F. *Inquiries into Human Faculty and Its Development* (London: Macmillan & Co., Ltd., 1883).

57. GERARD, R. W. "Physiology and Psychiatry," *Am. J. Psychiat.*, 106:161, 1949.

58. GRABER, G. H. "Carl Gustav Carus: Ein Vorläufer der Psychoanalyse," *Imago*, 12:513, 1926.

59. GROTJAHN, M. "Psychoanalysis and Brain Disease: Observations of Juvenile Paretic Patients," *Psychoanalyt. Rev.*, 25:149, 1938.

60. GROTJAHN, M. "Psychoanalytic Contributions to Psychosomatic Medicine: A Bibliography," *Psychosom. Med.*, 6:169, 1944.

61. GROTJAHN, M. "Psychoanalytic Investigation of a 71-Year-Old Man with Senile Dementia," *Psychoanalyt. Quart.*, 9:80, 1940.

62. GROUP FOR THE ADVANCEMENT OF PSYCHIATRY. *Psychiatric Social Work in the Psychiatric Clinic* (Report No. 16, September, 1950).

63. GROUP FOR THE ADVANCEMENT OF PSYCHIATRY. *The Psychiatric Social Worker in the Psychiatric Hospital* (Report No. 2, January, 1948).

64. HARTMANN, H. "Technical Implications of Ego Psychology," *Psychoanalyt. Quart.*, 20:31, 1951.

65. HARTMANN, H.; KRIS, E.; and LOEWENSTEIN, R. M. "Comments on the Formation of Psychic Structure," in *The Psychoanalytic Study of the Child*, 2:11, 1946.

66. HARTMANN, H., and KRIS, E. "The Genetic Approach in Psychoanalysis," in *The Psychoanalytic Study of the Child*, 1:1, 1945; also *Psychoanalytic Yearbook*, 2:1, 1946.

67. HERMANN, I. " 'Der Mensch und seine Welt'; aus der Psychologie des ungarischen Philosophen Karl Böhm," *Imago*, 11:147, 1925.

68. HOFFMAN, F. J. *Freudianism and the Literary Mind* (Baton Rouge, La.: Louisiana State University Press, 1945).

69. HULL, C. L. *Principles of Behavior* (New York: Appleton-Century, 1943).

70. JEKELS, L. "Psycho-analysis and Dialectic," *Psychoanalyt. Rev.*, 28:228, 1941.

71. JELLIFFE, S. E. Foreword, in *Psychoanalysis Today*, ed. S. LORAND (New York: International Universities Press, 1944), pp. vii–ix.

72. KAUFMAN, M. R. "Psychoanalysis in Medicine," *Bull. Am. Psychoanalyt. Assoc.*, 7:1, 1951.

73. KAUFMAN, M. R. "The Role of Psychoanalysis in American Psychiatry," *Bull. Am. Psychoanalyt. Assoc.*, 6:1, 1950.

74. KIRBY, G. H. "Presidential Address: Modern Psychiatry and Mental Healing," *Am. J. Psychiat.*, 91:1, 1934.

75. KLUCKHOHN, C. "The Influence of Psychiatry on Anthropology in America during the Past One Hundred Years," in *One Hundred Years of American Psychiatry* (New York: Columbia University Press, 1944), pp. 589–617.

76. KLUCKHOHN, C. "The Limitations of Adaptation and Adjustment as Concepts for Understanding Cultural Behavior," in *Adaptation*, ed. J. ROMANO (Ithaca, N.Y.: Cornell University Press, 1949), pp. 96–113.

77. KNIGHT, R. P. "The Relationship of Psychoanalysis to Psychiatry," *Am. J. Psychiat.*, 101:777, 1945.

78. KOENIG-FACHSENFELD, O. F. VON. *Wandlungen des Traumproblems von der Romantik bis zur Gegenwart* (Stuttgart: F. Enke, 1935).

79. KRAPF, E. E. "A Clandestine Psychoanalyst of the Eighteenth Century," *Rev. psicoanal.*, 4:5, 1948.

80. KRIS, E. "Ego Psychology and Interpretation in Psychoanalytic Therapy," *Psychoanalyt. Quart.*, 20:15, 1951.

81. KRIS, E. "On Preconscious Mental Processes," *Psychoanalyt. Quart.*, 19:540, 1950.

82. KUBIE, L. S. *Practical and Theoretical Aspects of Psychoanalysis* (New York: International Universities Press, 1950).

83. LANGER, S. K. *Philosophy in a New Key* (New York: Mentor Books [No. M25], 1942).

84. LEE, R. S. *Freud and Christianity* (New York: A. A. Wyn, 1949).

85. LEEPER, R. "Dr. Hull's Principles of Behavior," *J. Genet. Psychol.*, 65:3, 1944.

86. LENIN, V. I. *Left Wing Communism: An Infantile Disorder* (New York: International Publishing Co., 1940).

87. LEVIN, A. J. "Maine, McLennan, and Freud," *Psychiatry*, 11:177, 1948.

88. LEWIS, N. D. C. "General Considerations in Therapeutic Failures," in *Failures in Psychiatric Treatment*, ed. P. H. HOCH (New York: Grune & Stratton, 1948), pp. 1–8.

89. LEWISOHN, S. A. *Human Leadership in Industry* (New York: Harper & Bros., 1945).

90. LIEBMAN, J. L. *Peace of Mind* (New York: Simon & Schuster, 1946).

91. LIEBMAN, J. L. (ed.). *Psychiatry and Religion* (Boston: Beacon Press, 1948).

92. LOEWENSTEIN, R. M. "The Problem of Interpretation," *Psychoanalyt. Quart.*, 20:1, 1951.

93. LORAND, S. "A Survey of Psychoanalytic Literature on Problems of Alcohol: Bibliography," *Yearbook of Psychoanalysis*, 1:359, 1945.

94. McKINLEY, J. C. (ed.). *An Outline of Neuropsychiatry* (St. Louis: J. S. Swift, 1944).

95. McNEILL, H. "Freudians and Catholics," *Commonweal*, 46:350, 1947.

96. MANN, T. *Freud, Goethe, Wagner* (New York: A. Knopf, 1936), pp. 3–45.

97. MANN, T. "Freud's Position in the History of Modern Culture," *Psychoanalyt. Rev.*, 28:92, 1941.

98. MARMOR, J. "Psychoanalysis," in *Philosophy for the Future: The Quest of Modern Materialism*, ed. R. W. SELLERS, V. J. McGILL, *et al.* (New York: Macmillan Co., 1949), pp. 317–39.

99. MEADE, M. "Educative Effects of Social Environment as Disclosed by Studies of Primitive Societies," *Suppl. Ed. Monogr.*, No. 54, pp. 48–61, 1942.

100. MENNINGER, W. C. "Individualization in Prescriptions for Nursing Care of the Psychiatric Patient," *J.A.M.A.*, 106:756, 1936.

101. MENNINGER, W. C. "Psychiatric Hospital Therapy Designed To Meet Unconscious Needs," *Am. J. Psychiat.*, 93:347, 1936.

102. MENNINGER, W. C. *Psychiatry in a Troubled World* (New York: Macmillan Co., 1948).

103. MILLER, J. G. *Unconsciousness* (New York: John Wiley & Sons, Inc., 1942).

104. MISBACH, L. "Psychoanalysis and Theories of Learning," *Psychol. Rev.*, 55:143, 1948.

105. Moore, T. V. "A Century of Psychology and Its Relationship to American Psychiatry," in *One Hundred Years of American Psychiatry* (New York: Columbia University Press, 1944), p. 447.
106. Moore, T. V. *The Nature and Treatment of Mental Disorders* (New York: Grune & Stratton, 1943).
107. Mowrer, O. H., and Kluckhohn, C. "Dynamic Theory of Personality," in *Personality and the Behavior Disorders*, ed. J. McV. Hunt (New York: Ronald Press Co., 1944), 1, 69–135.
108. Murray, H. A. "Sigmund Freud, 1856–1939," *Am. J. Psychol.*, 53:134, 1940.
109. Osborn, R. *Freud and Marx: A Dialectical Study* (New York: Equinox Co-op. Press, 1937).
110. Overholser, W., and Richmond, W. V. *Handbook of Psychiatry* (Philadelphia: J. B. Lippincott Co., 1947).
111. Pannekoek, A. "Society and Mind in Marxian Philosophy," *Sci. & Soc.*, 1:445, 1936–37.
112. Plant, J. S. *Personality and the Cultural Pattern* (New York: Commonwealth Fund, 1937).
113. "The President's Page," *Bull. Am. Psychoanalyt. Assoc.*, 4:30, 1948.
114. "Psychoanalysts in World War II," *Bull. Am. Psychoanalyt. Assoc.*, Suppl., May, 1950.
115. Rapaport, D. "The Autonomy of the Ego," *Bull. Menninger Clin.*, 15:113, 1951.
116. Rapaport, D. "The Conceptual Model of Psychoanalysis" (unpublished manuscript).
117. Rapaport, D. *Emotions and Memory* (Baltimore: Williams & Wilkins, 1942).
118. Rapaport, D. "On the Psychoanalytic Theory of Thinking," *Internat. J. Psycho-Analysis*, 31:161, 1950.
119. Rapaport, D. "Consciousness: A Psychopathological and Psychodynamic View," in *Problems of Consciousness*, ed. H. Abramson (New York: J. Macy, Jr., Foundation, 1951), pp. 18–57.
120. Rapaport, D. "Toward a Theory of Thinking," in *Organization and Pathology of Thought*, ed. D. Rapaport (New York: Columbia University Press, 1951), pp. 689–730.
121. Rathbun, C. "On Certain Similarities between Spinoza and Psychoanalysis," *Psychoanalyt. Rev.*, 21:1, 1934.
122. Redl, F., and Wattenberg, W. W. *Mental Hygiene in Teaching* (New York: Harcourt, Brace & Co., 1951).
123. Reik, T. *From Thirty Years with Freud* (New York: Farrar & Rinehart, 1940).
124. "Review of Psychiatric Progress, 1946," *Am. J. Psychiat.*, 103:513, 1947.
125. Rickman, J. *Development of Psycho-analytical Theory of the Psychoses, 1893–1926* (London: Baillière, Tindall & Cox, 1928) (*Internat. J. Psycho-Analysis*, Suppl. No. 2).
126. Rickman, J. "Reflections on the Function and Organization of a Psychoanalytical Society," *Internat. J. Psycho-Analysis*, 32:218, 1951.

127. SACHS, H. "The Prospects of Psycho-analysis," *Internat. J. Psycho-Analysis*, 20:460, 1939.
128. SAPIR, E. "Cultural Anthropology and Psychiatry," *J. Abnorm. & Social Psychol.*, 27:229, 1932.
129. SCHILDER, P. "The Social Neurosis," *Psychoanalyt. Rev.*, 25:1, 1938.
130. SCHILDER, P. "Sociological Implication of Neuroses," *J. Social Psychol.*, 15:3, 1942.
131. SCHNEIDER, D. E. *The Psychoanalyst and the Artist* (New York: Farrar, Straus & Co., 1950).
132. SCHNEIDER, L. *The Freudian Psychology and Veblen's Social Theory* (New York: King's Crown Press, 1948).
133. SEARS, R. R. "Experimental Analysis of Psychoanalytic Phenomena," in *Personality and the Behavior Disorders*, ed. J. McV. HUNT (New York: Ronald Press, 1944), pp. 306–32.
134. SEARS, R. R. *Survey of Objective Studies of Psychoanalytic Concepts* (Social Science Research Council Bull. No. 51 [1943]).
135. SHAKOW, D. "Psychology and Psychiatry: A Dialogue," *Am. J. Orthopsychiat.*, 19:191, 381, 1949.
136. SMITH, M. H. "Spinoza's Anticipation of Recent Psychological Developments," *Brit. J. M. Psychol.*, 5:257, 1925.
137. STONE, J. T. "The Theory and Practice of Psychoanalysis," *Sci. & Soc.*, 10:54, 1946.
138. SULLIVAN, H. S. *Conceptions of Modern Psychiatry* (Washington, D.C.: William Alanson White Psychiatric Foundation, 1947).
139. TRILLING, L. *The Liberal Imagination* (New York: Viking Press, 1950).
140. WAELDER, R. "The Structure of Paranoid Ideas," *Internat. J. Psycho-Analysis*, 32:167, 1951.
141. WATSON, F. "The Father of Modern Psychology," *Psychol. Rev.*, 22:333, 1915.
142. WERTHAM, F. *Dark Legend: A Study in Murder* (New York: Duell, Sloan & Pearce, 1941).
143. WHITE, W. A. "Presidential Address," *Am. J. Psychiat.*, 82:1, 1925.
144. WILBUR, G. B., and MUENSTERBERGER, W. (eds.). *Psychoanalysis and Culture* (New York: International Universities Press, 1951). This book includes a full bibliography of Roheim's writings.
145. WITTELS, FRITZ. "Freud's Correlation with Josef Popper-Lynkeus," *Yearbook of Psychoanalysis*, 4:21, 1948.
146. WOLF, S. "Effect of Suggestion and Conditioning on the Action of Chemical Agents in Human Subjects—the Pharmacology of Placebos," *J. Clin. Investigation*, 29:100, 1950.
147. WORTIS, J. "Freudianism and the Psychoanalytic Tradition," *Am. J. Psychiat.*, 101:814, 1945.
148. YELLOWLEES, H. *The Human Approach* (London: Churchill, 1946).
149. ZILBOORG, G. "The Future of Psychoanalysis and Religion: A Response," *Psychoanalyt. Quart.*, 13:93, 1944.
150. ZILBOORG, G., and HENRY, G. W. *A History of Medical Psychology* (New York: W. W. Norton & Co., 1941).

# INDEXES

# INDEX OF NAMES

# SUBJECT INDEX